“The second edition of *Becoming an EFT Therapist: The Workbook* extends and updates an exceptionally useful book. Not only is this the definitive workbook for learning emotionally focused couple therapy, it also covers the recent developments of Johnson’s attachment theory in practice treatment model in individual and family therapy. It provides the kind of hands-on how to do it information that therapists need and look for. A wonderful resource either in conjunction with a training program or as part of a therapist’s individual development, this workbook has great value not only for those who wish to become practitioners of EFT but also for all therapists.”

Jay Lebow, Ph.D., ABPP, *senior scholar and clinical professor; editor,* Family Process; *The Family Institute at Northwestern and Northwestern University, Evanston, IL*

“If you want to internalize the feel and the craft of EFT, this is your book. It takes you inside sessions, making you think about how you would respond and how you can go deeper. And this updated workbook shows the power of EFT to heal individuals and families as well as couples. Any therapist on the planet will benefit from reading it.”

William J. Doherty, Ph.D., *professor of family social science at the University of Minnesota and co-author of* Helping Couples on the Brink of Divorce: Discernment Counseling for Troubled Relationships

“Whenever I teach or supervise EFCT, I always use the Workbook. I have not found a better book to help EFT therapists learn how-to-do-it. This second edition only intensifies that recommendation. In some ways the new edition is essentially a whole new book. There are new chapters on EFT with individuals (EFIT); the family chapter (EFFT) has been expanded; the approach of the EFT Tango is explicated; and the application of EFT to trauma is more in-depth. However, this second edition has maintained the central strength of its predecessor—its ongoing involvement with the reader as an active learner—asking the reader to state what they are learning while they are learning it, to apply various procedures to imagined cases, and to reflect on the personal ramifications of the material. The Workbook makes the learning come alive and shortens the bridge between theory and practice. For any therapist who is floundering with, ‘but what do I say now?’ this is a must-read.”

Hanna Levenson, Ph.D., *professor, Wright Institute, Berkeley, CA*

Becoming an Emotionally Focused Therapist

This second edition of *Becoming an Emotionally Focused Therapist: The Workbook* has been fully revised by expert therapists with advances in attachment science and emotionally focused therapy (EFT) practice, the integration of the "EFT Tango"—a guide to the EFT process—and new chapters on working with both individuals and families.

Suitable as a companion volume to *The Practice of Emotionally Focused Couple Therapy* or as a standalone learning tool, it provides an easy road-map toward mastering the ins and outs of EFT with practice exercises, review questions, and compelling clinical examples.

Invaluable for clinicians and students, this workbook takes the reader on an adventure: the quest to become a competent, confident, and passionate emotionally focused therapist.

James L. Furrow, Ph.D., is contributing author and editor of *Emotionally Focused Family Therapy, The Emotionally Focused Casebook, Becoming an Emotionally Focused Couple Therapist,* and *Emotionally Focused Couple Therapy for Dummies.*

Susan M. Johnson, Ed.D., is the leading developer of EFT. She is professor emeritus of clinical psychology at the University of Ottawa, distinguished research professor in the Marital and Family Therapy Program at Alliant University in San Diego, and director of the International Centre for Excellence in EFT.

Brent Bradley, Ph.D., is president of the Couple Zone, with counseling offices throughout Texas. He is contributing author of *Emotional Focused Couple Therapy for Dummies, The Emotionally Focused Casebook,* and *Becoming an Emotionally Focused Couple Therapist.*

Lorrie L. Brubacher, M.Ed., is founding director of the Carolina Centre for EFT and author of *Stepping Into Emotionally Focused Therapy: Key Ingredients of Change.* She is a certified EFT supervisor and trainer.

T. Leanne Campbell, Ph.D., is a registered psychologist and co-director of the Vancouver Island Centre for EFT and Campbell & Fairweather Psychology and is an honorary research associate of Vancouver Island University. She is a certified EFT supervisor and trainer.

Veronica Kallos-Lilly, Ph.D., is a registered psychologist and co-director of the Vancouver Couple & Family Institute and Vancouver Centre for EFT Training. She is a certified EFT supervisor, trainer and co-author of *An Emotionally Focused Workbook for Couples* The Two of Us, Second Edition.

Gail Palmer, M.S.W., is co-director of International Centre for Excellence in EFT (ICEEFT). Gail is co-author of *Emotionally Focused Family Therapy, Becoming an Emotionally Focused Couple Therapist* and leads trainings in EFT internationally.

Kathryn Rheem, Ed.D., is director of the Washington Baltimore Center for EFT and co-founder of The EFT Café. She is a certified EFT supervisor and trainer and leads trainings in EFT internationally.

Scott R. Woolley, Ph.D., holds the rank of distinguished professor at Alliant International University. He has trained therapists in EFT in Asia, Europe, and the Americas for over 20 years.

Becoming an Emotionally Focused Therapist

The Workbook

Second Edition

James L. Furrow and Susan M. Johnson
With
Brent Bradley, Lorrie L. Brubacher, T. Leanne Campbell,
Veronica Kallos-Lilly, Gail Palmer, Kathryn Rheem,
Scott R. Woolley

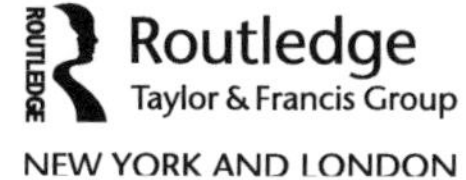

NEW YORK AND LONDON

Cover image: © Getty Images

Second edition published 2022
by Routledge
605 Third Avenue, New York, NY 10158

and by Routledge
2 Park Square, Milton Park, Abingdon, Oxon, OX14 4RN

Routledge is an imprint of the Taylor & Francis Group, an informa business

First edition published by Routledge 2005

Library of Congress Cataloging-in-Publication Data
A catalog record for this book has been requested

ISBN: 9780367483470 (hbk)
ISBN: 9780367483425 (pbk)
ISBN: 9781003039457 (ebk)

DOI: 10.4324/9781003039457

Typeset in Melior
by Apex CoVantage, LLC

Access the Support Material: www.routledge.com/9780367483425

This workbook is dedicated to the creativity, passion, and heart of our EFT community, including therapists, supervisors, and trainers whose inspiration and efforts have been a source of hope, healing, and growth to those who seek their care in love and life.

CONTENTS

PREFACE

Welcome to an emotionally focused therapy (EFT) experience! This workbook provides therapists and counselors with a "hands-on" approach to deepening EFT practice through insight, examples, and exercises. This new edition of *Becoming an EFT Therapist* updates and expands the original EFT focus on couples (EFCT) and families (EFFT) to individuals (EFIT). This workbook offers a practical resource for getting inside EFT, an empirically supported approach is based on over three decades of clinical practice including research on the outcome and process of EFT. Becoming an EFT Therapist includes exercises that complement the core EFT texts, including *The Practice of Emotionally Focused Couple Therapy: Creating Connection*, 3rd ed. (Routledge, 2019); *Attachment Theory in Practice: Emotionally Focused Therapy with Individuals, Couples, and Families* (Guilford); *Emotionally Focused Family Therapy: Creating Connection and Restoring Resilience* (Routledge); and *EFIT—A Primer: On Target Intervention for Emotional Disorders* (Routledge). For a list of up-to-date EFT references and training resources, explore the International Centre for Excellence in Emotionally Focused Therapy website (www.iceeft.com).

The first edition of *Becoming an Emotionally Focused Couple Therapist: The Workbook* was designed by seven practicing EFT therapists and is now revised and expanded by additional EFT practitioners, who share lessons learned from their practice with individuals, couples, and families. The original team included early innovators in EFT Alison Lee, and Douglas Tilley, who generously shared from their EFT expertise and clinical wisdom. We are indebted to Alison and Doug for their poignant contributions to the original workbook and the many ways their insights live on in this current edition.

This workbook provides readers with a next step into EFT practice. To gain confidence in EFT and effective use with individuals, couples, and families, most therapists should read the EFT treatment manuals and additional chapters and articles, attend training with an EFT trainer, and obtain clinical consultation or supervision from a certified EFT supervisor (listed at www.ICEEFT.com). Such diligent training is required for any form of psychological intervention but especially one in which a therapist is intervening in an ongoing, multidimensional and emotionally powerful intrapersonal and interpersonal drama. Becoming fluent in EFT is an ongoing process and cannot be learned by simply reading a book or watching an expert therapist.

This workbook is divided into three sections. Chapters 1 through 3 present a theoretical overview and summary of EFT interventions. Chapters 4 through 8 focus on the use of EFT with couples, including following a single case through a full course of EFT treatment. Chapters 9 through 12 expand the couple focus of the EFT model to its use with individuals, families, and clients working through trauma and attachment injuries. The appendix and online eResource page provide additional resources to further your success in bringing EFT.

Online resource can be found at www.routledge.com/9780367483425.

Everyone who reads this book will likely have their own way of conducting EFT and will bring their own styles and strengths to the model. In the era of pragmatic approaches to intervention, it is tempting to try to reduce interventions to four or five invariant quick fixes and to teach therapists in this way. We believe that you do not have to move to a simplistic level to be efficient and incisive in individual, couple, and family therapy. Instead, you must learn to create a safe, collaborative environment; know how to focus on what matters; and help people work with the powerful emotional and attachment dramas in which they are caught.

There are certain elements of EFT that are very difficult to learn from any printed page. For example, we find that students of EFT learn about key issues of pacing from watching their own video recordings of therapy. Often the difference between an experienced EFT therapist and a novice therapist is not the number of EFT interventions used but rather that the more experienced therapists go more slowly, repeat themselves, and circle again and again through the same territory until clients can hold a tangible new emotional reality in their hands. The more experienced therapist knows the emotional process that a client engages with their EFT therapist is intimate by nature, and the therapist can slice risks thin, structuring new responses again and again until powerful bonding events emerge and transformative growth is realized.

In light of this, an explicit structure exists to support those who wish to become registered as EFT couples' therapists. This structure includes training, supervision, and case review (see EFT certification www.ICEEFT.com). EFT is now taught in many graduate programs in North America and in many other parts of the world. We hope that those who teach these programs will also find this workbook useful and supportive.

You cannot practice EFT without also using it as a lens for your own relationships and as a path into your own attachment issues—we all have them. We hope that this book will help you use this lens in a positive way for your personal and your professional life. Most of all, we hope you find your journey through this book stimulating, powerful, and emotionally engaging.

SECTION I

THEORETICAL OVERVIEW AND INTERVENTION SUMMARY

1

INTRODUCTION: THE NATURE OF EFT

Emotionally focused therapy (EFT) is a short-term, systematic, and tested intervention to reduce distress and dysfunction in individuals suffering from the emotional disorders of depression, anxiety, and post-traumatic stress; couples struggling with love relationships; and families dealing with distressed adolescents. It is an **experiential attachment-based intervention** that can be used across modalities with single clients, dyads, and family groups (Johnson, 2019). The title reflects the priority given to emotion as a key organizer of inner experiences and key interactions in attachment relationships. A focus on emotion is seen as the essential transforming element in effective psychotherapy. The word "emotion" comes from the Latin word "to move." EFT uses the power of emotion to "move" clients, evoking new realities and new responses in the recurring inner process of constructing self and experience, and in key interactions that make up the key dramas in people's relationships with significant others. When we speak of being emotionally "moved," we are usually talking of being touched, stirred up, compelled to respond to a powerful cue that evokes action in us. Emotion pulls for and organizes key responses in the dance with self, in close relationships, and our way of engaging with the world we live in.

EFT has always been used in clinical practice across the three modalities mentioned above. However, it is best known as a couple intervention (EFCT), and much of EFT training and research has focused on therapy in which the relationship between two people is the client, and the therapist works with both individuals; the dance between them to change this relationship. The creation of individual change in models of self and other and affect regulation patterns, has always been part of EFCT, as has the shifting of specific relationship patterns between individuals to change the culture of a distressed family. Individual- and family-focused EFT has now been made more specific in the outlining of EFIT and emotionally focused family therapy (EFFT), both of which are part of this workbook. Many exercises in this book still focus on couple therapy examples given that this modality explicitly combines intra- and interpersonal, within and between levels of change, change in self and relational system.

THE EFT PROCESS

If you were to watch an EFT therapist work, what would you see? You would see the therapist creating a safe, egalitarian relationship with clients. This is often somewhat easier in EFIT than when making an alliance with both members of a warring couple or family who want you to pick sides. You would see the therapist, guided by attachment theory, always moving within and between with clients. This involves tracking and exploring how

DOI: 10.4324/9781003039457-2

emotions organize how a client tells their life story to the therapist; how emotional signals direct a couple's dance into predictable patterns; and how the relational dance, whether in the imaginary conversation an individual client reports with an attachment figure or between intimates in your therapy room, then in turn shapes key emotions. You would see the therapist noting how the client's habitual ways of dealing with difficult emotions actually maintains these emotional dilemmas and expanding emotional responses to include core implicit fears and needs.

The therapist then helps to create a new dance with parts of self, such as a fearful withdrawn part of self, or with attachment figures based on these expanded emotions. *Constriction and rigidity in processing experience and engaging with others is gradually replaced by expansiveness and flexibility.* The therapist shifts from questions such as, "What happens to you when your partner moves away, as he did just now?" to formulations such as, "Your desperate anger takes you over and also scares your partner—and it is so hard for you to feel or show the loneliness and longing underneath," to requests such as, "Can you look at me? Can you tell me again how small you feel and tell me what you see in my face—whether you see the contempt that you 'know' you will see?" or "Can you tell him 'Please, I need you to hold and reassure me.'"

We have attempted to present the model in small steps and to build these steps gradually to the point where readers will sense that they have a compass and a map to improving their clients' lives and relationships and will know the road to take with clients at key moments in therapy. The model offers a foundation in a coherent, developmental, and very well researched theory of adult personality, including a clear guide to the core elements of health and of emotional disorders, a map to the structure of love relationships, an outline of the process of change, and a clear guide to intervention across three modalities. EFT and the attachment framework it is based on help therapists see the terrors and vulnerabilities underlying reactive or less than functional responses and the process patterns in relationships that trap people in constant aloneness and insecure bonds.

AN EVOLVING MODEL

EFT has evolved in the past two decades from a little recognized approach to working with couples focusing on the power of working directly with emotion from an attachment perspective into a mainstream model of couple therapy that is accepted all over the world as a cutting-edge, empirically validated intervention in this field. Recently, its systematic application to individuals with emotional disorders and to distressed families has been further outlined (Johnson, 2019; Furrow, Palmer, Johnson, Faller, & Palmer-Olsen, 2019), and this is reflected in the pages of this workbook. This attachment-based model of intervention is taught in many different cultural contexts and is used for many different kinds of clients, for example, for Christian and orthodox Jewish couples and families, for gay and straight couples, for less educated and more intensely educated populations, and as an individual therapy intervention, for nearly every diagnosis and designated problem in mental health, except for schizophrenia and antisocial personality disorder. The treatment of clients with various levels of post-traumatic stress disorder (PTSD) and of those designated with borderline personality disorder has become a particular focus in EFIT.

When EFT was first formulated in the 1980s, actively working with emotion was not generally popular in the couple and family field. Emotion itself was most often seen as a troublesome intrapsychic variable that was not part of an interpersonal systemic perspective. Emotion was viewed as part of the problem rather than as a potent part of the solution. Attachment theory, the model of adult love and close relationships used in EFT, has also been more clearly articulated and researched in these two decades, and the need for a model of adult love as a map for couples' intervention has become more obvious. Part of the present popularity of EFT rests with the greater recognition of the positive power of working with emotion and that adult attachment has generated a large following and a vibrant body of associated research and literature. In addition, the need for treatment models to be able to demonstrate positive and lasting outcomes has become increasingly more compelling. The outcomes on EFT for couples can be seen as the most positive and promising in the field of couple therapy (see www.iceeft.com for a list of outcome, follow-up, and process of change studies with different populations). This research has also documented individual change in the context of couple therapy sessions, for example, studies showing that EFT interventions impact individual partners' depression levels and is able to shift levels of attachment security.

EFT reflects the priorities and recent foci of the present general psychotherapy and couple therapy context in the following nine ways:

1. EFT is a brief treatment focused on key factors in emotional disorders and relationship distress so it can be used in a brief therapy environment. It targets the core organizing variables in the drama of distress—emotion and its regulation, models of self and other, and patterns in the drama of engagement with key others and levels of attachment security.
2. EFT has been systematically described and rigorously tested and found to be effective with consistently positive results. It must be noted, however, that only one study exists for EFFT as yet. Current research is focusing on demonstrating the effects of EFIT on depression and anxiety.
3. Relapse is a significant concern in psychotherapy in general but in the couple therapy field in particular. Research with high-risk couples and other studies suggest that relapse is not a significant issue with EFT. Shaping positive bonding interactions has palpable power in sessions that focus on relationship repair. Attachment science also supports that such interactions build positive models of self and other that continue to impact positive adaptation.
4. The need for studies of how change occurs and exactly how therapists should intervene at key times is an ongoing issue in the field of psychotherapy. Substantial process research exists that supports the clinical wisdom of EFT with couples (see Greenman & Johnson, 2013, for a summary), elaborating on how change occurs, specific processes, and change events in therapy. We expect these results to generalize to change processes in EFIT as well.
5. The EFT general perspective fits with recent research: on the nature of relationship distress and satisfaction within the developing science of personal relationships; on the nature of emotion and other neuroscience findings; and, of course, on the model of personality health and dysfunction offered by attachment. For example, the findings of Gottman and colleagues have emphasized the significant role of emotional communication in the development of relationship distress. Research also suggests that rather than help couples resolve content issues, therapy should help couples develop soothing interactions and maintain emotional engagement during disagreements. The process of change

in EFT mirrors this research in that it structures small steps toward safe emotional engagement so that partners can soothe, comfort, and reassure each other. The work of James Gross (Gross & Levenson, 1997) on factors such as the cost of suppression as a coping technique and of Nancy Eisenberger (Eisenberger & Lieberman, 2004) on how the brain encodes rejection in much the same way as physical pain, all fit with EFT interventions used with individuals, couples, and families (Johnson, 2019). Many different lines of research are coming together and creating a coherent picture of who we are and how we relate to others, and the EFT model is part of this new consilience or coming together.

6. There is an increasing focus in psychotherapy on issues of diversity. EFT is used with many different individuals, couples, and families; with people of different social classes; with different kinds of problems; and across cultural groups. The attachment framework, which is a biologically based model of generic human functioning, aids in this regard. Also, the therapeutic alliance in EFT is collaborative and egalitarian. The experiential roots of EFT generally promote a therapeutic stance of respect for differences and an openness to learning from clients what is meaningful for them and how they view themselves and intimate relationships. Every individual, every couple, and every family system is a culture unto itself, and the therapist must learn about and adapt interventions to this unique culture. But EFT also assumes that there is a certain universality that tends to cut across differences of culture, race, and class. For example, Tomkins (1986) lists what appears to be a small set of universal basic emotions: interest/excitement, joy, surprise, distress/anguish, disgust/contempt, anger/rage, shame, and fear/terror. Considerable evidence also suggests that attachment needs and responses are universal.
7. EFT shares a number of characteristics with gender-oriented and feminist approaches to couple therapy. The EFT attachment perspective on relationships parallels the work of feminist writers (Jordan, Kaplan, Miller, Stiver, & Surrey, 1991) who de-pathologize dependency. EFT and other feminist-informed therapies examine the impact of gender-based constraints and work to increase personal agency and to develop egalitarian relationships in which reciprocity, intimacy, and interdependency can flourish.
8. EFT fits with the present climate of humanistic psychotherapy in that it takes a postmodern stance, promoting a collaborative alliance in which clients are the "experts" on their reality and therapists discover with their clients how inner and outer realities are constructed in the moment. This stance parallels the humanistic perspective of Carl Rogers (1961), whose main concern was to honor his clients' constructions of reality. Like John Bowlby, he believed in discovering the logic and attempting to adapt less than functional behaviors. Bowlby saw all dysfunction as a distortion of adaptive behaviors that fit a specific survival goal but have then become rigidified and generalized. EFT can be thought of as a postmodern therapy in that EFT therapists help clients deconstruct problems and responses by bringing marginalized aspects of reality into focus, probing for the not-yet spoken, and integrating elements of a personal or relational reality that have gone un-storied. However, EFT does not fit with the more extreme postmodern position that there are no common existential conditions or processes, that reality is arbitrary and random, and that problems generally exist only in language and can therefore be "dis-solved" in language.

9. Last, but not least, the growth of the EFT model reflects the increasing pressure for clinicians to find an integrative framework for human functioning, dysfunction, and change that unifies and brings clarity to their endeavors. The growth of adult attachment and the hundreds of studies associated with it (see Mikulincer & Shaver, *Attachment in Adulthood*, 2016) offers order and coherence—an overarching understanding of who we are as humans and what dilemmas we all face—and provides direction in the chaos of more and more diagnoses and therapy models.

EFT PRINCIPLES AND ATTACHMENT THEORY

Attachment theory, epitomized by EFT, offers guidance for the conduct of effective psychotherapy. The following five areas illustrate how the lens of attachment theory brings focus to the EFT process.

Focus on Emotion: The primacy of emotion as the organizer of our inner world and the music that structures our most important relationships brings to the forefront the necessity of actively focusing on and finding new ways to regulate emotion in therapy. Significant change is always a corrective emotional experience which further processes, "frightening, alien and unacceptable emotion" (Bowlby, 1988). In session, safety is essential to effective psychotherapy, so the therapist attempts to be emotionally present, that is accessible, responsive, and engaged, as any good attachment figure would be. The therapist joins with and validates the client's emotional reality and then expands this reality with the client, titrating risks within the client's window of tolerance.

Growth and Exploration: It is a central tenet of attachment that emotional safety fosters exploration and growth. Change always involves the intrapsychic and interpersonal—within and between change—a shift in the self of the client and the relational system that is the context in which the process of the definition of self is embedded. The dance with others defines the dancer and vice versa. The therapist systematically shapes new more constructive dramas with real or imagined/mental images of important others in session. The goal of therapy is not just to improve coping with symptoms of distress but also to create growth and more healthy models of self and other to foster the secure dependency that we all need to thrive.

Emotional Balance: The securely attached style offers us a clear picture of health characterized by emotional balance, a coherent and integrated sense of self, positive models of others, and the ability to reach for them when needed. Vulnerability is accepted and seen as manageable, needs are embraced, and the self is seen as competent and worthy of love and care. Growing toward health is an organic process that then follows the natural development of human children who live with safe haven and secure base relationships. The therapist identifies and confronts the blocks in this natural process of growth in the client. Progress in therapy occurs by encountering new experiences or new levels of experience in the present in session, and examining how experience is shaped and colored to foster rigidity and constriction or openness and growth.

Present Experience: The therapist focuses on the how of experience as it is encoded in the present rather than the content itself. Emotional realities are then rendered more concrete and specific, so rather than teaching a client or offering skills to deal with the fact that she cannot let others close, the therapist will ask her to reveal her vulnerability and let herself be seen, and guide how she processes this experience. Attachment is firmly grounded in empiricism, that is, in the observation and demarcation of patterns of inner and interpersonal responding.

Experiential Map: The EFT therapist has a map to the universal ways of formulating emotions and emotional needs, to the universal longings that are wired into our nervous system, and the universal strategies we use to get others to respond to us or deal with rejection and abandonment. Attachment provides therapists with a "map of common human misery and basic human motivation" (Johnson, 2019, p. 31). This fosters attunement on the part of the therapist and allows the process of change to be predictable. What we understand we can shape. When we understand that fear consumes us and blocks empathy for others, we can normalize this process and help a client with overwhelming fear knowing that when the client has his or her balance, empathy for others can be evoked with ease.

THE EFT WORKBOOK

This workbook is designed not to stand alone but to be used in conjunction with other EFT resources, including *Attachment Theory in Practice* (Johnson, 2019), *The Practice of Emotionally Focused Therapy*, 3rd edition (Johnson, 2020), and *Emotionally Focused Family Therapy* (Furrow et al., 2019). This book is designed to help therapists and counselors learn the EFT model and apply it with confidence. Given the difficulty of learning any therapy approach simply from descriptions of ways to see problems and ways to intervene, this book offers examples and exercises to involve the reader and to bridge the gap between reading words on a page and being part of the evolving drama of a therapy session. Training videos/DVDs of actual sessions of EFT can be found on the website, www.iceeft.com, and will help readers tune into this model, and an extensive literature base that describes the breadth of EFT practice and its effectiveness. The goal of this book is to take readers by the hand and walk them through the EFT model.

Some of the answers to the questions asked in the exercises, especially in the first few chapters, are found in the EFT literature rather than in the text of this book. We assume that readers will allow themselves to guess at answers—to play—to follow hunches and then discover how accurate their hunches were from the answers given in the back of the book, especially if their exposure to the EFT literature is only preliminary. We hope this engagement in the process of discovery will allow the EFT model to come alive. As in the model itself, the point is not to focus on performance (on getting the right answer) but on presence (on engaging in the process of discovery that occurs when you consider options or, in later chapters, draft your own responses).

EFT PRACTICE RESOURCES

As stated previously, EFT references and resources can be found on the EFT website (www.iceeft.com). The main resources are the following:

1. a) *The Practice of Emotionally Focused Couples Therapy: Creating Connection* (Johnson, 2020). This manual for EFT with couples was first published in 1996, then revised in 2004 and again in 2019;
   b) *Emotionally Focused Family Therapy: Creating Connection and Restoring Resilience* (Furrow et al., 2019) is the treatment manual for EFFT:

c) *Attachment Theory in Practice* (Johnson, 2019).
d) *A Primer in Emotionally Focused Individual Therapy (EFIT)* (Johnson & Campbell, 2021).

2. The EFT training videos demonstrate EFT practice with couples and individuals, including *EFIT: Emotionally Focused Individual Therapy (EFIT)—Working with Anxiety and Depression* and *EFIT: Creating Core Change in Emotionally Focused Individual Therapy*. These videos highlight the EFIT process of working with distressed and anxious individual clients.
3. In-person or online supervision or consultation from ICEEFT-certified EFT supervisors, who are listed on the ICEEFT website.
4. General reading on EFT—articles, chapters, and books listed on the ICEEFT site. Most chapters have transcripts of therapy, which can help less experienced EFT therapists understand how the process of therapy unfolds.
5. General reading on topics such as emotion, experiential and systemic models, and attachment theory, as well as the books for the public on EFT, *Hold Me Tight* (2008) and *Love Sense* (2013).

REVIEWING THE ESSENTIAL NATURE OF EFT

Respond to the following questions by checking the correct answer or answers from the options provided. As with all the exercises, the answer key is found at the end of this chapter. Often more than one of the possible answers given will be correct.

Question 1.1. The theoretical basis of EFT can best be described as: (Mark the correct answer.)

a. A Bowenian view of close relationships and a solution-focused approach to intervention in therapy. ____
b. An attachment view of identity and close relationships and a traditional insight-driven psychodynamic approach to intervention. ____
c. A CBT/exchange theory view of close relationships and a skill-building approach to intervention in couple and individual therapy sessions. ____
d. A relational attachment view of individual functioning and close relationships, and a humanistic/experiential approach to intervention that combines Rogerian and systemic oriented approaches. ____
e. A differentiation of self-focused view of identity and close relationships, including a constructivist/narrative approach to intervention. ____

Question 1.2. The core organizing variables that define and order self and relational systems from the EFT perspective are: (Mark all that are correct.)

a. How emotion is habitually regulated. ___________
b. How orienting cognitions about self and other are structured and processed. _____
c. How response protocols for engaging with others are structured. ___________
d. How a, b, and c interact and feedback into and confirm each other. __________

Question 1.3. From an EFT or attachment perspective, the principal feature of effective personality functioning and mental health is: (Mark the correct answer.)

a. The ability to define the self as separate from others—maintain boundaries and negotiate intimacy with others. ____
b. The capacity to make intimate bonds with others, in care-seeking and care-giving roles in which co-regulation of emotion can occur to create emotional balance. ____
c. The ability to gain insight into unconscious drives and how a person projects these onto present reality. ____
d. The ability to self-regulate and control one's emotion with reason and find effective coping skills for difficult situations. ____

Question 1.4. The neuroscience of attachment tells us just how relational we are as humans. Connection is about physiology rather than sentiment or cultural context. Evidence says that close others: (Mark all that are correct.)

a. Are incorporated into neural representations of self as vital resources. ____
b. Provide emotional connection that promotes survival and dilutes risk. ____
c. Flood the brain with dopamine and oxytocin, allowing us to ride out trauma. ____
d. Promote pragmatic load sharing, the regulation of negative emotion, and buffer stress. ____
e. Have enormous existential significance, fostering the ability to deal with the dilemmas of life. ____

Question 1.5. Which of the following is not a goal of EFT? (Mark the correct answer.)

a. To offer corrective emotional experiences that impact model of self and other and shape constructive dependency with loved ones. ____
b. To address frightening or alien emotions and to render them acceptable, owned and a compass in a client's life and existential dilemma. ____
c. To create a more secure bond between distressed partners or family members. ____
d. To restructure interactions with real or internalized attachment figures characterized by a sense of agency and, when possible, accessibility, responsiveness, and engagement. ____
e. To de-escalate arguments so that a couple or a family become effective negotiators. ____

Question 1.6. A prototypical scene or slice from EFT in process would look like: (Two correct answers.)

a. The therapist cognitively linking clients' present responses to childhood conflicts. ____
b. The therapist encapsulating a key emotional response with a client and asking the client in turn, to share this with the other partner or imagined attachment figure in a congruent, open way. ____

c. The therapist suggesting another, more skilled way to express anger and helping partners practice this in the session. ____

d. The therapist tracking and validating emotional responses, and putting them in the frame of patterned cycles of interaction and attachment needs and fears. ____

Question 1.7. EFT is a multi-modal approach. This means that: (Mark the correct answer.)

a. It can be used to address all distressed relationships in couples and families, and there is a separate protocol that can be used for depressed individuals. ____

b. It is a couple therapy that can be used with different kinds of clients. ____

c. It is a relational attachment approach that integrates self and system, and uses the same concepts and macro and micro interventions whether one person, a dyad, or family members are in the room. ____

d. There are three different EFT therapies, but they all use a de-pathologizing attachment orientation. ____

Question 1.8. Coding studies and theory tell us that the key elements of significant change events in EFT across all modalities are: (Mark all that apply.)

a. The ability to tune into, accept, and actively engage with core vulnerabilities and needs. ____

b. The construction of clear coherent messages that assert these needs with specificity. ____

c. The ability to take in comfort and affirmation from a supportive other or the mental representation of a supportive other. ____

d. The ability to turn back and give attuned congruent support to another. ____

Question 1.9. EFT focuses on couple interventions but intervenes with individual partners and on the level of dyadic interaction. It fits with the present zeitgeist of couple and family therapy in the following ways except: (Mark the one that doesn't fit.)

a. It is brief and constructionist. ____

b. It is integrative (integrating systems and experiential approaches). ____

c. It is empirically validated. ____

d. The alliance in EFT is collaborative and egalitarian. ____

e. It is used with many different kinds of clients and to address different kinds of problems. ____

f. Its reliance on the process of change has been systematically studied and outlined. ____

g. Its focus fits with recent research on the nature of attachment, emotional regulation, and relational distress and satisfaction. ____

h. It echoes extreme postmodern positions that view all realities as arbitrary and random. ____

Question 1.10. The EFT perspective on couple and family therapy fits very well with the recent body of research on the nature of relational distress and satisfaction, and predictors of divorce. The most obvious points of convergence are: (Mark all correct answers.)

a. The expression and regulation of emotion are noted as key factors in the definition of close relationships, e.g., fear and contempt on the face of partners predict divorce, according to Gottman's (1994) research, and attachment fears are a primary focus in EFT. ____
b. Conflict is not seen as the best predictor of dissolution. Emotional disengagement is noted as being more dangerous for close relationships. ____
c. Rigid, patterned interactions, such as criticize/complain or defend/distance, that preclude safe emotional engagement are toxic for close relationships. ____
d. The power of soothing emotionally connected interactions to define and redefine relationships is considerable. ____
e. Elements such as give–get equity or problem-solving skills do not seem as crucial as the ability to create safe emotional engagement. ____
f. Secure attachment is associated with greater levels of empathy and assertiveness, and with less reactive anger and less negative attributions for another's behavior. ____

Question 1.11. In terms of empirical validation, the status of EFT is: (Four correct answers.)

a. EFT has a few promising but very preliminary studies. ____
b. A solid and rigorous empirical basis for the effectiveness of EFT exists, but research has been focused until now on couple interventions. ____
c. EFT for couples is associated with lack of relapse, positive effect stability, and in some studies with post-therapy improvement. ____
d. Process studies have outlined EFT change events and key interventions that predict success in therapy. ____
e. Empirical validation is considered unnecessary in a postmodern world and by EFT therapists. ____
f. Only weak studies of EFT (studies without control groups) exist. ____
g. The percentage of clients who recover from relationship distress and who significantly improve found in the meta-analysis of the best EFT studies are impressive in terms of psychotherapy outcomes generally and for couple therapy, in particular. ____

Question 1.12. Which of the following is not an essential role of the EFT therapist?

a. Process consultant. ____
b. Creator of a safe haven and secure base in each session—surrogate attachment figure. ____
c. Collaborative processor of emerging experience in the moment with the client. ____
d. Guide and attuned validating partner in the change process and in key change events. ____
e. Coach in the practice of specific new communication skills. ____

Question 1.13. In the naming of EFT: (Four correct answers.)

a. The title EFT arose out of the originators, respect for catharsis, and distrust of emotional repression. ____
b. The title EFT was assigned to reflect the originators' understanding of the key importance of emotional signals in the processing of experience and sense of self, and in the drama of close attachments. Emotion organizes dancer and dance. ____
c. The title was assigned to stress emotion as a key agent of change in a field that was focused mostly on cognition and behavior. ____
d. The title reflected the humanistic experiential perspective of EFT and the recognition of the role of emotion in the creation of meaning. ____
e. The title is a statement of the usefulness of ventilation as a way out of repression and inhibition. ____
f. The title reflects a view of emotion as an adaptive rapid response system that has a unique power to "move" people into new ways of seeing and acting. ____

Question 1.14. In EFT, emotions are not viewed as:

a. Adaptive responses, providing a rapid and compelling response system that organizes behavior in the interests of security, survival, and the fulfilment of needs. ____
b. A powerful focusing and orienting force; a compass that directs attention to needs and specific environmental cues. ____
c. A major element in the creation of meaning, especially in social interactions in which many responses tend to be ambiguous and we have to "fill in the blanks." ____
d. A prime "mover" and organizer of responses in attachment relationships. ____
e. An activator of key cognitions concerning the nature of the self and others. ____
f. Arising from the more primitive part of the brain that is ruled by cognition in mature adults. ____
g. The primary signaling system in interactions with key others (the music of the dance of intimacy). ____

Question 1.15. Which of the following are primary tasks of EFT? (Three correct answers.)

a. To prevent all occurrences of negative interactions between partners', cycles, such as blame/defend, and within person emotion regulation cycles such as increased vigilance/more agitation and flooding/more frequent triggering of distress. ____
b. To assemble, reprocess, and expand clients' key emotional responses. ____
c. To structure and shape new kinds of interactions, including accessible and responsive interactions with key others. ____
d. To foster secure emotional bonds between partners in EFT with couples. ____
e. To help partners choose marriage over divorce. ____

Question 1.16. Change occurs in EFT primarily through which two ways?

a. New corrective emotional experiences. Core attachment vulnerabilities and needs then take on a new shape and color. ____
b. New emotional moves create new relational events that redefine the nature of the bond between partners in EFT for couples, and between individuals and their representations of attachment figures and parts of self in EFIT. New dramas recast models of self and other. ____
c. Revision of the dominant story of a distressed relationship and the externalizing of problems. ____
d. Creating new problem-solving and communications skill sequences. ____
e. Insight into past childhood dynamics and unconscious wishes. ____

Question 1.17. The three stages of EFT are:

a. De-escalation of conflict, the step of clarifying underlying feelings, and promotion of positive narratives. ____
b. De-escalation/stabilization of overwhelming negative emotional states and negative interactions with key others; changing/restructuring interactional positions and so core existential dilemmas and sense of self; and consolidation and integration. ____
c. Position restructuring, emotional engagement, and consolidation. ____
d. Alliance creation, behavioral contracting, and the change event entitled "blamer softening". ____

Question 1.18. The four contraindications for EFT with couples and individuals include:

a. In couple therapy, ongoing abusiveness/violence in a relationship, especially if the "victim" expresses fear or the "perpetrator" does not take responsibility. ____
b. The inability to create any kind of collaborative alliance. ____
c. Obvious, active addiction that is unacknowledged and untreated and will undermine progress in EFIT and EFT with couples. ____
d. Depression or posttraumatic stress in an individual or one partner. ____
e. An "inexpressive" style in one partner in couple therapy. ____
f. In EFIT, antisocial personality disorder or schizophrenia. ____

Question 1.19. Check the following statements to see if you can identify the two best predictors of success in EFT for couples. This information is not included in the brief information on EFT given at the beginning of this workbook. If you have not read the EFT literature in detail, see which ones make the most sense to you and then compare your answer with the ones given at the end of this chapter.

a. Initial relationship distress level accounts for almost 50% of the variance in behavioral couple therapy outcome. As might be expected, this is also the best predictor of success in EFT. ____

b. The traditionality of the couple predicts success in EFT: It is hard to get traditional couples to talk about feelings. ____
c. The faith of the one partner that their partner still cares for them is the best identified predictor of success in EFT for couples. ____
d. Higher income and length of marriage predict success in EFT. ____
e. The quality of the alliance with the therapist is a significant predictor of success in EFT. ____

Question 1.20. Of the three elements of the therapeutic alliance—bond with the therapist, agreement about goals of therapy, and the perceived relevance of therapy tasks—the element of the therapeutic relationship found to be the most predictive of outcome in studies of EFT for couples and in clinical experience with individuals is: (Mark the correct answer.)

a. The bond aspect of the alliance between each partner and the therapist. ____
b. The goal agreement aspect of the alliance between each partner and the therapist. ____
c. The task aspect of the alliance: how relevant and engaging processes and tasks feel in the sessions. ____

Question 1.21. The usual number of sessions in early EFT studies and in EFT clinical practice are: (Two correct answers. Again, if you are just beginning to read the literature, go with your hunch about the answer and see how it compares with the one we give at the end of this chapter.)

a. In studies and in practice, the usual number of sessions is 15. ____
b. In studies, the usual number has been 10 to 12, whereas in practice, it is 10 to 20. ____
c. In studies, the usual number of sessions is 20, whereas in practice, it is 30. ____
d. In EFT for couples with clients who have PTSD, the average number of sessions is 30 to 35. ____

Question 1.22. Health in attachment science and in experiential models of therapy is viewed as: (Mark the answer that does not fit.)

a. Being able to be open to new experience and explore and discover this experience and its meaning so that models of self and other can be ongoingly revised and change. ____
b. Being able to stay present with and process core emotions in a coherent manner that results in emotional balance. ____
c. Being able to differentiate from others and keep strong boundaries so as to always feel in control of one's life. ____
d. Being able to attune to and engage authentically with others and respond to their emotional cues in a way that build secure connection. ____

Question 1.23. In EFT, the focus is on present process as it comes alive in the session. The main way a focus on the past is used is to: (Mark the correct answer.)

a. Explain the developmental delays of the clients and their need for re-education. ____
b. Make unconscious desires and conflicts conscious. ____
c. Validate and empathize with each client's present ways of seeing and dealing with distress and insecurity. ____
d. Contrast past negative responses with the unique positive responses of the present. ____

Question 1.24. Which of the following is a core assumption of EFT? (Mark all correct answers.)

a. Emotion is the music of the couple's dance. Rigid, constricted, or "stuck" emotions evoke constricted patterns of responses or interactions and vice versa. ____
b. On-target change requires focusing on the core organizing variables of a phenomena (e.g., vigilance for threat and compulsive avoidance is a key part of the emotional disorders that EFIT addresses). ____
c. The alliance and the safety it provides is the most significant change ingredient in EFT; it is sufficient to create change in and of itself. ____
d. Clients are stuck in less than functional ways of dealing with emotional needs and fears and in negative patterns of interaction with key others. Significant change is always within and between. ____
e. Close connection with others is the ecological niche in which the human brain, nervous system, and key behavioral patterns evolved. ____
f. Often, habitual ways of regulating emotion and engaging with others that offered protection from vulnerability without solution become prisons that block growth. ____
g. Effective couples' therapy addresses emotional accessibility, responsiveness, and engagement—the security of the bond between spouses. ____
h. Secure attachment is a major resource and a potent source of individual growth, positive identity, and resilience in the face of stress. ____
i. Attachment science provides the therapist with a map of common human misery and motivation. ____

Question 1.25. In each session, an EFT therapist might be expected to: (Mark all correct answers.)

a. Monitor and maintain the collaborative alliance with each client. ____
b. Discover, assemble, deepen, and distil with each client new elements of his or her emotional experience or responses, making such elements less frightening and alien. ____
c. Track and reflect on the sequence or patterns of interactions with real or imagined others in the session and in narratives told in the session. ____
d. Lead the client or clients into the five moves of the EFT Tango again and again. ____
e. Generally, frame responses or realities in terms of attachment needs and fears and existential dilemmas, such as emotional isolation versus the risk of relying on others. ____

f. Assemble specific emotional responses and create an enactment where partners share these responses with one another or individuals share with the therapist or imagined others. ____
g. Across therapy modalities, titrate risks by "slicing them thinner," reflecting on clients' strengths, and validating their responses whenever possible. ____
h. After the clients have left, the therapist notes the present stage of therapy, the current blocks to engagement with experience, and key themes and emotional *handles* to use and repeat in upcoming sessions. ____

Question 1.26. The main differences between EFCT and EFFT are: (Mark all correct answers.)

a. There is always a group—all family members in every session. ____
b. The main point of couple sessions is to de-escalate negative cycles to the point where the couple can be an effective parenting team, not building intimacy per se. ____
c. There is less focus on mutuality in sessions; the goal is to help the parent move into becoming more responsive and providing secure attachment for the child. ____
d. The therapist focuses specifically on regulating the parents' sadness and shame at failing as parents so they can look at their difficulties in a coherent way that allows them to see the negative cycles they and their child are caught in. ____

SUMMARY

This chapter has offered a general overview of EFT. The next chapter reviews the theoretical basis of EFT in more detail. A key reference for a recent general overview of all modalities of EFT is *Attachment Theory in Practice* (Johnson, 2019). Short chapters on EFT for couples can also be found in the *Encyclopedia of Couple and Family Therapy* (Lebow, Chambers, & Breunlin, 2019).

ANSWERS

1.1 **Answer: D.** Emotionally focused therapy (EFT) is informed by the humanistic tradition of Rogers and the systemic formulation of Minuchin and family systems theory.

1.2 **Answer: All responses.**

1.3 **Answer: B**. Secure attachment and the capacity to form and sustain close bonds resulting in greater emotional balance and relational responsiveness is essential in human resilience and well-being.

1.4 **Answer: A, B, D, and E**. Attachment science underscores the ways in which emotions are embodied and intrinsic to growth and resilience in human development.

1.5 **Answer: E**. The EFT therapist is not focused on negotiating relationship compromises; rather, the therapist engages individuals, couples, and families in working through relational blocks that drive distress, disengagement, and intra- and interpersonal conflict.

1.6 **Answer: B and D**. The EFT therapist focuses and engages specific emotional responses through exploring and enacting these experiences. The therapist reflects and validates the emotionally informed patterns that inform individual and relational interactions.

1.7 **Answer: C**. Applications of EFT to individuals, couples, and families are rooted in a common theory of change and emotionally focused interventions targeting attachment processes within individuals and across relationships.

1.8 **Answer: All responses**. Each response describes a critical aspect of an EFT change event based on theory and process research studies of EFT.

1.9 **Answer: H**. The EFT stance is that there are common existential conditions and processes, emotion, and attachment.

1.10 **Answer: All responses**. Each response highlights EFT's relevance to factors associated with relational distress and satisfaction.

1.11 **Answer: B, C, D, and G**. For answer G, the results for EFT are a significant improvement over other results reported for couples' therapy and over most results reported for individual therapy in the literature.

1.12 **Answer: E.** The EFT therapist facilitates the sharing of new experience through focusing on the accessing and engaging of attachment-related emotion, rather than teaching and practicing communication skills.

1.13 **Answer: B, C, D, and F**.

1.14 **Answer: F**. EFT recognizes that emotions are a core facet to human experience, and inform and motivate understanding and actions across individuals and relationships.

1.15 **Answer: B, C, and D**. In answer A, it is impossible to prevent all occurrences of negative cycles and they will inevitably occur. But they do not have the same ability to define the relationship once partners can exit from them; secure bonding interactions also occur. In answer E, the experiential therapist does not pressure clients to make any choice. His or her job is to make implicit choices explicit and help clients make them with awareness and responsibility.

1.16 **Answer: A and B**. EFT promotes change through corrective emotional experiences informed by accessing and engaging attachment vulnerability and related needs, leading to new emotional moves with self and significant others (e.g., partners, parents, children).

1.17 **Answer: B.** The stages describing the process of change in EFT include: de-escalation/stabilization; restructuring of interactional positions and self-understanding; and consolidation/integration.

1.18 **Answer: A—C, and F**. EFT has been used extensively and successfully with depressed and traumatized partners. EFT has been found in a study of predictors of success to be particularly potent in couples in which the female partner identifies the male partner as being "inexpressive." EFT has been shown to be effective in clients with low socioeconomic status (Denton, Burelson, Clark, Rodriguez, & Hobbs, 2000).

1.19 **Answer: C and E**. Answer C was the most powerful predictor of success in EFT in the Johnson and Talitman (1997) study. Level of distress was found to account for only 4% of the variance in outcome three months after treatment termination. This is a very small percentage compared with that found in the psychotherapy literature in general, which implies that EFT can be used successfully with very distressed couples. Alliance was found to account for 20% of variance in outcome. In other studies of psychotherapy outcome, it has been found to account for 10%. Predictors noted in Answers C and E are presumed to impact outcome by influencing the level of engagement in therapy.

1.20 **Answer: C**. This response identifies the task aspect of the alliance, which has shown to be most predictive of successful outcomes in EFT (Johnson & Talitman, 1997).

1.21 **Answer: B and D**. Research studies involve intense supervision that enhance the amount accomplished in each session.

1.22 **Answer: C**. This answer does not fit the health assumptions of attachment science and experiential therapy.

1.23 **Answer: C**. This answer highlights the EFT therapist's focus on honoring the client's distress and insecurity in reflecting and validating these experiences in the present moment.

1.24 **All answers** describe assumptions of the EFT approach.

1.25 **All answers** describe actions an EFT therapist would take.

1.26 **Answer: B, C, and D.** Each indicate key differences between emotionally focused couples therapy (EFCT) and emotionally focused family therapy (EFFT).

2

THEORETICAL BACKGROUND TO EFT

Emotionally focused therapy (EFT) espouses a specific, empirically based developmental theory of personality and close relationships—attachment theory (Bowlby, 1969, 1988; Milkulincer & Shaver, 2016). This theory has "spawned one of the broadest, most profound and most creative lines of research in 20th and 21st century psychology" (Cassidy & Shaver, 2016). A literature search on the topic of attachment will access thousands of studies, hundreds of which are about adult attachment, which has only really been addressed in recent decades, with approximately 30,000 entries since 1975. No matter whether the therapist is working with an adult depressed client, a distressed couple, or a chaotic family, attachment offers the therapist a map to grasping the core of dysfunctional intrapsychic and interpersonal processes, a pathway to individual and relational health, and a systematic pathway to moving from one to the other. The EFT couple therapist uses attachment theory as a guide to the territory of adult love and the process of bond disruption and repair. The individual therapist is able to use the attachment perspective to hone in on core organizing variables, such as affect regulation strategies that define how inner experience and relational steps are constructed, and to systematically create change in session. Attachment theory attunes the therapist to primary emotional realities and patterns of key signals sent to others in a way that makes profound sense to clients and empowers the therapist.

The following overview provides a brief synopsis of attachment theory and experiential methods of intervention associated with this theory that form the basis of EFT in general, and with the modalities emotionally focused individual therapy (EFIT), emotionally focused couple therapy (EFCT), and emotionally focused family therapy (EFFT). Imagine that Carl Rogers, Ludwig von Bertalanffy or Salvador Minuchin, and John Bowlby, with comments from emotion theorists, neuroscientists, and culture commentators, have come to visit and offer their perspective on the task of being a psychotherapist in the 21st century, when most therapists see individuals and couples or families in session, and all deal in one way or another with the demons of individual depression, anxiety, post-traumatic stress, and insecure attachment to others.

The essence of any brief therapy intervention is focus. The attachment perspective and the integration of experiential and systemic perspectives on intervention provide a focus for each therapy session and a guide to change processes for individuals and partnered and family relationships. The goal for the EFT therapist, no matter how many clients are in the room, is the same, namely, to help clients move into what Rogers (1961) called "existential living" and into the accessibility, responsiveness, and engagement with others that foster secure bonding and potentiate individual growth and resilience. Existential living is characterized by openness to the flow of experience and living the moment fully,

DOI: 10.4324/9781003039457-3

organismic trusting that involves affirming the validity of inner experience and using it as a guide to action, experiential freedom that enables choice and taking responsibility for choices made, and creativity that opens up the possibility of constant growth.

ATTACHMENT THEORY

Attachment theory provides a guiding organization for the conceptualization and practice of EFT across modalities. As stated by Johnson in *Attachment Theory in Practice* (2019, pp. 6–10), these ten core tenets illustrate the importance of attachment to mental health and human development.

Core Tenets

1. From the cradle to the grave, human beings are hard wired to seek not just social contact but also physical and emotional proximity to special others who are deemed irreplaceable. The longing for a "felt sense" of connection to key others is primary in terms of the hierarchy of human goals and needs. Humans are most acutely aware of this need for connection at times of threat, risk, pain, or uncertainty. Threats that trigger the attachment system here include both outer and inner sources of threat, for example, troubling construals of rejection by loved ones, negative images or concrete reminders of one's own mortality (Mikulincer, Birnbaum, Woddis, & Nachmias, 2000; Mikulincer & Florian, 2000). In relationships, shared vulnerability builds bonds precisely because it brings these needs to the fore and encourages reaching for others.
2. Predictable physical and/or emotional connection with an attachment figure, often a parent, sibling, long-time close friend, mate, or spiritual figure, calms the nervous system, and shapes a safe haven where comfort and reassurance can be obtained and emotional balance can be restored or enhanced. The responsiveness of others, especially when we are young, tunes the nervous system to be less sensitive to threat and creates expectations of a relatively safe and manageable world.
3. This emotional balance shapes a grounded, positive, and integrated sense of self, and the ability to effectively organize and structure inner experience into a coherent whole. This grounded sense of self also facilitates the congruent expression of needs to attachment figures that are likely to result in more successful bids for connection, which then continue to build positive models of close others as accessible sources of support.
4. A felt sense of being able to depend on a loved one creates a *secure base*—a platform from which to move out into the world, take risks, explore, and develop a sense of competence and autonomy. This *effective dependency* is a source of strength and resilience, while the denial of attachment needs and pseudo self-sufficiency are liabilities. Being able to reach out to and depend on reliable others and internalize a "felt sense" of secure connection with others is the ultimate resource that allows our species to survive and thrive in an uncertain world.
5. The key factors that define the quality and security of an attachment bond are the perceived *accessibility, responsiveness*, and *emotional engagement* of

attachment figures. These factors can be translated into the acronym A.R.E. (In clinical work, I use A.R.E as shorthand for the key attachment question that arises in couple's conflict, "Are you there for me?")

6. Separation distress arises when an attachment bond is threatened or secure connection is lost. There are other kinds of emotional bonds based on shared activities or respect, and when these are broken, a person may be distressed. But that distress does not have the same intensity or significance as when an attachment bond is called into question. Emotional and physical isolation from attachment figures is inherently traumatizing for human beings, bringing with it a heightened sense, not simply of vulnerability and danger, but also of helplessness (Mikulincer, Shaver, & Pereg, 2003).
7. Secure connection is a function of key interactions in bonded relationships and how individuals *encode patterns of interaction into mental models* or protocols for responding. One's sense of general attachment security is not a fixed character trait; it changes when new experiences occur that allow one to revise cognitive working models of attachment and their associated emotion regulation strategies. It is possible, then, to be insecure in one relationship but secure in another. Working models are primarily concerned with the trustworthiness of others and the entitlement to care—that is the acceptability of the self. They ask both, "Can I count on you?" and, "Am I worthy of your love?" They involve sets of expectations, automatic perceptual biases that trigger emotions, episodic memories, beliefs, and attitudes, and implicit procedural knowledge about how to conduct close relationships (Collins & Read, 1994). These models, in their most unbending and automatic form, can distort perceptions in interactions and so bias responses. They are experienced as reality, as "just the way things are," rather than as constructed.
8. Those who are securely attached are comfortable with closeness and their need for others. Their primary attachment strategy is, then, to acknowledge attachment needs and congruently reach out (e.g., matching verbal and nonverbal signals into a clear whole) in a bid for an attachment figure to make or maintain contact. When this figure responds, this response is trusted and taken in, calming the nervous system of the person who reached out. By providing one with such an effective strategy, attachment security appears to buffer stress and potentiate positive coping throughout life.
9. If others have been perceived as inaccessible or unresponsive, or even threatening, when needed, then secondary models and strategies are adopted. These secondary models can take the form of vigilant, hyperactivated anxious ways of engaging with others and regulating attachment emotions, or of avoidant, dismissing, and deactivated strategies. The first of these secondary models, anxious attachment, is characterized by sensitivity to any negative messages coming from significant others and by "fight" responses designed to protest distance and get an attachment figure to pay more attention and offer more reassuring support. On the other hand, deactivating avoidant responses are "flight' responses designed to minimize the frustration and distress through distancing oneself from loved ones who are seen as hostile, dangerous, or uncaring. Attachment needs are then minimized, and compulsive self-reliance is the order of the day. Vulnerability in the self or perceived vulnerability in others triggers distancing

behaviors. All people use all these fight-or-flight strategies at times in relationships; they are not dysfunctional per se. However, they can become generalized, habitual, and rigid into a style that ends up constraining a person's awareness and choices, and limiting their ability to engage constructively with others.

A third kind of secondary model arises when a person has been traumatized by an attachment figure. He or she is then in a paradoxical situation in which loved ones are both the source of and solution to fear. Under these circumstances, this person often vacillates between longing and fear, demanding connection and then distancing, and even attacking when connection is offered. This type of response is called disorganized attachment in children but is termed fearful avoidant attachment (Bartholomew & Horowitz, 1991) in adults, and is associated with especially high distress in adult relationships.

The psychodynamic concepts of inner ambivalence, conflict, and defensive blocks are central to understanding the secondary models (and insecure strategies) described above. Avoidant children in infant research look calm and contained but are, in fact, highly aroused by separation from their mother. Similarly, avoidant adult partners show little explicit emotional distress or need for others, but the evidence is that high levels of attachment distress exist for them at deeper or less conscious levels (Shaver & Mikulincer, 2002). Avoidant individuals are also less able to trust and benefit from the greatest resource we have for dealing with our vulnerability to stress and threat, safe connection with special others (Selchuk, Zayas, Gunaydin, Hazan, & Kross, 2012).

10. Compared to child–parent attachment, the bonds between adults are more reciprocal and not so dependent on physical proximity; cognitive representations of an attachment figure can be evoked to create symbolic proximity. Bowlby also identified two other behavioral systems in intimate relationships (particularly adult relationships) besides attachment: caretaking and sexuality. These are separate systems; however, they act in concert with attachment, and attachment is considered primary—that is, attachment processes set the stage for and organize key features of these other systems. Secure attachment and the emotional balance resulting from this security are associated with more attuned attention to another adult and more responsive caregiving. This security is maintained, of course, on a continuum and is not a constant steady state but varies somewhat in specific relationships and situations.

    Security is also associated with higher levels of arousal, intimacy, and pleasure, and more sexual satisfaction in relationships (Birnbaum, 2007). Sex, a bonding activity in humans, has an emotional signature that varies with different attachment styles and the strategies for dealing with emotions and engaging others that accompany those styles. More avoidantly attached individuals tend to separate sex and love, focusing on sensation and performance in sexual encounters, while those who are more anxiously attached focus on affection and sex as a proof of love, rather than on the erotic aspects of sexuality (Mikulincer & Shaver, 2016; Johnson, 2017).

From *Attachment Theory in Practice: Emotionally Focused Therapy (EFT) with Individuals, Couples, and Families* (pp. 6–10), by S. M. Johnson, 2019, New York, NY: Guilford Press.

ATTACHMENT SECURITY AND MENTAL HEALTH

Secure attachment, as a style or habitual engagement strategy, has been linked in systematic research to almost every positive index of mental health and general well-being outlined in the social sciences (Mikulincer & Shaver, 2007). On an individual level, these include resilience in the face of stress; optimism, high self-esteem, confidence, and curiosity; tolerance for human differences; a sense of belonging; the ability to self-disclose and be assertive; and the ability to tolerate ambiguity, regulate difficult emotions, engage in reflective meta-cognition, and grasp different perspectives. The essential elements of this picture are an ability to regulate affect effectively in a way that maintains emotional equilibrium, an ability to process information into a coherent integrated whole, and to maintain a sense of confidence in oneself that fosters decisive action. Even in the face of trauma, such as the events of 9/11, secure attachment appears to not only mitigate the effects of such experience but also to foster post-traumatic growth.

On an interpersonal level, these indices include capacity for sensitive attunement to others, empathic responsiveness, compassion, openness to people who are perceived as different from oneself, and a tendency to altruistic action. When we can maintain our emotional balance, the evidence is that we are simply better at sensitively picking up on other people's cues and need for support, and then responding in a caring way that they can take in and accept. When we are secure, we simply have more focused attention and more resources to offer to others. In contrast, more anxiously attached people tend to become preoccupied with managing their own distress, or they offer care that does not fit the needs of the other. Avoidant individuals dismiss their own needs and those of others, expressing less empathy and reciprocal support. They turn away from vulnerability in themselves and others.

When we have a safe haven and secure base with loved ones, we are also better at dealing with differences and conflict. The evidence is that secure connection shapes balanced adjusted human beings who then have better relationships with loved ones and friends, which then foster ongoing mental health and adjustment, and more ability to relate to others.

For the purposes of this book, it is especially important to note the impact of secure attachment on emotion regulation, social adjustment, and mental health. These were Bowlby's prime concerns. In terms of mental health, it is clear that attachment insecurity increases vulnerability to the two problems most commonly addressed in therapy: depression and anxiety. Exactly how this occurs will depend on individual clients but, in general, the process begins for the attachment scientist with the process of emotion regulation. Secure people are more able to attend to and stay engaged with distressing emotions without fear of losing control or being overwhelmed. They do not need to alter, block, or deny these emotions, and so can use them adaptively to orient to their world and move toward the fulfillment of their needs and goals. They can recover faster from negative feelings such as sadness and anger. I like to think of effective affect regulation as a process of moving with and through the emotion rather than reactively intensifying or suppressing it, and then being able to *use* this emotion to give direction to one's life.

On the other hand, it is clear that insecurity is a significant risk factor for maladjustment. Anxious and fearful avoidant attachment are particularly associated with vulnerability to depression and various forms of stress and anxiety disorders, including posttraumatic stress disorder, obsessive-compulsive disorder, and generalized anxiety disorder. The severity of depression symptoms has been linked to insecure attachment in over 100 studies. If we look more specifically at different forms of depression, anxious attachment seems to be related to more interpersonal forms characterized by a sense of loss, loneliness, abandonment, and helplessness, while avoidant attachment is associated with the achievement-oriented kinds of depression, characterized by perfectionism, self-criticism, and compulsive self-reliance (Mikulincer & Shaver, 2007; see tables of studies on pp. 380–382). Attachment insecurity is also related to many personality disorders, with borderline personality disorder being particularly associated with extreme anxious attachment, and schizoid and avoidant personality disorders with dismissing avoidant attachment. Insecurity has also been linked to externalizing disorders, such as conduct disorders in adolescents, and antisocial tendencies and addiction in adults.

REVIEWING THE EFT THEORY OF ADULT LOVE—ATTACHMENT THEORY

Question 2.1. Theorists of adult attachment espouse the idea that: (Mark all correct answers.)

a. The need to connect with and depend on key others is wired in by evolution. ____
b. Attachment is a universal primary survival motivation in human beings across cultures. ____
c. Recent understandings of attachment are that it involves, not just bonding but also caretaking and sexuality; these are not separate systems. ____
d. Attachment is only applicable to mother–child relationships. ____
e. Attachment is a systemic theory: it deals with key patterns of interaction and self-sustaining feedback loops of responses between intimates. ____
f. Attachment is also an intrapsychic theory: it deals with affect regulation and inner models of self and other. ____

Question 2.2. The attachment view of dependency assumes: (Mark all correct answers.)

a. Dependency on a few key others is a lifelong adaptive survival mechanism and promotes adaptation and growth. ____
b. Dependency is adaptive in childhood but adults should be self-sufficient. ____
c. The more securely interdependent we can be, the more separate and different we can be. ____
d. Autonomy and the ability to be separate, and a felt sense of secure connection are two sides of the same coin. ____________
e. Dependency and autonomy are dichotomous: they are opposite ends of a continuum. ____

Question 2.3. A positive secure attachment relationship has two basic elements, which are:

a. A set of procedures to minimize conflict. ____
b. A safe haven—an antidote to fear and helplessness. ____

c. A secure base from which to explore the universe with confidence. ____
d. A caretaking contract in the case of need. ____

Question 2.4. When distressed in a relationship or in life, a securely attached adult is likely to deal with her or his emotions by: (Mark all correct answers.)

a. Reaching for the comfort and caring of a significant other. ____
b. Using the representation of an attachment figure to soothe the self. ____
c. Asserting needs for care in a way that invites responsiveness. ____
d. Being optimistic about others' willingness or ability to respond. ____
e. Protesting any upsetting distance in hopeful, constructive ways. ____
f. Numbing and focusing on tasks, thereby increasing feelings of control and competence. ____
g. Being able to resist flooding with negative emotions, thereby being more able to reciprocate responsiveness. ____

Question 2.5. What element would you not typically see in a secure attachment relationship?

a. Both partners can reach for the other when vulnerable. ____
b. Both express needs for closeness and reassurance. ____
c. Both use the comfort offered to soothe the self. ____
d. Both feel wary of dependency needs and wish to put them aside. ____
e. Both find it rewarding to be able to calm and reassure the other. ____
f. Both feel basically safe and engaged, and can then play and explore the relationship. ____

Question 2.6. To increase a person's sense of attachment security, a partner or family member must become: (Mark all correct answers.)

a. More accessible, especially when the other is stressed, fearful, or uncertain. ____
b. More responsive on an emotional level to attachment requests, fears, and needs. ____
c. Less dependent on this person. ____
d. More morally committed to staying in the relationship. ____
e. More consistently reflective rather than emotional during difficult times. ____
f. More able to stay emotionally engaged when the less secure person protests distance or disconnection. ____
g. More comfortable with offering reassurance. ____

Question 2.7. When a person cannot get an attachment figure to respond or engage, separation distress occurs. The first two steps in this distress usually are:

a. Sulking followed by depression, if sulking is not effective in getting a response from an attachment figure. ____

b. Rage, contempt, and criticism, followed by defensive distancing. ____
c. Protest, often in the form of anger, and clinging or seeking closeness and connection. ____
d. Distancing and denial of attachment needs. ____

Question 2.8. In couple therapy, protest and seeking connection may show up or look like the following: (Mark all correct answers.)

a. Criticism and complaining. ____
b. Clear, logical negotiations as to exactly how the spouse should change. ____
c. Expressions of emotional anguish or hurt, and fear for the relationship. ____
d. Descriptions of grief, isolation, and loss, as in, "I am alone." ____
e. Calm and caring discussions about how problems can be solved. ____

Question 2.9. If there is still no emotional response from the partner, the last two steps of separation distress outlined in attachment theory are: (Mark all correct answers.)

a. Problem-solving as to how each partner can be more independent. ____
b. Spiraling into depression and despair. ____
c. Logically discussing and moving to friendly problem solving. ____
d. Grief beginning to evolve into detachment and true separateness. ____

Question 2.10. In couple therapy how do these last two steps of separation distress show up? (Mark all correct answers.)

a. Expressions of grief and hopelessness/helplessness. ____
b. Brief flares of angry contempt, as in, "I will make you respond to me." ____
c. Calm acceptance of the relationship as it is. ____
d. A feeling of letting go and a growing detachment from the relationship. ____

Question 2.11. Attachment concerns move to front and center, and become compelling at particular times. In what way can these times be summarized? (Mark all correct answers.)

a. Stressful conditions in the environment, or life transitions or challenges, such as parenthood, that increase attachment needs. ____
b. Conditions or shifts that appear to threaten the future—the status of the attachment relationship. ____
c. Conditions that increase personal fear and vulnerability, such as illness. ____
d. Unconscious projective identifications from the past are aroused and the partner is maneuvered into playing them out. ____

Question 2.12. In terms of individual responses, the four adjectives that Bowlby used to describe adult depression, which are consonant with recent research on the core features of depression are:

a. Lonely ____
b. Angry ____

c. Unwanted ____
d. Helpless ____
e. Unlovable ____
f. Agitated ____

Question 2.13. As well as universal elements, attachment theory focuses on individual differences in attachment responses. The two basic dimensions of attachment insecurity that vary among individuals are:

a. Anxiety ____
b. Disorganization ____
c. Avoidance ____
d. Self-sufficiency ____

Question 2.14. These dimensions have resulted in three categories of insecure adult attachment responses: (Mark the correct three categories below.)

a. Anxious attachment: when people are preoccupied with bonds and are vigilant for any threat to them. ____
b. Dismissing avoidant attachment: when people deny attachment needs and fears, especially when they are vulnerable. ____
c. Fearful avoidant attachment: when people are anxiously vigilant but also do not trust closeness and turn away when it is offered. ____
d. Disorganized chaotic attachment: when no pattern can be seen. ____
e. Detachment: when people become so mature that they do not need others. ____

Exercise 2.15. Attachment responses or strategies (e.g., secure, anxious, avoidant, and fearful avoidant) are best described by which of the following statements? (Mark all correct answers.)

a. Labels for set personality types or traits; people are the same across time and different relationships. ____
b. Habitual but changeable forms of engagement in close relationships. ____
c. Strategies for managing dependency in close relationships. ____
d. Scripts or default options for emotion regulation in close relationships. ____
e. Forms of engagement or strategies or scripts that can be different in different relationships, and at different times in the same relationship. ____
f. Models that can be coherent, elaborated, and open to revision, or relatively inaccessible, undifferentiated, and closed. ____
g. Strategies that are kept stable by confirmation processes in a relationship, rather than just as existing models that always bias perception. ____

Question 2.16. Secure attachment with at least one person has been found to impact models of self in the following ways: (Mark all correct answers.)

a. More security is associated with a more organized coherent sense of self. ________

b. More security is associated with a more positive sense of self in which flaws are accepted. ____
c. More security is associated with a more articulated sense of self. ____
d. Secure attachment is associated with higher levels of competence and efficacy. ____
e. In terms of self-disclosure, more avoidant individuals disclose less. While anxious and secure people tend to be willing to disclose, anxiously attached individuals disclose indiscriminately. ____
f. Individuals with a secure style are better at managing emotion and appraising or reappraising events in benign terms, short-circuiting threat. They remain open to their emotions and are less likely to distort or defend against them. ____
g. Secure individuals can sidestep the interfering or more dysfunctional aspects of emotions while benefiting from their functional adaptive qualities. ____

Question 2.17. In terms of dealing with their emotions in a distressed attachment relationship, more securely attached partners often: (Mark all correct answers.)

a. Ask openly and clearly for comfort and support. ____
b. Stay curious and open to new evidence and cues even when distressed. ____
c. Tolerate uncertainty and see whole cycles of interaction from a meta-perspective. ____
d. Discuss emotions and emotional events in a coherent, integrated way. ____
e. Empathize with and respond to their partner's disclosures. ____
f. Own their needs and fears, and ask for their needs to be met in a congruent way that pulls for a compassionate response. ____
g. Are unable to turn easily and trustingly to friends and other resources for comfort when partners are unavailable. ____

Question 2.18. It has been found that attachment style and strategies change and that therapy can foster this process: (Two correct answers.)

a. No, only years of new experiences can change attachment styles once set in childhood with parental figures. ____
b. Attachment style has only been shown to change in individual more psychodynamic therapy that focuses on reflective function. ____
c. Attachment style has been shown to change in partners after EFT couple therapy, with avoidant partners changing a little in every session and anxious partners only changing after key Stage 2 change events. ____
d. Attachment style can be expected to change with new emotionally loaded experiences such as getting married and has been shown to change in attachment oriented individual and couple therapies. ____

Personal Reflection. See if you can identify a person in your own life who could often be described as engaging with you or others in one of the ways described earlier, with a secure style or with an insecure style. What impact do you think their style had on you and the way you responded to them?

____

____

____

____

Question 2.19. An anxiously attached person will often: (Mark all correct answers.)

a. Amplify and become absorbed in the different elements of their own anxiety: cues, body sensations, negative meanings or attributions, actions. ____
b. Become reactively angry and desperate, critically pursuing the other. ____
c. Recall and obsessively recount specific incidents but be unable to articulate a coherent overall picture of their relationship. ____
d. Be difficult to soothe in that responsiveness or caring is not necessarily trusted. ____
e. Turn easily to inner representations of an attachment figure to soothe and regulate distress. ____
f. Speak of past attachment figures as being inconsistent and unpredictable. ____
g. Experience unpredictable, large, and rapid swings in attachment-related emotions. ____

Question 2.20. A dismissingly or avoidantly attached person will most often: (Mark all correct answers.)

a. Deny distress and focus on tasks—external events. ____
b. Speak in vague general abstract terms or idealized images. ____
c. Have difficulty focusing on their own or their partner's emotional signals. ____
d. Shut down, defend, and distance emotionally and physically when anxiety increases or the other partner protests. ____
e. Problem solve in a distant, detached manner when the partner becomes upset. ____
f. Express "incompetence" or "inadequacy" in relation to emotional closeness or responses. ____
g. Express cold, general hostility. ____

Question 2.21. Identify which of the following statements best fit the ways an anxious or avoidant attachment strategy may impact a relationship. Indicate whether each response is more likely for a partner with an anxious (ANX) or avoidant attachment (AVD) strategy.

a. Clinging, pursuit, and frequent bids for reassurance are the order of the day. ____

b. More likely to somaticize, to become hostile, and to engage in promiscuous sexuality. ____
c. Often vigilant for threat; for example, more jealous and distrustful. ____
d. Often make disparaging remarks about dependency and disown vulnerability as a form of "weakness." ____
e. Bids for attention often escalate into angry blaming and coercive demands. ____
f. May become very reactive and less than coherent in their presentation of the problem and the relationship. ____
g. Often state the goal of "just wanting the arguments to stop" rather than a change in the relationship, closeness, or caring. ____
h. Use rejection less and evocative requests for caring more. ____
i. Ambiguous cues about the other's dependability are likely to be taken negatively. ____
j. This way of engaging others has been called "closed," "diversionary," and "fragile" in that it does not deal with or really diminish distress. ____

Personal Reflection: See if you can think of a client who might be described as anxiously attached and list the letters from the descriptions above that might fit their responses toward their partner.

Question 2.22. Identify which of the following statements best fit the ways an anxious or avoidant attachment strategy may impact a partner's view of self or other, or how that partner might regulate their emotion. Indicate which strategy best applies: anxious (ANX) or avoidant (AVD).

a. They prefer to focus on objects and instrumental tasks, away from attachment cues and issues. ____
b. Attachment emotions or concerns go into hyperactivation or overdrive. ____
c. Attachment emotions and concerns are generally deactivated and suppressed. ____
d. Partners tend to see themselves as flawed and unlovable. ____
e. Deactivation is particularly employed when experiencing vulnerability or neediness. ____
f. Arousal is high, but awareness and expression of emotions are blunted and masked. ____
g. Partners actively worry about abandonment. ____
h. They are more likely to see others as unreliable and untrustworthy. ____

Personal Reflection. See if you can think of a client who might be described as avoidantly attached and list the letters from the descriptions above that might fit how they regulate emotions or their view of others or self.

Question 2.23. A fearful avoidantly attached person will often: (Mark all responses that apply.)

a. Demand reassurance, emphasizing their need and that the other is the only solution to their pain. ____
b. Refuse engagement when offered, stating that they cannot trust the other and that she or he is the source of their pain. ____
c. Become disorganized because many emotions—anger, shame, fear, and grief—arise together and become overwhelming. ____
d. Be unable to assert emotional needs, becoming caught in a sense of shame and unworthiness. ____
e. Flip between anxious pursuit and numb distancing and defense. ____

Question 2.24. Fearful avoidant attachment is not associated with: (Mark correct answer.)

a. Past trauma and violations by attachment figures. ____
b. A tendency to view oneself negatively, as unlovable or shameful. ____
c. A tendency to desire and pursue closeness but also to fear and distrust it. ____
d. A paradoxical view of others as both the source of and solution to fear. ____
e. The ability to openly trust and accept caring and reassurance when it is offered. ____

Exercise 2.25. In the face of a relationship threat—perhaps a sexy, ambiguous phone message from a partner's new office colleague—write out what a securely attached, anxiously attached, and avoidantly attached partner might say to their partner about the phone call when they came home. Note: How will each of these people tend to think about themselves as a result of this experience?

A securely attached partner might say:

____

____

An anxiously attached partner might say:

____

____

The avoidantly attached partner might say:

____

____

Exercise 2.26. Now imagine how the partner who received the phone call responds to the reaction of their partner. How would you describe each response, and how might this impact their negative self-dialogue?

Responding to the securely attached partner, this person might say:

____

____

Responding to the anxiously attached partner, this person might say:

____

____

Responding to an avoidantly attached partner, this person might say:

____

____

Exercise 2.27 In terms of acknowledging distress and needs, engaging with a partner, and seeking connection and support, read the following partner comments and label the pattern of responses as typical of secure (SEC), anxious (ANX), dismissing (DIS), or fearful attachment (FA).

a. "I don't care what you say. You are never around, never there for me. I just never feel really sure of this relationship, how much I matter to you. I might as well not be married. All you want is sex anyway. Even last week, on my birthday, when you promised..." She bursts into tears. She turns in her chair and her voice then becomes very biting, "But then, as you point out, I get 'unreasonable,' so how can you stay home with me? All I am is a maid. I am so alone." ____
b. "I refuse to speak with you when you get like this—there is no point. I don't know what gets into you when you get like this. I try to talk about our issues and come up with some solutions, but you just go off the deep end all the time. I think our relationship is fine—if you could just be more reasonable." ____
c. Wife: "I'd like you to talk to me more, to show me I am important to you." (Stares into the distance.) "Sometimes I think I am just too difficult to love—too difficult. I want more connection between us." Husband: "Maybe we can be closer. I liked holding you last night." He reaches and tries to take her hand, but she sighs and moves away. Wife: "Don't. I feel sick. Last night was too much for me. It got so I felt I couldn't breathe; you were looking at me all the time." ____
d. To therapist: "And it felt so different. We just held each other all night. And in the morning ... I just told him how safe I felt. I felt precious to him. Like we were going to be okay, even if we fight sometimes. And now—since then—it just feels like I can count on him. I can reach out and bring him close. I don't think I have ever felt this, even when we were first together." ____

Question 2.28. These patterns occur as the result of and are maintained by: (Mark all responses that apply—more than one correct answer.)

a. Past relationship history and the sensitivities it creates. ____

b. Present relationship interactions: confirming or disconfirming responses of the partner. ____
c. Models, beliefs, or expectations about others and relationships. ____
d. Negative or positive cycles of attachment responses in the present relationship. ____
e. How attachment-related emotions are regulated, communicated, and responded to in the present relationship. ____
f. The process of projective identification in which expectations are projected onto the partner in such a way as to confirm the worst fears. ____

Question 2.29. Attachment involves not only affect regulation but also cognitive models—expectations, needs, biases. Match the main models of self and other usually found in each kind of attachment style. (Indicate the correct style: SEC, ANX, AVD, or FA.)

a. The self is seen as lovable and competent. The other is basically dependable and trustworthy. This is a description of a(n) ____ person.
b. The self is seen as lovable, but others are basically untrustworthy. ____
c. The self is often seen as undeserving of care, and the other is mostly idealized and seen as lovable and desirable. ____
d. The self is seen as defective or deficient, and the other is seen as unreliable or dangerous. ____

Question 2.30. As a whole, attachment theory can be described as: (Mark all responses that apply—more than one correct answer.)

a. A systemic theory that focuses on patterns of interaction and their impact on how a relationship is defined, and how the experience of self and working models are shaped ____
b. A theory of affect regulation. ____
c. A theory of trauma—the trauma of isolation. ____
d. A constructivist theory focusing on the construction of inner and interpersonal attachment realities. ____
e. A theory of how the wounds of childhood are inevitably projected onto our partner. ____
f. A theory that offers a map of the defining elements in our closest relationships; childhood bonds predict adult bonds. ____
g. The most comprehensive and well-researched theory of adult love. ____

Question 2.31. In an EFIT and an EFCT session, EFT therapists find that attachment theory offers: (Mark all correct answers.)

a. A language; a frame; a way of making sense of the intense emotional dramas of depression, recurring anxiety, echoes of trauma, and relationship distress. ____
b. A guide through many client narratives and content issues and more surface emotional reactions to the core emotional longings, injuries, needs, fears, and dilemmas that shape self-definition and the nature of adult close relationships. ____

c. A compass in the territory of adult love, directing the therapist to pivotal defining moments in a relationship and to structuring key moments of connection. ____

d. A vision that tells the therapist what to target, what will make a difference, and what the steps are on the route from distress to emotional balance and efficacy, and to secure connection with others. ____

e. A guide to the patterns of affect regulation and meaning frames that maintain depression and anxiety (within variables) and how these patterns interact with levels of engagement with others (between variables) to maintain mental health problems or to begin to shape openness and growth. ____

Question 2.32. Once distressed individuals and/or partners become more open and optimally responsive to inner emotional cues and interactional cues, they feel more secure in themselves and in relationships. The theory suggests that these more secure individuals will be able to: (Mark all responses that might apply—more than one correct answer.)

a. Be curious and explore new information about self and others. ____
b. Solve problems more collaboratively and effectively with others. ____
c. Seek comfort and support from significant others. ____
d. Be separate and different from key others without overwhelming anxiety. ____
e. Be able to see the big picture in key relationships without getting reactively stuck in proving points or sorting emotions. ____
f. Name and explore fears and doubts that arise in the self and in relationships rather than assuming the worst. ____
g. Deal with stressful or painful situations with self-acceptance and self-compassion, and avoid making catastrophic attributions about self or others or life issues. ____
h. Listen to their own emotional needs for comfort and caring and clearly articulate them. ____
i. Consider a close other's perspective and tune in and respond empathically from a place of emotional balance. ____
j. Prevent all fights and negative cycles such as demand or defend. ____
l. Be more intimate, assuming intimacy is trusting self-disclosure and empathic responsiveness. ____
m. Protest to assert one's needs to another without using rejection or threat. ____
n. Hold a positive sense of self and feel entitled to care. ____
o. Be more resilient in the face of depression, anxiety (stress), and existential dilemmas since they do not face these alone but have a sense of connection to a loved one. ____

Question 2.33. From an attachment point of view, love relationships are primarily defined by: (Mark the correct answers.)

a. Equity of giving and getting so that each profits rather than loses. ____
b. The ability to negotiate and problem solve concrete issues together. ____

c. The companionship and friendship between partners. ____
d. Moments of emotional responsiveness when key vulnerabilities and attachment needs, and fears arise, and are responded to or not. ____
e. Times when one partner provides or doesn't provide, emotional and/or psychological "proximity" to the other when the other feels abandoned, rejected, or alone. ____
f. Key moments when people are able to be independent and differentiated, preventing fusion and allowing each person to go their own way. ____

Exercise 2.34. Here are the key moments of an experiment to assess attachment security between mother and child, called the "strange situation." In a securely attached child, the drama unfolds as follows:

Move 1. The child is in a "strange," that is, a stressful situation in an unfamiliar room with a stranger, and the mother has exited. But the child can handle her inevitable distress, believing the mother will return and come close to her.

Move 2. When the mother returns, the child is able to ask clearly and assertively for comfort and reassurance, most often desiring physical touch.

Move 3. When the mother responds, the child takes in the comfort and allows herself to be calmed and soothed.

Move 4. The child can then, feeling connected to the mother and trusting in her responsiveness if needed, turn and explore the environment.

Take the above four moves and write them out as they would likely occur between a securely attached couple when Shawn comes home after a very difficult day at work and greets Steve.

Move 1

____

____

Move 2

____

____

Move 3

____

____

Move 4

____

____

Exercise 2.35. In the scenario below that involves a distressed adult relationship, identify who is the anxiously attached, critical blamer and who is the avoidantly attached, distancing withdrawer.

A wife goes to a party with her husband. She knows no one there, and they have a fight on the way to the party. Then at the party, she finds her husband engrossed in a conversation with a beautiful new colleague. She feels small and unimportant, and remembers their fight on the way to the party. Her emotions explode. She feels anguish, and then, after a few moments, rage. She storms up to her spouse and taps him on the shoulder, insisting that he speak to her. She finds it difficult to be coherent but she accuses him of flirting and then asks to be taken home. He becomes very cold and distant, and refuses to talk about what is happening. He attempts to change the subject while implying that she has had too much to drink and should be more polite. When she asks, he refuses to introduce her to his colleague. He then points out that colleagues are often easier to talk to than "paranoid" spouses. She then insists on leaving and harangues him for his "inappropriateness" all the way home. She cannot concentrate on anything on the way home and then goes to sleep in another room.

a. Who is anxiously attached? ______________________________
b. Who is avoidantly attached? ______________________________
c. Write out what the wife might have been able to say to her partner if she had been in a happy stage in their relationship and had been securely attached, that is, had trusted that he would listen and respond to any vulnerabilities she might express.

____

____

____

Example 1:

Husband: You say I just want sex, but it's not true. I just feel like giving up when you say that, like we are doomed. How can it ever work?

Wife: (In a calm, flat voice.) I really don't know. But if you would just calm down and be less demanding. ... I just move away to stop the fights. I just think it is better if we don't get caught in these arguments ... the relationship is easier—calmer—that way.

Husband: How can things be easy when we never make love, when you are never close to me? Tell me that. It's like everything else comes first with you, but my feelings ... they never count. You just focus on the event, like all I want is an orgasm. But that is not all I want. I want to feel close to you—desired—like I am important to you. But first comes the kids, then the house, then your job, and then—maybe—if there is time left—maybe us. Sometimes I think if I were dying, you would tell me to hold on till you were less busy. You wouldn't be there for me. I might as well live alone.

Wife: I just get that whatever I do will never be good enough for you, I am a big disappointment ... so I just give up, I just shut down. It just doesn't feel safe in our house anymore. I am not sexy enough for you, not warm enough—not enough.

Example 2: (The same couple at the end of session 10 of EFT)

Wife: I am starting to feel a lot safer here. Like I am not on trial all the time, being tested. I just give up when I feel that. I just shut down and go numb. I am starting to get that we both get scared and insecure, and then we don't know how to reassure each other. (To spouse.) I do want this relationship, and you are important to me—very important. I feel lonely, too, you know. I just want to be held sometimes and talked to, paid attention to—not always asked to make love. Then I just feel like I am just a route to an orgasm, not like you want me. (She cries.) When we were first together, you made me feel like I was so special—so precious. I miss that—I do. But now you seem so mad at me all the time.

Husband: I know. I get desperate—feel like I am losing you—so I guess I come on all furious and pushy. But really it's just because I am so unsure of us—of you. And it's pretty risky to tell you this—guess it's easier to demand to make love.

Exercise 2.36. Take above interactions in Exercise 2.35 and underline the attachment language that the couple uses. This language often reflects the following themes:

1. Abandonment, loss, and aloneness: fears of finding the other unavailable and unresponsive.
2. Rejection and being unvalued or seen as inadequate by the other: feeling unworthy or unlovable.
3. Lack of safety and support: doubting that one would come first, that one can count on one's partner, and therefore being overwhelmed by stress.
4. Feeling that you do not exist in the mind of the other—that one is peripheral and dispensable—and how this impacts one's sense of self.
5. The risks involved in reaching out: fears of asking for attention and admitting need.

THE EFT THEORY OF INTERVENTION AND CHANGE—HUMANISTIC AND SYSTEMIC

EFT is an integration of the experiential/humanistic and systemic approaches to therapeutic change. It is a constructivist approach in that it focuses on the ongoing construction of present experience (particularly experience that is emotionally charged), and it is a systemic approach in that it also focuses on the organization and construction of patterns of interaction with intimate others. The EFT therapist's focus is constantly on patterns of experiencing, especially affect regulation and expression, and patterns of responses in interactions with intimate partners. These patterns define how the self, other, and relationship are experienced at any point in time. This integration is perhaps captured in the phrase by Rogers, "I enjoy discovering the order in experience." Experience is brought alive, made tangible, evoked, and ordered in session, and change occurs through new corrective experiences that are made manageable and coherent with the therapist.

The Basic Elements of an Attachment-Oriented Experiential/Humanistic Model

As discussed in the book *Attachment Theory in Practice* (pp. 26–32), the principles set out below are completely consonant with and reflect the wisdom found in attachment science.

1. *Alliance is key.* The experiential/humanistic perspective focuses on emotional responses and uses them in the process of therapeutic change. But to deal with emotions, a sense of safety is crucial. Therefore, humanistic therapies feature a strong focus on the quality of the therapeutic alliance, in which the therapist, like a good attachment figure, is emotionally present and actively helps clients regulate difficult emotions. EFT follows two basic premises: (a) that the therapeutic alliance creates a safety that is, to a certain extent, healing in and of itself, and that should be as egalitarian and collaborative as possible; and (b) that the acceptance and validation of the client's experience is a key element in therapy. Empathic responding, especially to vulnerability, is then perhaps the most basic building block of EFT. In couple therapy, this involves an active commitment to validating each person's experience of the relationship without invalidating the experience of the other. The therapist's empathy and acceptance allows each client's innate self-healing and growth tendencies to flourish. To be *seen* and *heard* allows people to reorganize and make new sense of their experiences. The scaffold of safety in each session is fostered by the authenticity, presence, and transparency of the therapist.
2. *An optimistic, non-pathologizing stance is essential.* Both Bowlby and Rogers believed in the logic behind problematic responses, that they were learned for good reason to meet and adaptive goal in a different context but are now applied in an out-of-context, general manner that narrows down the client's realities and leaves them trapped. The essence of the humanistic perspective is a belief in the ability of human beings to grow and make creative, healthy choices if given the opportunity. This approach is essentially non-pathologizing. The focus is the person, not the problem—the process of growth, what blocks it, and how to foster it, not the symptom, per se, or the offering of solutions by the therapist. The therapist helps to articulate the key moments when choices are made in the ongoing process of identity construction or in a relationship drama, or in an approach to existential dilemmas and stressors, and supports clients to formulate new responses. A humanistic therapist assumes that we find ways to survive and cope in dire circumstances when choices are few but then later, find those ways limiting and inadequate for creating fulfilling relationships and lifestyles. In this framework, all ways of responding to the world can be adaptive, but problems arise when these ways become rigid and cannot evolve in response to new contexts. Therefore, a therapist must first accept where each client starts from—the present nature of his or her experience and coping strategies—and understand how each client has done his or her best to survive and adapt given the options open to them.
3. *Health is openness and engagement.* The humanistic model of health for individuals and relationships is one that stresses openness to experience and engagement with others. As laid out in attachment theory and in systems theory, health is flexibility and the ability to learn from experience and adapt to new situations. Health is also seen as an inherent acceptance and prizing of self and others, and a sense of responsibility for our construction of experience and our responses. The fostering of this is then the ultimate goal of therapy, whether the client unit is an individual, couple, or family.
4. *Sessions focus on moment-to-moment process—the HOW of things—in the present.* Experiential therapies encourage an examination of how inner and outer

realities define each other. *The therapist is a process consultant who follows this moment-to-moment shaping of these realities the way a dancer follows music.* The inner construction of experience evokes interactional responses that organize the world in a particular way. These patterns of interaction then reflect back and, in turn, shape inner experience. The EFT therapist moves between helping individuals and partners recognize and reorganize their inner world and their interactional dance. The focus of sessions is on the here and now rather than on the past or future. In emotional moments, the therapist may use the past to validate present responses, and emotion may also bring past events alive in the session.

5. *There is a privileging of emotion.* Humanistic therapists encourage the integration of affect, cognition, and behavioral responses. But they tend to privilege emotions as sources of information about needs, goals, motivation, and key meanings. They help clients change how they regulate and shape emotions, especially anxiety and fear, that constrict information processing, and use emotions to create change events. Emotion is seen as intelligent and as a primary mover and organizer of action. Emotion is discussed further in the next chapter.
6. *Significant change requires a new corrective emotional experience.* Experiential approaches attempt to foster new corrective emotional experiences for clients that emerge as part of personal encounters with others, the therapist, mental representations of attachment figures, or attachment figures who are present in the room, in the here and now of the therapy session. In EFIT, emotional dialogues are used to connect with disowned parts of self as well, as in, "I can keep my balance and talk quietly to my small, scared self here and calm down rather than struggle to numb it out all the time." Cognitive insight or superficial behavior change is generally not viewed as optimal or as having sufficient impact. New choices and perspectives rise out of new emotional experiences.

The Systemic Model

The other half of the EFT synthesis is the contribution from family systems theory. In systems theory, the focus is on the circular, self-maintaining feedback loops that occur between members of a relational system, therefore organizing this system, giving it stability. The hallmark of all family systems therapies is that they call attention to and interrupt negative repetitive cycles of interaction that include problem or symptomatic behavior. However, we can think of inner processes in systemic terms as well. The EFT therapist focuses on the interaction of process variables in the construction of experience, for example. The therapist might say, "So you are used to shutting down and shutting out your softer emotions, and the more you do this, the harder it becomes, and the more overwhelming they are when they erupt and take you over, and the more they scare you. And the more you struggle to shut them down. This way you have of staying "together," which you needed when you were little to feel hidden and safe, has become like a wheel you are always stuck on and which now is just 'exhausting.' The protection has become a prison—yes?"

EFT draws on Minuchin's structural systemic approach (Minuchin & Fishman, 1981) with its focus on the enactment of "new" patterns of interaction. In terms of systemic therapies, the unique contribution of EFT is the use of emotion in breaking destructive cycles of interaction and creating new patterns. Systemic therapies have also traditionally focused on certain elements, such as power hierarchies and boundaries, whereas EFT focuses more on nurturance and connection. Consonant with systems theory, the EFT therapist helps the couple to develop new responses to each other and a different, more process-oriented, relational "frame" on the nature of their problems and opens up the system to new possibilities. The same thing occurs when the therapists talks to an individual about interacting processes in affect regulation as discussed earlier.

EFT follows the basic premises of systems theory, including:

1. Causality is circular, so it cannot be said that action A "caused" action B. In distressed couples, demanding by one partner creates and maintains withdrawal in the other and vice versa. Both partners' responses are shaped by a feedback loop, a cycle of interaction.
2. We must consider behavior in context. To understand the behavior of one partner, the therapist must always consider this behavior in the context of the behavior of the other partner. The system as it is organized, not the behavior of any one partner or any one element, is the problem.
3. The elements of a system have a predictable and patterned relationship with each other. *These patterns have a life of their own and tend to remain stable.* Couples' relationships are characterized by the presence of regular, repeating cycles of interaction, as are systems of affect regulation. The more narrow and rigid these cycles, the more *stuck* they are, the more likely the relationship—the system—is to be distressed.
4. All behavior has a communicative aspect. What is said and how it is said define the role of the speaker and the listener. Turning away and saying nothing is a communication. As we avoid emotions more, we become more sensitive to what we are avoiding and more terrified of doing anything but avoiding.
5. The task of the systems therapist is to interrupt negative cycles of interaction so that new, more adaptive patterns can begin to emerge and offer alternative ways to relate to others.

It is also important to point out here that Bertalanffy (1956) stated that not all elements in a system are created equal. To shift a living system, you have to know what the key variables are that organize a system and change them. In EFT, we assume that the key organizing element in a relational system and in constructing inner realities is emotion. Emotion is the music of the dance with key others, and colors and shapes inner processes.

The Experiential–Systemic Synthesis in EFT

The experiential and systemic approaches to therapy share important commonalities. Both focus on present experience rather than historical events. Both view *people as process rather than product*, as fluid rather than as possessing a rigid core or character structure that is inevitably resistant to change.

The two approaches also bring something to each other. Experiential approaches have often focused within the person to the exclusion of a consideration of external relationships. The systemic therapies, on the other hand, traditionally focus on the interactions between people to the exclusion of a consideration of the emotional responses and associated meanings that organize such interactions.

To summarize the experiential–systemic synthesis of EFT, there is a focus in both the circular cycles of interaction between people, as well as the process—the structuring of the emotional experiences of each person or partner. The word "emotion" comes from the Latin word meaning "to move." As mentioned earlier, emotion moves the individual and communicates to others, thereby organizing the dance between intimates, and readies us for action; it is part of our motivational system. In EFT, emotions are identified and expressed as a way to help people move into new stances toward elements of self or processes such as affect regulation, and partners move into new stances in their relationship dance, stances that they then integrate into their sense of self and their definition of their relationship. This results in a new, more open, flexible and satisfying cycle of processing or interaction that does not include the presenting problem, and, more than this, promotes integration of self and secure bonding with others.

THE HUMANISTIC NATURE OF EFT

Question 2.37. The therapist in EFT is best thought of in the following terms: (Mark all responses that might apply—more than one correct answer.)

a. As a skills coach. ____
b. As an expert who can offer unique insight and direction. ____
c. As a creator of safety—a secure base—in the therapy session. ____
d. As a process consultant for inner and interpersonal processes. ____
e. As a collaborative consultant who learns from and with the clients. ____

Question 2.38. The EFT therapist strives to be: (Mark all responses that might apply—more than one correct answer.)

a. Attuned to and emotionally engaged with individual clients, both partners in couple therapy, and all family members in EFFT. ____
b. Active—directing the process of the session, choreographing interactions, titrating risks, and promoting safety. ____
c. Nonjudgmental—accepting and validating clients' experiences and finding the logic in less functional responses. ____
d. Genuine and transparent. ____
e. Primarily a teacher and coach about skills of affect regulation and the nature of relationships. ____
f. Approving and endorsing all responses. ____

Question 2.39. The most basic building block of EFT, one that reflects its humanistic perspective, is:

a. Empathic reflecting on and validating each client's emotions. ____
b. Structuring new interactions to teach communication skills. ____
c. Promoting catharsis. ____
d. Allowing for the safe ventilation of emotions. ____

Question 2.40. The therapist's empathy, in which imagination plays a key role, allows people to: (Mark all responses that might apply—more than one correct answer.)

a. As Rogers said, explore and discover "the order in experience." ____
b. Place aside defensiveness, vigilance, and the need to avoid. ____
c. Regulate difficult and sometimes overwhelming emotions. ____
d. Focus on, assemble, and thereby distil or make granular the complex meanings—the whole—from the parts in their experience. ____
e. Accept and integrate elements of their experience that they judge themselves for or find difficult to deal with. ____
f. Tolerate ambiguity and uncertainty. ____
g. Take responsibility for how they construct their experience and their responses. ____

Question 2.41. Which of the following is not an essential humanistic stance?

a. People have good reasons for their ways of seeing and responding (paralleling Bowlby's belief that all responses, even if distorted, are reasonable if the context they evolved in is taken into account), and if supported, they can grow and learn. ____
b. Emotion colors perception and plays a key role in the formation of meaning. ____
c. The task of therapy is to enhance awareness, thereby creating an expanded sense of agency. ____
d. All the therapist needs to do is create a good alliance and empathize. ____
e. Adaptive defenses become chronic and begin to constrict awareness—experience—and, therefore, choices. ____

Question 2.42. The focus of the humanistic EFT therapist is: (Mark the two correct answers.)

a. On the present and the past as it becomes present. ____
b. On past events and how they defined the individual client. ____
c. On the structure of personality and psychodynamic understandings. ____
d. On present process and the ongoing construction of reality and interaction patterns. ____

Question 2.43. In what way is emotion *not viewed* in humanistic interventions?

a. Providing the organism with rapid, compelling, and vital information about what matters, such as survival, and answering basic needs; alerting people to the significance of events for their well-being. ____
b. Focusing attention and priming, and organizing appropriate action responses. ____
c. Playing a crucial role in the construction of meaning. ____

d. Communicating with others; emotional expression is the primary signaling system between primates, and pulls for specific responses. ____
e. Needing to be ventilated without reflection, thereby discharging tension. ____

THE SYSTEMIC NATURE OF EFT

Question 2.44. EFT adds to or departs from the usual structural systemic approaches in that it: (Mark all responses that might apply—more than one correct answer.)

a. Focuses on emotion, not just behavior and cognition, as a key organizing factor in relational systems. ____
b. Focuses on nurturance and vulnerability, not only on power, hierarchy, and boundary issues. ____
c. Focuses on change in a particular direction, toward a secure bond, not just change in itself. ____
d. Focuses on patterns of interaction in a system, and the self-reinforcing circular nature of these patterns. ____

Question 2.45. EFT is systemic (fits with the original formulation of systems theory) in the following ways: (Mark all responses that might apply—more than one correct answer)

a. Reality is seen as a set of circular feedback loops, rather than in terms of linear cause and effect. ____
b. It is the organization of elements within any system, in couple and family therapy particularly, the interpersonal system (patterns of interaction) that is the focus of therapy rather than simply change in one element, such as inner cognition ____
c. Each element is seen in the context of others, and each partner's behavior is continually seen in the context of the other partner's responses. ____
d. Emotions are seen as being what Bertalanffy (1956) (the father of systems theory) called "leading" or organizing elements in a relationship. ____
e. Dysfunction is seen in systemic terms as narrow, stuck patterns that cannot be revised and updated. ____

Exercise 2.46. Identify the following interventions as systemic or as not fitting with a systemic orientation. See if you can say why each one is systemic or not systemic.

a. The therapist says, "So, I can really see here how the more distant you see your partner as being, the more you naturally begin to push to get his attention. And then he begins to see you as pressuring him and tends to move away. Is that it?"
   Is this systemic? (Yes/No) ____ How is it systemic? ____
b. The therapist says, "So, you are both caught in this cycle of demand and defend. It has taken over your relationship."
   Is this systemic? (Yes/No) ____ How is it systemic? ____

c. The therapist says, "Can we just hold off on the details of this issue for a moment? I was noticing how, again, you, Mum, were taking your 'I will make you listen to me' stance, while your kid, Will, you were getting back into what you call your 'Can't get me, I'll put up a wall' stance. Is that right?"

   Is this systemic? (Yes/No) ____ How is it systemic? ____

d. The therapist says, "Can you put down your wall for a moment, Will? Can you do what you just spoke about and come out and meet your wife? Can you tell her 'I want to let you in?' I think perhaps if you can do that, she may be less 'frantic' and act less angry and scary for you."

   Is this systemic? (Yes/No) ____ How is it systemic? ____

e. The therapist says, "So, you see yourself as quite retiring and naturally withdrawn, Will, but when your wife becomes soft and shows you her softness and how she needs you, as she did just now, you really come out of your shell and take her hand and show yourself. You are right out there."

   Is this systemic? (Yes/No) ____ How is it systemic? ____

LINKING EXPERIENTIAL AND SYSTEMIC PERSPECTIVES

John Bowlby (1973, p. 180) spoke of inner and outer rings of a system. The inner ring (processes within a person's skin) and the outer ring (relationship interactions with others) complement each other and maintain each other in a homeostatic way. John Bowlby knew Bertalanffy, and it is clear that *attachment is a systemic theory*. Experiential approaches have tended to focus on inner processes (the construction of inner experiences). Systemic approaches have focused on interpersonal processes (the construction of relational patterns). The EFT therapist puts them both together.

LINKING EXPERIENTIAL AND SYSTEMIC PERSPECTIVES

Question 2.47. Experiential and systemic approaches both: (Mark all responses that might apply—more than one correct answer.)

a. Focus on process, inner and outer. Inner and interpersonal realities are fluid systems constantly in the process of being constructed, not fixed entities. ____
b. Focus on the present more than on how the past determines the present. ____
c. View people and systems as stuck rather than deficient or sick. ____
d. Espouse joining with clients in a respectful, collaborative alliance. ____
e. Have in traditional practice, focused on triangulation and hierarchies. ____

Exercise 2.48. Write out in the space below, in your own words, what experiential and systemic approaches add to each other that helps the EFT therapist.

____

____

____

Question 2.49. In summary, when experiential and systemic perspectives are put together in an attachment framework, the primary theoretical assumptions of EFT are: (Mark all responses that might apply—more than one correct answer.)

a. All relationship behavior is about attachment. Secure attachment ensures that no difficult conflicts occur in a relationship. ____
b. Emotion is key in organizing the inner construction of models of self and other, and relational experience and interactions with loved ones, making it an essential target of intervention. ____
`d. People's needs and desires are essentially healthy and adaptive. It is the disowning and constriction of these needs that becomes problematic. ____
e. Change involves new emotional experience, shifts in models of self and other, new ways to assemble and distil emotional realities, and new attachment-oriented interactions. ____
f. The most powerful route to change is through catharsis, insight, or negotiation skills. ____

Exercise 2.50. To stress the non-pathologizing nature of EFT, please link up the following quotes to the forerunners of EFT. Are these the statements of Rogers, the father of experiential approaches; Minuchin and colleagues, systemic therapists; Henry Stack Sullivan; or John Bowlby, the father of attachment theory? Link each statement with a person. Choose between: Rogers, Minuchin, Bowlby, or Stack Sullivan.

a. Most often, even negative attachment models, in which the self is seen as unlovable and/or others are seen as untrustworthy, are not neurotic "projections" but "perfectly reasonable constructions" that are adaptive in a particular context. Hopefully they are then updated and revised. Who said this? ____
b. If the therapist is accepting and empathic, then the client finds that he is "daring to become himself." This results in clients becoming "more self-directing and more self-confident" and open to emotion that leads to the "discovery of unknown elements of the self." Who said this? ____
c. "Different contexts call forth different facets of self. ... Expanding contexts allow for new possibilities to emerge." Changing people's "position" in a system changes their subjective experience. Who said this? ____
d. "When I accept myself as I am, then I change." Who said this? ____

We have now reviewed the basic theory base of EFT. The next chapter is a synopsis of the basic EFT therapeutic tasks and interventions. A brief list of the references given in the chapter can be found in the EFT Workbook eResource Page found at (www.routledge.com/9780367483425).

As you work through this workbook, you will become clearer and more comfortable about the theories presented and how they translate into effective interventions with distressed clients. You will become more confident about working with clients' emotional experiences, using these experiences as a compass and a guide, and working with patterns of interactions to create new steps in a relationship dance. For additional personal reflection exercises, see the EFT Workbook eResource Page at (www.routledge.com/9780367483425). Many resources—books, articles, chapters, research studies, talks, and training videos—can be found on the International Centre for Excellence in EFT website (www.iceeft.com), as well as on Dr. Sue Johnson's website (www.drsuejohnson.com). These sites will help you access the theory, research, and practical interventions that are the basis of EFT.

I hope you will appreciate the relevance of attachment theory as a map to the terrain of personality structure and function, and to adult love and family bonds.

Sue Johnson.

ANSWERS AND SUGGESTED RESPONSES

2.1 Answer: A, B, C, E, and F.

2.2 Answer: A, C, and D. Secure interdependence and the ability to be autonomous and separate are two sides of the same coin, not dichotomies.

2.3 Answer: B and C.

2.4 Answer: All but F.

2.5 Answer: D.

2.6 Answer: A, B, F, and G.

2.7 Answer: C. The expression of contempt usually occurs when protest becomes more desperate and hopeless.

2.8 Answer: A, C, and D.

2.9 Answer: B and D.

2.10 Answer A, B, and D.

2.11 Answer: A, B, and C. Bowlby states in the second book of his trilogy, *Separation* (1973), that the concept of projection is not helpful in that it directs attention away from a person's real experiences and treats him as a closed system, as little influenced by his environment.

2.12 Answer: A, C, D, and E.

2.13 Answer: A and C.

2.14 Answer: A, B, and C.

2.15 Answer: B–G. Styles are explicitly interpersonal and relational, and are better predictors of relationship variables than traits (Shaver & Brennen, 1992). They are predispositions but are also shaped by current relationship events. (See Johnson & Whiffen, 1999; Johnson, 2019, for a general academic discussion of attachment styles, strategies, and forms of engagement.)

2.16 Answer: All answers are correct.

2.17 Answer: A–F. Describe responses of individuals in more secure relationships.

2.18 Answer: C and D.

2.19 Answer: A, B, C, D, F, and G. Describe responses of individuals with more anxious strategies.

2.20 Answer: All answers are correct. These responses are typical among individuals responding with a dismissing attachment strategy.

2.21 Answers: a. ANX; b. AVD; c. ANX; d. AVD; e. ANX; f. ANX; g. AVD; h. ANX; i. ANX; j. AVD.

2.22 Answers: a. AVD; b. ANX; c. AVD; d. ANX; e. AVD; f. AVD; g. ANX; h. AVD.

2.23 Answer: All answers are correct. Even if they have never seen or experienced secure attachment, fearful avoidants will fight for a connection, and will risk needing and wanting if the EFT therapist cuts those risks fine enough. As Bowlby suggests, attachment needs and longings are wired in.

2.24 Answer: E.

2.25 Answer: The secure partner is more likely to openly ask about the call and the relationship, and be able to express concern or discomfort and ask for reassurance. The anxious partner is more likely to accuse, catastrophize, demand, and criticize or become extremely distraught in ways that annoy or alienate her spouse. The avoidant partner might become hostile without ever really addressing what upset her or simply mention the message in passing but stay very distant.

2.26 Answer: The secure partner is then most likely to get reassuring feedback. The other two are likely to evoke feedback that confirms their fears.

2.27 Possible responses listed for each example.

- **a. ANX:** Anxious blaming pursuer.
- **b. DIS:** Dismissing avoidant husband who distances and defends.
- **c. FA:** Fearful avoidant wife who pursues and distances.
- **d. SEC:** Wife describing secure attachment after a key change event in EFT. Attachment strategies or forms of engagement tell you how partners engage with their attachment needs and fears—their emotions and their partner—that is the basic position they take in the relationship dance. How you handle your attachment emotion is how you emotionally engage your partner in this dance.

2.28 Answer: All but F. Childhood adversity creates sensitivities, but these can be reversed by more secure attachment experiences; secure attachment can be "earned."

2.29 Answer: a. SEC; b. AVD; c. ANX; d. FA.

2.30 Answer: All are correct except answer E.

2.31 Answer: All are correct. Think of a couple you are working with or even your own relationship. Use attachment theory as outlined to make sense of a response, suggest a need or fear, or suggest a key move or moment that shaped the relationship or tells you what response would make a difference.

2.32 Answer: All but J. In couples who have successfully concluded EFT and say they feel more secure, fights and cycles such as demand/withdraw still occur, but they do not take over and define the relationship, and can be managed more effectively.

2.33 Answer: D and E. In attachment terms, marriage and romantic relationships are more than friendship. Research suggests that only distressed couples become caught in issues of equity and profit. The Bowen perspective (reflected in answer F) is discussed in relation to EFT in the EFT manual *Creating Connection* (3rd ed., 2019).

2.34 **Answer: Move 1:** Shawn thinks on the way home of confiding in Steve and of how good it will feel to have a hug. **Move 2:** Shawn comes in and asks for a hug and if they can talk about his day—he needs his support. **Move 3:** Steve responds, and Shawn sighs and relaxes and, as they talk and hold each other, Shawn feels calmed and soothed. **Move 4:** After confiding in Steve, Shawn feels better and can go and make a stressful phone call he needs to make.

2.35 **Answer: A**. Wife is anxiously attached, pursuing, and critical. **B**. Husband is distancing avoidant. **C**. She would have been able to wait, would not have been so overwhelmed by her fears, and would not have become angry. Then she would have been able to say something like, "I guess I just got to feeling scared and a little vulnerable when I watched you with your colleague. I realize I am not quite sure of us—of how you feel about me right now. Maybe I need a little hug."

2.36 **Suggested examples** of the following themes:

Abandonment and loss: "I just feel like giving up when you say. ..." "You wouldn't be there for me. I might as well live alone."; "I get desperate—feel like I am losing you."

Rejection: "... you are never close to me." "I am a big disappointment." "It's just because I am so unsure of us—of you."

Lack of Safety: "I just move away to stop the fights." "It just doesn't feel safe in our house anymore."

Fail to Exist: "Sometimes I think if I were dying, you would tell me to hold on till you were less busy."

Risk of reaching: "I am starting to get that we both get scared and insecure, and then we don't know how to reassure each other." "It's pretty risky to tell you this—guess it's easier to demand to make love."

The EFT Theory of Intervention and Change—Humanistic and Systemic

Exercises: The Humanistic Nature of EFT

2.37 **Answer: C, D, and E.**

2.38 **Answer: All but E and F.** Acceptance is not the same as approval or endorsement.

2.39 **Answer: A.**

2.40 **Answer: All answers are correct.**

2.41 **Answer: D.**

2.42 **Answer: A and D.**

2.43 **Answer: E.** It is interesting to note for EFT therapists that it seems easier to promote assertive responses by providing validation of hurts and fears, and supporting the natural move toward assertion of needs to the partner, than to formally "teach" and "coach" assertive behavior even if such assertion seems to be very "out of character" at the beginning of therapy. Emotion tells us and others what we need.

The Systemic Nature of EFT

2.44 **Answer: A, B, and C.** Answer D is not an addition or departure but a feature that structural systemic and EFT interventions share.

2.45 Answer: All answers are correct. Answer D is compatible with systems theory but different from how this theory was traditionally applied in family therapy. Traditional applications left emotion out of the picture and have been accused of being impersonal and mechanistic in their focus on "external" variables only.

2.46 Answer:

A. **Yes**. It places responses into a whole, a pattern, into context. A circular pattern of interactions and how it self-reinforces is laid out.

B. **Yes**. The process of interaction/communication (feedback loops) are set out as the problem.

C. **Yes**. Individual responses are reframed as part of feedback loops.

D. **Yes**. The therapist sets up a new task and an enactment designed to change the way interactions are organized/structured. This task can bring the husband closer to his partner and place him on a more equal, active footing.

E. **Yes**. Systems theorists believe that different contexts activate different parts of self. A change in one person's way of engaging pulls for a change in the other.

Linking Experiential and Systemic Perspectives

2.47 Answer: All but E. Certain less recent systemic approaches have focused almost exclusively on these elements, but a focus on these elements is not a large part of EFT. Traditional systemic interventions for child problems would often focus on "de-triangulating" the child from a parent, and assume that the parents would then repair/enhance their own relationship. More recent systemic approaches (see Johnson & Whiffen, 2003) focus on the attachment security/nurturance between parent and child.

2.48 Possible response: Experiential perspectives offer a map to emotion regulation and information processing, and how to work with that in therapy. Systems theory offers a map to charting and restructuring interpersonal interactions. In a therapy in which the client is in a relationship, both are needed.

2.49 Answer: All but A and F. In recent versions of attachment theory, attachment behaviors and concerns are integrated with caretaking and sexuality; previously, these had been thought of as separate systems. Even so, a long-term love relationship is a complex, multi-layered drama, and no theory can encompass all elements of this drama. A basically secure attachment in a relationship also does not preclude conflicts and prevent that relationship from running into difficulties. Security is on a continuum, and all can become anxious or avoidant when distressed.

2.50 Answer: A. Bowlby (1979); **B.** Rogers (1961); **C.** Minuchin and Fishman (1981); **D.** Rogers (1961).

3

EFT INTERVENTIONS

The practice of emotionally focused therapy (EFT) involves mastering a set of basic systemic and experiential practices that guide the therapist to transform attachment processes using emotion as an agent of change. While reading this chapter, you will observe, practice, and differentiate the essential practices that are used throughout the change processes of EFT. First, we review the three tasks of EFT which provide a framework for reviewing the relationship of EFT micro-interventions to each task. Then we lead you through the language and process of these interventions as they relate to each task, highlighting key ways the EFT therapist accepts, expands, and engages emotion to promote change. The EFT meta process, or EFT Tango, is summarized, focusing on the five moves of this macro-intervention. Mastery of these in-session practices enables the therapist to effectively engage couples, individuals, and families through the five EFT Tango Moves to create the stages of change that will be explored in more detail in the following chapters.

EFT THREE TASKS

Three tasks summarize the focus and function of EFT. These tasks are intertwined through the EFT process. The therapist is fostering new emotional experience to create new meaning and dialogue that are used to engage new interactional events that impact self and important others in one's life. The experience of safety promotes vulnerability. When engaged, this vulnerability transforms relational experiences and one's understanding of self in that relational world (Table 3.1).

Table 3.1
Summary of the Three Tasks of EFT

Task 1	Creating and maintaining a therapeutic alliance. EFT is effective when the therapist's rapport with clients is characterized by accessibility, responsiveness, and genuine emotional engagement. This secure base allows clients to explore interactional processes and the emotions underlying them. The early stages of therapy require therapists to foster a secure connection and to assure alliance on therapeutic goals and tasks. The therapist actively monitors the therapeutic alliance throughout the EFT process to maintain the constancy of a trusting bond, ensure that clients sense the relevance of the therapeutic tasks, and repair ruptures when they occur.
Task 2	Accessing, assembling, and reformulating emotion. A therapist's ability to access and engage clients' emotional experience is essential to promoting change. The therapist must learn to facilitate the expression of new or expanded emotional experience that, in turn, forms the basis for restructuring clients' problematic patterns of engaging. New emotional experience opens clients to new ways of interacting. A therapist must be skilled in helping clients identify, assemble, express, and experience these emotions in session.

DOI: 10.4324/9781003039457-4

Table 3.1
(Continued)

Task 3	Restructuring key interactions. Restructuring patterns of interaction through shaping affiliative encounters in session is a primary treatment goal in EFT. The therapist uses a number of systemic interventions to track the pattern, reframe ineffective patterns in light of unexpressed attachment fears and needs, and shape new ways of interacting. These corrective emotional experiences lead to more positive, loving connections and responses. The completion of this task results in prototypical bonding events that form a new basis for secure attachment and growth.

These three tasks can be remembered with the acronym TEA: T for Therapeutic alliance; E for Engaging and deepening emotion; A for shaping affiliative interactions. (Brubacher, 2018; Brubacher & Wiebe, 2019).

Task 1. Creating and Maintaining a Therapeutic Alliance

Task 1 highlights the therapist stance in EFT in which the therapist provides a personal and emotional presence that is accessible, responsive, and emotionally engaged (ARE). This relational stance is foundational and fundamental to the EFT process of change. The interventions most often associated with Task 1 include empathic attunement, acceptance, genuineness, and alliance-related skills (e.g., forming and monitoring the alliance).

Empathic Attunement

The EFT therapist immerses in each client's world and uses inner experience as a reference point to resonate with and get a felt sense of each client's experience. Focusing on the client's verbal and nonverbal messages, the therapist uses imagination and personal reflection to empathically connect to each client's experience and to the therapeutic alliance. Attunement is what happens within the therapist and between the client and therapist before the therapist formulates any words to express out loud. Consider the following example.

Jamal and Rosa begin therapy, caught in their typical distressed interaction. Rosa, an anxious pursuer, complains that Jamal is never available—always too busy. She protests, "I can never get Jamal's attention in the most dire moments of need—like when the baby was sick—once again I was alone!" Jamal, in exasperation, pleads, "Can't you see how hard I am trying to show you that you are important—to make up for that?" He suddenly flips into frustration that Rosa never remembers or gives him credit for anything.

In this example, the therapist pauses before finding words to respond and empathically attunes to Rosa's complaints and story of being alone and to Jamal's failing efforts to please her. The therapist also attunes to the rapid interactional responses each partner makes to one another.

Now, notice in your own body how you feel as you tune into Rosa's exasperation and loneliness, then notice what you feel as you tune into Jamal's frustration with his failing attempts to make Rosa happy, and finally notice how you experience the push-pull-push dynamic between them. Draw on your personal experience and use your imagination to get a felt sense in your own body of what you imagine each is experiencing. In emotionally focused individual therapy (EFIT), it is the same process: While a relevant *other* is not physically present in the room, an individual's emotional struggle is invariably relational, and the therapist attunes to the client's story of distress.

Exercise 3.1. Empathic Attunement

In the following examples, practice attuning to the underlying emotions of the client. Name the client's possible underlying emotion and view of self or other you experience in stepping into these clients' experiences.

Hugo sighs with exasperation, "My boss is on my case all the time. I achieve more than any of my colleagues, and yet I'm monitored like a hawk. It's totally unfair, and I'm just fed up!"

Underlying emotion: ______________________________

View of self/other: ______________________________

Exercise 3.2. Empathic Attunement Failures

An attachment perspective provides the EFT therapist with a great ally when facing the challenge of attuning to multiple realities in couple and family relationships and identifying the relational impact of disconnection. Imagine a session with Bob and Marie, in which Marie characterizes Bob's indifference as his preoccupation with work to which Bob responds by turning away, folding his arms, and crossing his legs, saying, "You just don't understand. You have no idea what this is like for me."

Choose the therapist response below that fails to attune or capture the partner's experience. _____

a. Therapist notes a tone of defeat in Bob's voice and senses Marie's agitation.
b. Therapist senses a look of dismay on Marie's face while Bob turns away.
c. Therapist wants to help Bob understand that Marie truly wants to understand him.
d. Therapist senses Bob is closing off from Marie while he describes his frustration of wanting to be understood.

How did the therapist fail to attune?

____

____

Acceptance

The EFT therapist takes a non-pathologizing stance, actively resisting the tendency to see clients as deficient or defective. The attachment frame guides a therapist's understanding of a client's problematic behaviors and how they may make sense in the context of the client's world, including their need for connection. The therapist avoids fixed terms of character disorders, such as narcissist or borderline, promoting an acceptance that validates a client's experience and action as a potentially adaptive and "reasonable" response to an unmet need or fear.

Exercise 3.3. Expressing Acceptance

Choose from the following responses, one that best promotes a therapeutic stance of acceptance and de-pathologizing when a client fidgets continually in her chair, doodling on a pad of paper, rarely making contact, saying, "I can't concentrate if I am not doing something." _____

a. "I am wondering if your ADHD medication may need to be adjusted."
b. "I appreciate you need to be doing something active to remain in this conversation."
c. "Could you please put that pen and paper away so we can get some work done here together? It is far too distracting."
d. "I've seen you take a few glances at me and at your partner, but mostly it looks like you'd rather not be in this room."

Genuineness

An EFT therapist is available for a real human encounter with the client. This may include the therapist admitting missteps and privileging the client's experience over the therapist's understanding and genuinely respecting times a client expresses dissatisfaction or mistrust. A therapist's genuine care and concern is a clear expression of their accessibility and responsiveness to the client.

Exercise 3.4. Therapist Genuineness

A client says in a slightly demanding, anxious tone, "We want tools to make change," adding. "Aren't you going to give us tools?" (Brubacher, 2018, p. 99). All but one of the following therapist responses below illustrates therapist genuineness and transparency in the context of empathic attunement. Choose the response that *does not* illustrate therapist genuineness and prepare to describe how it is different from the other choices. ______

a. "I understand you are eager to make change as quickly as possible and want tools to get out of this painful place you are in. Absolutely, I will be helping you with this."
b. "Absolutely, we will be giving you tools—tools to send clearer message to your partner so that your best attempts for the relationship don't end up pushing your partner further away or firing them up in anger. Before we can learn the tools, we are going to explore together how it is that your relationship keeps getting stuck in the same old ruts."
c. "The first tools I want to help you with are those of discovering what keeps blocking you from being the sort of parent you want to be to your son and then finding how to make the changes you are longing for in your relationship with him."
d. "I was hoping you wouldn't ask that! EFT therapists do not teach tools. We help you create corrective emotional experiences in each session, so you don't need to learn skills and tools. Just trust me!"

What is different in the therapist response that does not illustrate therapist genuineness?

____

____

Self-Disclosure and Transparency

A therapist's openness to being impacted by the client and sharing this impact through self-disclosure extends the felt sense of security a client experiences through his or her alliance with the therapist. Self-disclosure can include a therapist's brief sharing of a personal experience to intensify validation of a client's experience; therapist transparency about their own sadness to build alliance; or therapist openness about their confusion to show genuine curiosity.

Therapist transparency builds and maintains alliance, conveys hope and belief in the client, and conveys confidence in the EFT map as a reliable path forward. The therapist discloses in early sessions, "This is how we will be working together . . . " and invites clients to talk about how they feel about the session before the end or potentially during sessions. Such invitations require therapist courage, openness, and vulnerability. Therapist transparency is primarily used in Task 1, but it can also be used to resonate with and acknowledge the difficulty of experiencing fears of being vulnerable and fears of trusting (pertinent to Task 2) as well as fears of doing encounters (pertinent to Task 3).

Exercise 3.5. Therapist Self-disclosure and Transparency

Choose which of the following responses are examples of self-disclosure or transparency that an EFT therapist might use in building and maintaining alliance and inviting transparent dialogue with client(s): _____

a. "I feel the heaviness in my heart for the frustration you are both describing and also get the strong sense of how very important you are to each other and how much you want to get out of this negative pattern."
b. "Together we will explore how this negative pattern takes over your relationship so automatically, and we will learn to listen to the music of softer emotions and best attempts—playing in the background—that keep getting drowned out by the noise of your frustrations."
c. "Ben, I am wondering what is going on for you now; I seemed to have lost you. Was that too strong or off the mark for you?"
d. All of the above.

Active Monitoring the Alliance

A therapist takes active steps to monitor his or her engagement with each partner. This involves tracking clients' responses to interventions and checking to make sure that the therapist is still in tune with the clients' experience and that the clients are engaging with the therapeutic process and trusting it is relevant to their concerns. The therapist invites direct responses from clients about their experience in the session or in treatment as a whole and encourages and responds fully to client concerns. Active monitoring underscores the value of clients' experience and the need for a therapist to pay conscious attention to pacing and to inviting clients' feedback. Monitoring enables the therapist to empathically respond to possible ruptures in the therapeutic alliance

Exercise 3.6. Continuous Alliance Monitoring

Choose the responses that best conveys a therapist's attempt to monitor and assure a strong alliance with the clients. If the therapist sensed they had offended the client, the therapist could respond to repair the rupture by saying:

a. "So, it seems like that was too strong. The word fear doesn't quite fit what you are going through. Help me better understand what it is like for you." ____
b. "It seems like it is difficult for you to see that what you are doing might be pushing your daughter away." ____
c. "Could you tell me when you were less afraid of the influence of your daughter's friends than you are now?" ____
d. "What is it like for you when I raise these questions about your typical responses as a mother?" ____

Joining the System

In conjoint sessions, the therapist actively joins the couple or family's experience as a relational system. A therapist validation of different family or partner experience is crucial in reflecting and processing the varied experiences within a family system. In reflecting and validating the different experiences and tracking interaction patterns, the therapist is better able to hold a meta-perspective that affirms individual experiences without solely organizing around them. The EFT therapist invites a collaborative stance as a process consultant who is able to acknowledge and validate differences and their shared impact on other relationships.

Task 2. Accessing and Reformulating Emotion

The EFT therapist's focus on emotion includes shaping experience, making meaning, and mobilizing action and social connection. Emotion points us to salient desires and needs that are made available through assembling, expanding, and expressing emotion within internal and interactional patterns. The task of accessing and reformulating emotion is pivotal to the restructuring of interactional patterns for individuals, couples, and families. In this section, we ask you to identify core emotions and explore emotion as a process. We review the key assumptions informing our work with emotion and practice common interventions used in accessing and reformulating emotion.

Exploring Emotion

EFT therapists are reminded of the powerful role emotional experience has in shaping relationships and present moment experience. Emotion motivates and signals key interactional moves. The word "emotion" comes from the Latin "emovere," meaning, literally, "to move." Johnson (2019, 2020) describes how emotions are conceptualized in the EFT approach, as much more than *feeling words* but as a dynamic active process of rapidly unfolding elements. This impact of this powerful process can be seen in the following example.

Tom and Susan have grown increasingly dissatisfied with their relationship. Susan senses that Tom is no longer willing to work on their relationship, and she assumes his frequent silence and withdrawal are evidence of his rejection of her and their relationship. Tom doesn't understand why Susan questions his commitment. He explains his occasional distance as a coping response to her incessant nagging. The EFT therapist who immediately hears a simple pattern of *the more Susan pushes and questions, the more Tom explains and withdraws*, can use a number of EFT interventions to help this couple access the emotions that drive their interactions and inform the meaning that they are making about this relationship. The process of accessing and assembling underlying emotions leads clients to:

- Experience underlying emotions that may have been outside of awareness. Tom is able, through focusing on the loneliness that results from his withdrawing actions, to identify his fear of not being good enough for Susan. Clarifying his core fear will give him more access to his attachment needs.
- Create new meaning about one's own or another's behavior. As Tom is able to talk about his fear of rejection, Susan sees Tom's withdrawal from her not as his rejection of her but as his own fear of being inadequate in her eyes.

- Mobilize new responses toward others. Susan begins to see Tom's withdrawal as a sign that he might be feeling threatened by her responses to him. Rather than challenging him, she eases up on her pushing and questioning and invites him to talk about his concerns when he is ready.

Emotions are viewed as action tendencies that arise from preconscious (pre-cognitive) perceptions of the relevance of situations to a person's basic concerns and needs (Arnold, 1960; Frijda, 1986; Johnson & Greenberg, 1994). Emotion is anything but a primitive, irrational response. It is a high-level information processing system that integrates innate biological and emotional needs with past experience, present perceptions of the environment, and anticipated interpersonal consequences (Frijda, 1986). Emotion can be understood as a stepwise process that unfolds across aspects of human experience (Arnold, 1960).

Exercise 3.7. Emotions Common to Human Experience

A number of basic emotions are considered common to human experience (Ekman, 1992; Izard, 1977; Plutchik, 2001; Tomkins, 1991). They are recognizable by common patterns of verbal and nonverbal expressions. Match the emotions on the left with the compelling forces for action that each emotion mobilizes on the right.

1. Anger	to seek comfort and nurturance
2. Joy	to fight, flee, seek protection
3. Sadness	to disappear, to hide, to retreat
4. Fear/anxiety	to move towards, to explore
5. Shame/disgust	to move towards, engage, connect
6. Surprise/curiosity	to fight, attack, defend

Note: Hurt/anguish is a complex emotion of anger, sadness, fear of loss, and shame (Vangelisti, 2009). The specifics of the experience of hurt need to be assembled and distilled to access the core experience, meanings made, action impulse, and embedded longings and need.

Exercise 3.8. Identifying Basic Emotions

Match the following statements to one of the following emotions (anger/rage, joy/elation, sadness/despair, fear/anxiety, shame/disgust, surprise/curiosity):

1. "My world falls apart when I hear you talking about leaving." ________________
2. "I can't talk about this. No, I don't want to even look at him. I don't want him to see me like this." ____________________
3. "I know it's my fault. I try my best, but it's really not good enough. It's not what she is looking for." ________________
4. "It just felt so good—to have him come down and ask me for a hug. It felt like we really turned a corner last night." ______________
5. "It's too much. I can't do it. I feel so fragile." ______________
6. "Yeah, I say those things just to get a response out of you. I know you can't handle it. You're emotionally dead." ________________

Typical action tendencies for core emotions are: Explore/approach; assert/attack; flee/escape/avoid; mourn/shut down/evoke a response from others; hide/retreat; engage/connect.

Exercise 3.9. Linking Interpersonal Triggers, Action Tendencies, and Experienced Emotion

Now apply these emotions and action tendencies to the following situations.

1. When a father and son get in a heated argument, the son withdraws from the argument by disengaging from the intensifying escalation. What feeling would typically lead him to withdraw? ____________________
2. As the father finds his son less and less responsive to his concerns, his anger escalates, and he senses he cannot get through to him. What is the cue triggering his anger? ____________________
3. How will his anger typically prompt him to respond? ____________________

Remember emotions inform the actions people take and the meanings made of others' actions. They function like a compass guiding internal responses and interactions to others and the larger social world. Emotions serve an important role in organizing adaptive responses to a person's environment.

Distinguishing Core Emotions From Surface Emotions

Core emotions are direct responses to a present situation. They are typically visceral and non-conscious. When core emotions are in awareness, they guide a person to adaptive actions: Fear in response to a threat from another compels one to move away to safety or to respond with assertion; hurt and sadness in response to a loss compel one to seek comfort and solace.

To cope with difficult core emotions, people in distress without secure attachment bonds frequently replace core emotions with surface or reactive emotions. These responses typically obscure the initial emotional response that a person has to a given situation. Anger at violation may be masked by depression or anxiety; hostility may cover over a sense of shame. Surface or reactive anger or numbness often blocks access to the underlying core emotion and related needs. These reactive responses reinforce physiological arousal and negative appraisals and keep a person in a cycle of ineffective actions. For example, *Armando is reluctant to express his anger; instead he becomes numb and disconnects to avoid a possible escalation of hostility.*

Exercise 3.10. Distinguishing Core and Reactive Emotions

Identify the emotion illustrated in each example. Name the emotion and mark if it is either an immediate/core or surface/reactive emotion.

1. When he told her that he did not want to make love, she flew into a rage and began to list all of his mistakes and shortcomings. Emotion: ___________ Core ______ Reactive_____
2. When his son said, "You don't even know me!" he felt a pang of anguish and peaked with curiosity. Emotion: ___________ Core ______ Reactive_____
3. As she saw her smiling at her friend, she felt sick, and a sense of dread and hopelessness overcame her. Emotion: ___________ Core ______ Reactive_____

4. "I'm fine. My brother's suicide wasn't my fault. I will not let myself feel guilty."
   Emotion: ___________ Core ______ Reactive_____

Exercise 3.11. Attuning to Core Emotions and Longings Underlying Reactivity

Identify the surface/reactive emotion in each of the following client statements and conjecture at the underlying core emotion hinted at or on the leading edge. When clients are caught up in reactive emotion, the core emotion is usually outside of their awareness.

1. "I numb out; it just feels better than hearing I can't do anything right." Then quietly, "I know I am not perfect, not what you need."

   Reactive emotion: __________ Possible underlying emotion: ___________

2. "It's beyond frustration. I get exasperated when he just sits there. Not reacting. Not responding. It is like no one is home. I think to myself, 'I can get him to respond.' Then I show my anger."

   Reactive emotion: __________ Possible underlying emotion: ___________

3. "I get so upset. He says I don't parent the children right. And when I try to talk about it with him, he will just lecture me. I never get it right. So, I just pull away and don't try."

   Reactive emotion: __________ Possible underlying emotion: ___________

4. "I feel kind of trapped, like my efforts are futile. When I try to open up to her, it doesn't work. I just don't know how to talk about how I feel."

   Reactive emotion: __________ Possible underlying emotion: ___________

Clients are often stuck in reactive spirals of emotions, perceptions, and behaviors. This results from a lack of awareness and failure to express core emotions that signal to their core needs and longings. The EFT therapist tracks and responds to the clients' presenting pattern and works with them to attend to and assemble and distil the core emotions underlying their ineffective patterns. The therapeutic process promotes the processing, regulation, and expression of difficult emotions that define and inform problematic behavior. The therapist leads clients to new levels of emotional engagement by working with them to experience and express their core emotions.

Exercise 3.12. Focusing on Core Emotions

The following exercises will help you clarify your understanding of core emotions and will provide you with practice exercises in reflecting surface, reactive emotion or underlying, core emotional responses.

1. Core (or primary) emotions are
   a. The emotions most often or primarily witnessed in interactions.
   b. The primarily reactive emotions.
   c. The primary, most infantile emotions.
   d. Direct core emotional responses to external stimuli.

2. EFT therapists focus on core emotions related to
   a. Blocks to effective communication skills.
   b. Individuation.
   c. Attachment needs and bonds.
   d. Unresolved hurts from the past.
3. Core emotions in distressed relationships are often
   a. Disorienting.
   b. Pushed out of awareness.
   c. Unconscious.
   d. Here and now.

Emotion as a Process

Emotions can be understood in terms of a process that unfolds in a series of steps described by Arnold (1960). The steps of this process include:

- Perception: A rapid preconscious assessment of an environmental cue involving limbic system of brain, indicating warning of a potential danger or threat. Is it good or bad? Threatening or safe?
- Body arousal: Physiological activation, preparing to respond (fight, flight or freeze).
- Meaning making: Re-evaluation of initial assessment of an environmental cue involving more cognitive processes.
- Action tendency: Behavioral response to stimuli or impulse to action.

Now consider the example of a mother who becomes triggered when her son becomes silent in a discussion about her concerns regarding his schoolwork. Her internal response or appraisal is a global assessment indicating a warning of possible danger or distress. As a result, her response at a physiological level is to go hot—the pace of her breathing increases, and her face flushes. In her cognitive appraisal or meaning making of the situation, she interprets his silence as indifference and responds by getting his attention by lashing out with criticism and complaints.

Exercise 3.13. The Role of Assembling Emotion in Shaping Experience

The case of Will provides another example of the role of emotion in shaping experience and the significance of Task 2. Match the impact of assembling emotion with examples of an individual client, Will. Choose the example that best describes Will's evolving experience. List the corresponding letter on the line after each impact listed.

1. Assembling emotion mobilizes new responses _____
2. Assembling emotion creates new meaning _____
3. Assembling emotion to access core, underlying emotion reveals longings and needs ____

Will is in a committed relationship with his partner. Each partner has a successful career, and they are parents to active adolescent twins. Despite many positives in his life, Will has depression, which he finds at times can be immobilizing.

a. As Will explores the heaviness and darkness of his global depression, he accesses fears of being rejected and unwanted and discovers longings to belong in the center of the family.
b. As Will explores his pattern of stepping back when family tensions escalate and his underlying fear of fueling the fire if he were to step in, he begins to see that he is not being pushed out or being excluded because he is inept but rather because the family simply carries on without him when he "disappears."
c. As Will is able to access his underlying fear of rejection, he discovers motivation to reach more to his wife and ask for support instead of fighting his depression alone.

Exercise 3.14. Tracking and Assembling Elements of Emotion

Track the underlying process of emotion through each of these scenarios. Take note of how each cascade of emotion begins with an interpersonal trigger or cue that signals some attachment threat.

Jack tells his wife Sabrina that he does not want to comfort her. She stiffens in her chair and flushes red as she gestures by wringing her hands. The therapist reflects, saying: "When Jack says he doesn't want to comfort you (the cue), your back stiffens, and you begin to wring your hands. This is very difficult to hear, yes?" (evocative response, with empathy). She looks down and says, "I can't hear that—I just can't bear it." She stares out the window and sighs.

1. Identify the emotion she may be experiencing. ________
2. Now label the steps leading from her initial perception of threat to her action.

   Cue: *He refuses to comfort her.*

   Initial Perception: ____________________

   Bodily Arousal: ____________________

   Meaning Making: ____________________

   Action Tendency: ____________________

   How could you assemble this process in a way that matches Sabrina's present moment experience?

   ____

   ____

   ____

Marcy becomes very still and presses her lips together as her depressed and withdrawn partner, Jane, expresses that she has become "difficult and demanding" and says that she is no longer willing to put up with her criticism. Marcy moves forward, raising her voice and, with a challenging tone, says, "Oh, so it's my problem, I am the bad one? This has nothing to do with your affairs! You're just trying to shift the responsibility away from your lies. You blame me when it's your weakness that you can't handle. I will not stand for this. Do you hear me?"

3. Identify the emotions she may be experiencing.

   Validate her apparent, surface emotion: ____________________

   ____

What underlying attachment threat do you attune to? ______________________

____

4. Now label the steps of her emotion from Marcy's initial perception to her action. *Cue: Jane's criticism and labeling Marcy as "difficult and demanding."*

   Initial perception: ______________________________________
   Bodily arousal: ______________________________________
   Meaning making: ______________________________________
   Action tendency: ______________________________________

Key Issues in Working With Emotion

The EFT therapist's work with emotions is guided by three key principles that characterize the therapist's present process focus on reactive or core emotion.

- Involvement: Working with emotions requires the direct engagement and experience of those emotions. The Client Experiencing Scale (Klein, Mathieu-Coughlan, & Kiesler, 1986; Brubacher & Wiebe, 2019) shows levels of involvement that EFT therapists strive to elicit in clients. The therapist uses simple, concrete words and images that help a person connect to their experience with increasing depth of and where emotion becomes more vivid, alive, and specific. The therapist also helps the client to work at a "safe distance" from their emotion, so they do not become overwhelmed or numb.
- Exploration: Helping clients to assemble an emotion enables them to put words to the granularity of emotional experiences that has come to be represented by one emotional label such as frustration or fear. It brings coherence to the trigger, feeling, meaning, and action aspects of the emotion. It allows for new ways to engage with and regulate an emotional response.
- Discovery of new emotion: Task 2 of EFT involves the discovery and expansion of previously unrecognized or unformulated emotional experience. Supporting clients to engage with core emotions facilitates a new level of engagement that changes the pattern of distress.

In exploring and engaging emotion, the EFT therapist is guided by the qualities of emotion that they encounter in the moment. These qualities include a focus on:

- The most poignant or vivid aspect of experience, sometimes seen in a subtle nonverbal gesture or tear or a potent image.
- Emotions that are most salient to attachment needs and fears.
- Emotions that play a role in organizing distressing interactions. These emotions that are present in the typical problematic pattern are then explored and expanded.

The process of engaging emotional experience begins with the therapist acknowledging and validating the surface, reactive emotions expressed by the client. The therapist gradually begins to touch on the underlying fears and insecurities that spark these reactive emotions, placing them in the context of normal needs for safe and secure attachment. Even when the therapist may be aware of core, underlying emotions, she works with the clients to clarify and express their emotions at the surface level rather than immediately pursuing underlying, core emotions. The therapist joins each client where they are. Accepting and validating the surface emotion is the first step forward. Only gradually can a person begin to access pain, fear, and longing underlying the reactive self-protective responses. A client's numbness and lack of feeling will also be explored, named, and placed in the context of coping patterns.

In session, the EFT therapist focuses on emotion through:

- Accessing and evoking emotions that inform an understanding of individual's needs and fears and patterns of interacting with self and others.
- Helping clients shift their habitual ways of processing and regulating their emotions. This may include helping clients discover see how they are expressing reactive emotions and disregarding core emotions such as fear.
- Assembling and restructuring key emotional experiences that may be marginalized in a person's awareness, such as the experience of loss and abandonment that fuels expressions of apathy or numbness.
- Enabling clients to respond from core emotions to shape new responses—responses that are crucial to secure attachment, such as the ability to express needs or ask for comfort and caring.

Importantly, the EFT therapist assumes that it is not simply reframing negative emotions or naming emotions that is crucial for change, but a new experience of emotion that then organizes new interactional responses. The therapist's goal in Task 2 of EFT is then to explicate, expand, and reformulate key attachment emotions; use newly formulated emotions to expand meaning and to "move" into new responses; and enhance the ways clients are able to engage with others and their own experience through these expanded emotions.

EFT INTERVENTIONS AND TASK 2

In working with emotion, the EFT therapist relies on key experiential interventions of reflection, validation, evocative responding, redirecting, heightening, and empathic conjecture. This section highlights each of these skills, including examples and practice opportunities to clarify the formulation and use of each intervention. In reviewing these practices, we must first consider the therapist's tone used to deepen emotional experience. Working with emotion in EFT involves focusing on salient experience and also connecting with the experience itself.

Deepening Emotional Engagement With RISSSC

RISSSC, an acronym that represents the core, nonverbal practices of the EFT therapist, enables the therapist to hold and keep a client in the present moment with the therapist's own voice. These therapeutic responses invite the client into a deeper engagement with his or her emotional experience.

R: The therapist intentionally REPEATS key words and phrases for emphasis.

Example. "So it's painful to stay here, to feel the hurt, sadness; the pain is just too much to handle."

Note: Each repetition invites a client to further engage with and process an emotional u. experience.

I: The therapist uses IMAGES or word pictures that evoke emotions more than abstract labels tend to do.

Example. "He shuts you out, and you are on the other side of the door, knocking, hoping he will come out, but only getting silence in return. As you say, reaching for him is like 'jumping off a cliff.'"

S: The therapist frames responses to clients in SIMPLE and concise phrases.

Example. A therapist who wants to help a client understand her experience within the context of an attachment frame would frame a client's need for responsiveness: "So, part of you just wants someone to be there for you." The therapist does not explain the attachment concepts, just simply reflects the concept in the everyday language of the client.

S: The therapist will SLOW the process of the session and the pace of speech to allow for a client's deepening of emotional experience.

Example. "It's so quiet and lonely there (pause), you're alone (pause), all alone."

S: The therapist will use a SOFT and soothing tone of voice to encourage a client to deepen his or her experience.

Example. The therapist softens her voice and responds to the client's tears and his underlying fears. "It hurts, and this is hard. [pause] It's hard to sit with this, not knowing whether your mom will really be there for you."

C: The therapist uses CLIENT words and phrases in a supportive and validating way.

Example. A teenager characterizes his parents as "nagging and critical." He states: "They are never happy with a thing I do." The therapist later in the session provides the following reflection based on his telling of a recent experience of their criticism. "So, it almost sounds like that was one of those 'They're not happy with what I do' experiences, is that it?"

Note: These key phrases can be recorded by the therapist and used from session to session to evoke emotion and create continuity.

RISSSC is important to performing many EFT interventions effectively and to increasing client level of experiencing. Use the following exercises to practice a combination of verbal and nonverbal responses to hold and highlight clients' present moment experiences.

Empathic Reflection

Empathic reflection is foundational to the EFT process and serves as a building block for other EFT interventions. The therapist attends to, focuses on, and finds words to capture the most poignant emotion of the client's present moment experience. It is not mere echoing and paraphrasing; rather, it requires the therapist to find words from within his or her empathic absorption in the client's experience. Repetition and empathic reflection intensify the power and the function of every intervention. Empathy promotes engagement in the following ways:

- Provides a mirroring of present process.
- Clarifies the attachment emotional core of the message.
- Makes the leading edge of experience explicit.

- Orders and distills experience.
- Builds and maintains the therapeutic alliance.
- Slows down the moment-to-moment processing.

What do we reflect?

- Clients' words with most poignancy.
- Surface, reactive emotions.
- Bodily movements, expressions, tears, clenches fists, swallows, lip biting, gestures, breathing, etc.
- Voice tone, pace.

Empathic Reflection and Interaction Patterns. In tracking patterns of experience, the EFT therapist combines a focus on a reactive emotion and its place in an interactional pattern. The reflection links the emotional experience to the pattern. Here is a brief reflection of reactive emotion within the context of the cycle.

> *"So, then you back away, Tom, going flat and numb, when you see Betsy's anger. Her anger is way too much to handle."*

Here the therapist reflects to Tom that his response is to withdraw and go numb when he sees Betsy's anger that is too much for him to manage.

Exercise 3.15. Reflecting Surface Emotions in the Context of the Distressed Cycle

In this exercise, respond to each client statement by answering the questions that follow.

1. "I can't take it anymore. Jake raises his voice and demands an answer, and I don't have one. It drives me nuts! I get so angry at him. I just launch right back into him."

   List the reactive emotions stated or described in the example.

   ____

   Now create a brief reflection of reactive emotion within the context of the cycle.

   ____

   ____

   ____

2. "Lara just doesn't care. She could hurt me and just walk away, not thinking about it again. She hurls these accusations at me, and I just tune them out. I've heard it all before. At that point, I just shrug it off, like, 'Yeah. Whatever.'"

   List the reactive emotions stated or described in the example.

   ____

Now create a brief reflection of reactive emotion within the context of the cycle.

____

____

3. "Jake is always too irritable. I can feel it coming. I get tense . . . like I prepare for the onslaught. I fear that I won't be able to appease him. I won't measure up to his demands of me. I don't know what to do; it's awful. I try to respond, and he just gets more irritable. So, I try again, and he gets angrier. I keep trying to explain, but at some point, there's just no use. I can only take so much, so I end up either going cold, shutting down, or going off alone."

   Create your own reflection of reactive emotion within the context of the cycle.

   ____

   ____

   ____

4. Choose the best reflection of reactive emotion that also includes reference to the couple's reactive pattern.

   a. "So, she doesn't care, and this is clear from her accusations, so why listen?"
   b. "I can understand that. It makes sense to me that you'd see her that way."
   c. "When she is angry and attacks you, you tune her out. It's like, 'Whatever. You can't get to me." Is that how it goes?"
   d. "What's it like for you to feel attacked, all the while believing that she doesn't care? What happens inside when the battle rages hot?"

Validation

Validate present moment experience (feelings, meanings, action tendencies) as legitimate, understandable in the context of client's emotional and relational experience, and the increasingly negative feedback loops of ways of dealing with emotion. Begin with: "It makes sense you feel/you do . . . " and link experience to meanings made or to responses received from others or from within.

Main Functions of Validation:

- Builds and maintains the therapeutic alliance.
- Legitimizes client responses and experience.
- Supports further exploration of client's experience.

As a primary intervention in EFT, validation is used to communicate acceptance, recognize the legitimacy of clients' emotional experience, and normalize their perceptions in the context of the pattern in which they are caught. The EFT therapist uses validation to honor a client's description of their present moment experience. This often includes linking triggers, meanings made, and reactive emotion.

Example: A client, Janet, may express her frustration with her father's passivity when there is family conflict. Imagine that the therapist in the early stages of therapy hears Janet complain.

Janet: I just don't get it. My dad just checks out. He's in the room, but he's just ignores the fighting that's right in front of him. He doesn't care.

Therapist: Yes, and that makes sense why you feel so frustrated when you see him not responding to the trouble you all are in. It is so frustrating that it seems like you don't matter, and so you say he must not care.

Janet's complaints turn to tears of frustration, disappointment, and hurt. Now, the therapist may also use validation to respond to a Janet's newly experienced emerging emotion. As the therapist reflects her emerging core emotion, Janet's tears turn to sobs, and patiently the therapist responds.

Therapist: So, it's really tough to not get a response, when you feel alone and afraid in these moments, like there is no one here that you can count on. And when you get nothing back from him, it's like you don't matter to him, yes?

The following phrases provide a way of opening a validating response. It is important for the therapist to validate each client's unique experience, which may be very different from the intention or experience of an important other—partner, or family member.

- "Yes, I hear what you are saying. . . . "
- "That makes sense to me that you feel. . . . "
- "Okay, from your point of view. . . . "
- "Yes I can see how . . . "

Exercise 3.16. Practicing Validation

Practice validation with the following couple scenarios. Explore different ways you can form validating responses according to the client's in-session experience.

After Leo's affair, Sara found it difficult to resist checking up on Leo if he was late returning home. In Sara's words: "I feel better calling him, even if it annoys him. I just can't stand not knowing if he is where he said he would be."

a. Now form a statement to validate Sara's experience.

____

____

____

Soon after, Leo responds: "I know I have to earn her trust, but her calls get me so frustrated. I start thinking about why she has to call me and all the efforts I make to show her that I am committed, but nothing seems to convince her she can trust me again!"

b. Now form a statement to validate Leo's experience.

____

____

____

Check your responses: Do your responses communicate acceptance? Do they normalize each partner's experience, reflecting and validating their present experiences?

Leo's sense of futility and fear builds as he reflects on this. He wonders if they have reached a point of no return and he has lost Sara. Tearfully, he shares, "I hoped if I tried harder that things would eventually get better, but now I am afraid that I have ruined what we had. It's broken beyond repair."

c. Focusing on the present moment, validate Leo's new experience of this core fear that is coming forward in this moment.

____

____

____

Sara distrusts this show of Leo's vulnerability and responds: "Well, I don't see how I can say everything will be better. I can't make promises; after all, he is the one who broke this."

The EFT therapist could use validation to respond to Sara's response by saying: "Right, Sara, it's like you can't reassure him right now. You can't respond to his fear and say everything will be okay because that would take trust that is still uncertain. And it makes sense that you would want to back away from his fear, not knowing what to say."

Leo reacts by retreating into contempt. "See why it's hard to have hope and to keep trying when she doesn't give me a chance?"

d. Now normalize Sara's defensiveness and validate how her response impacts Leo.

____

____

____

A well-timed validation can be an effective intervention for containing the anxious and defensive response common between distressed couples. Communicating empathy and understanding of threatening emotions responses offers an alternative to the invalidation that often defines these moments. The therapist validating into their experiences and fears demonstrates an awareness of the different experiences of each partner.

Validating a client's present response can also serve to confront self-protective responses with empathy and understanding. Consider a father who avoids any discussion of his son's complaints about his absence from the family by minimizing these concerns in the face of his work demands. The therapist can respond to his problematic behavior by validating his action as a coping response that makes sense in an attachment frame.

Therapist: Conflict was not safe in your family, especially between your parents, and it makes sense that when you read the potential for trouble with your son, you pull back and keep your distance. It's like second nature to move away from these hard feeling and difficult moments, almost like it happens without thinking about it, without seeing your son's concerns.

e. Keeping these things in mind, form a validation statement for the following parent who is a "chronic criticizer." She seeks a closer relationship with her son, yet her concerns about his choices are often shared by critically pointing out areas that he could change. When he pushes back, she redoubles her criticism until he backs down or walks out. How might you validate this mother's experience given that she has shared that in her family of origin, harsh words were the only way to be heard or seen?

____

____

____

Evocative Responding

Evocative responding involves the use of questions and prompts to call up emotions into the conversation and to assemble the different elements of the rapidly unfolding sequence of the process of emotion. Evocative questions identify and intensify emotions that are often marginal to the partner's everyday experience. The therapist may use evocative responding to help clients express emotions that are being communicated nonverbally through somatic indications or physical cues. The use of imagery helps the client experience the emotion that is being elicited. Evocative responding directs the client to the "leading edge" of their experience. Rice elaborated on the function of accurate empathic reflections or as she called it, *evocative empathy* (Rice, 1974). It is important to remember as an EFT therapist that evocative responding can involve soft, tender basic reflections that may well serve more effectively to keep the client engaged in a deeper level of experiencing questions than questions do. Evocative questions can also very specifically call the client to explore and process a newly formulated emotional experience with more granularity and more specificity.

Review the following examples of evocative questions and responses.

- "What is it like for you when Mark turns away and won't give you eye contact?"
- After a period of silence, the therapist asks the silent partner, "What is going on for you *now?*
- "Phil, how does it feel when your wife says to you that she's afraid she's not special enough? That she's going to be too much trouble. That she thinks you are going to get fed up. What do you feel when she says that?"
- "What is going on for you right now as you look at him and see his sadness?"
- A client says: "I just don't need anything from this relationship." The therapist responds: "How are you able to do that? There is nothing you need from your wife?"

The therapist will use questions to explore the edges of the emotional experience of a client often building from a nonverbal emotional expression, bodily arousal, apparent interpersonal cue, sudden reaction in session, new experience, or information shared in the session. The therapist will focus on the how, what, where, and when of a person's experience, to expand on the elements of emotion. For example, the process of emotion begins with "when" (an environmental cue). "*When* does this feeling of regret or embarrassment arise? (evokes what cued the emotion). "*Where* in your body do you feel that weighty pain?" (evokes the bodily felt sense of emotion) "*What* does your sinking stomach say?" (evokes the meaning made). "*What* do you feel like doing? or "What do you typically do . . . ?" (evokes the action tendency). The use of a "why" question is not an evocative response in that it usually calls forth more abstract cognitive responses (Table 3.2).

Table 3.2
Evocative Questions

Therapist Focus	Possible Evocative Response
Ask about the impact of an event:	What is it like for you when . . . ? What is happening for you as you hear him say that?
Focus on bodily response related to a partner's response:	What happens inside of you when she turns away?
Focus on level of bodily arousal:	So, is the tightness you feel in your shoulders when he talks about his affair an anxious tightness or an angry tightness? What would that tightness say if it had words?"
Evoke the voice or speak as an attachment figure:	So, you said your aunt was there for you. You felt safe with her. What would she say to you now? What would she say to your fear?
Ask a client to repeat a poignant phrase:	Can you say that again, Paul, how lost you feel that she has pulled away?

Exercise 3.17. Evocative Responses that Expand a Client's Experience

Practice forming an evocative statement or question to evoke the client's experience in the following examples. You may form your response to the nonverbal cues that are underlined.

1. Your client has a *pained expression on his face* when describing what happens when he tries to talk with his partner about the way he makes financial decisions.

____

____

2. Felicia has *tears in her eyes* as she describes her angry pursuit of Jose when he ignores her, preferring to talk to his friends rather than her.

____

____

3. Jane looks at Stephanie after explaining the couple's most recent fight. Stephanie glares back at her with disgust, and *pain flashes across Jane's face* as she looks away.

____

____

4. Now form an evocative response for Stephanie.

____

____

Exercise 3.18. Forming Evocative Responses

Consider how you might use an evocative response to expand and bring to life the client's less obvious experience.

1. "I feel sick when she talks about leaving me."

____

____

2. "After our fight, I had to go and lie down. I was exhausted."

____

____

3. Sheri stumbles, struggling to find words to describe her sadness when she hears Paul talk about leaving the relationship.

____

____

4. Shawn describes his grandfather as the one person in his life he has always trusted and turned to for support. How might the therapist form an evocative response to address Shawn's fears of inadequacy in his relationship with Karen?

____

____

Heightening

Heightening intensifies a client's emotional experience creating a more vivid emotional engagement with this experience. The therapist's response crystallizes and deepens key elements of this emotional experience. It is out of this heightened engagement that the therapist will facilitate deeper experiencing, new engagement with core emotion, toward shaping *corrective emotional experiences* in Task 3. Heightening can take many forms, including the use of repetition, the manner of presentation, metaphors, images, interpersonal encounters, and refocusing.

- Repetition: So you're saying to Phil, 'I'm scared, and I find it hard to believe that you really, really want to be with me. I'm so afraid; I am scared to let you in, to rest in your arms.'
- Presentation: The therapist can heighten emotion by how they respond to the client. The therapist can intensify the experience by leaning forward and matching their pace and volume to the emotion being heightened: A slow and soft voice for more vulnerable emotions or a louder, more abrupt voice for assertive responses.
- Metaphors and images: And I'm scared to let you in. I start to doubt that if I open the door and start to count on him, how do I know that he won't find me too scared . . . or too depressed . . . or too 'sick'?
- Sharing internal experiences in interpersonal encounters: "Can you tell her that? Can you say that to her again? Can you say, 'I am so alone, I can't find you.' Can you turn to her and say that?"
- Refocusing: Therapist maintains the emotional intensity of the session by blocking a client's exits from experience and staying focused on the present moment.

EFT therapists heighten emotional depth by using repetition; images; a simple, soft, slow voice; and the client's words. They stay with, linger, and intensify newly emerging emotional experience to facilitate increased depth of depth of emotional experiencing. Heightening functions to highlight key experiences that organize actions or can reorganize new actions or new formulations of experience (Table 3.3).

Table 3.3
Common Metaphors and Images

The following list summarizes common metaphors and images used by EFT therapists to symbolize a client's emotional experience.

Edge of cliff	Light, darkness
Alarm going off	Desert—dying of thirst, parched
Door—come out from behind, closed	Dance, loop, cycle, merry-go-round
Dragon or fear in facing something	Water—deep, shallow, drowning, flooding
Little child, boy, or girl	Passing the test, litmus test, on trial, condemned
Paralyzed or numbing	Bleeding, starting, suffocating, can't breathe, being destroyed, trapped
Bomb is ticking or may go off	Empty, hollow, a puppet
Military—foxhole, fire, run for cover, minefield	Hot, boiling, simmering Cold, freezing or frozen, iced over

Reminder: Often the most powerful images are found in the client's own description of their experience.

Exercise 3.19. Images or Metaphors to Heighten

Use an image or a metaphor to form a heightening statement in response to the following situations.

1. A withdrawer's loneliness at her partner's disengagement in the relationship.

   ____

   ____

2. A pursuer's fear that his partner will never respond to his needs.

   ____

   ____

3. A daughter's frustration about not getting a meaningful response from her father.

   ____

   ____

4. An individual's surprise at the support he experiences from his previously estranged sister.

   ____

   ____

Exercise 3.20. Heightening Client Experiences

Select the therapist response that would most effectively heighten the following client experiences.

1. "I find it so hard to keep reaching when I know there will be no response!"
   a. "So, you protect yourself from his distance by staying away?"
   b. "Of course, this makes sense give he hasn't been there for you for years."
   c. "Should I risk? Should I dare to hope? Should I risk being left out in the cold again?"
   d. "Are you feeling afraid about what it might be like to be hurt again?"
2. "In the end, I don't see what difference it will make. My dad doesn't care. He's too wrapped up in his own world. I might as well be invisible. No one seems to care what I am going through."
   a. "Can you let him know that you feel invisible?"
   b. "No one cares. No one listens. I am invisible. No one sees me. No one really cares about me—that's how it seems?"
   c. "You feel invisible, like no one cares, right? So, talking to your dad about this would just go nowhere, right?"
   d. "It's hard because we all need to matter, especially to those who are supposed to love us the most."

3. "It sounds gross to admit, but since my husband committed suicide, I feel like I wasn't worth sticking around for."
   a. "Yes, it makes sense that you do not understand why he left you in that way!"
   b. "What's it like for you to not be able to make any other sense of this tragedy?"
   c. "He left you alone. Cuts so deep—feels like sheer abandonment. What about me? Aren't I worth struggling for?"
   d. "It's safer to explain it that way; at least you acknowledge you somehow feel responsible."

Exercise 3.21. Heightening by Reflecting and Tracking

Please form a heightening response of your own to the following client statements. It is important to remember that the effect of heightening is determined by *how* it is said as much as what is said. The RISSSC manner is essential to the heightening of emotional experience. After creating your responses, say them out loud in the simple, soft, slow, low tone of the RISSSC manner.

1. James is afraid to tell his partner Joe that underlying his withdrawal is a fear of not being good enough the way he is and a fear of losing his sense of himself if he keeps trying to please him.

   ____

   ____

2. Kris describes feeling safe with her father for the first time in months. Talking about his care brings tears to her eyes.

   ____

   ____

3. Lucinda fears that she is a disappointment to her son and hides her fear in being overly positive and placating her son's frequent demands.

   ____

   ____

4. Shannon shares how much better she feels about herself when she is immersed in work compared with the insecurity she feels in her relationship with Chris.

   ____

   ____

Empathic Conjectures

This intervention could be called *best guesses on the leading edge of client's experience*. Conjectures are more than cognitive interpretations; rather they are formed by the therapist's immersion in the client's attachment story, including their experience of being caught in negative patterns, and self-protective strategies used to cope with others, with their own emotional experiences, and with life in general. Conjectures are formed by the therapist's understanding of basic attachment processes, through the therapist's attunement to a client's core emotions (e.g., fears of abandonment, rejection, or engulfment) and to attachment longings implied in client's fears. They are similar to what Rice (1974) calls evocative empathy, in that the therapist attunes on the leading edge of what the client has not yet been able to put into words. The therapist attunes to the edges of emotional experience implied by and hinted at through clients' verbal and nonverbal expressions and clients' relational context. They are offered with tentativeness and an invitation to be corrected. (e.g., "Does that fit for you?")

Empathic Conjecture for Attachment Longings and Fear. In this example, the therapist uses an empathic conjecture to frame a client's underlying attachment longing.

> *"You are telling me that it is lonely, and the loneliness is overwhelming like a complete rejection, and you respond with an attack because it hurts. And I hear that it hurts—that you feel lonely and rejected. I also wonder if the hurt contains a longing for connection—a longing to be held and comforted—that a part of you longs to be with him, to make that connection, to be with him, really with him. Does that fit for you?"*

The next example shows how a therapist can work with a client's fear in a similar way.

> *"You are angry with him even though he has opened up to you. He says he wants to be with you, but that is confusing because he hasn't been like this before. I am not sure if this fits for you, but it seems like there is a part of you that wants to embrace this openness because it is what you have always wanted, but there is this other part that doesn't trust it. So, if you reach out to meet him, you may fear that he'll change his mind and pull away? That deep down you are afraid that maybe you do not really matter to him. Is that close?"*

Seeding Attachment. A variation of empathic conjecture builds on a therapist's skill to validate and heighten a partner's emotional engagement. This intervention is used to bring to light the attachment needs and longings that are blocked by client fears and to paint an evocative picture of these longings and needs being met by a significant other. The intervention helps clients see beyond the fears to the needs that ultimately underlie their stuck patterns. Seeding attachment opens up new possibilities for connection by making explicit the blocked attachment longing and behaviors and the antidote to unmet needs. Seeding attachment helps clients to see beyond the fear to a more secure interaction.

Framing the seeding attachment intervention:

1. The intervention sequence begins with the phrase: "So, you could never . . . "

   "So, you could never turn to her and say, 'I need you and I need to come first. I want to be important.'"

2. Then the therapist addresses the fear that keeps the client from a more engaged stance with his or her partner. "So, you could never . . . " (disclose attachment-related fear or need)

   "So, you could never turn to him and tell him that the criticism hurts you too much, and it makes you question your worth? What you really want is to feel safe and valued in his heart."

Disquisition. A disquisition is a special type of empathic conjecture most often used when clients are reluctant to explore their experience. It is used when other evocative strategies are not effective in promoting emotional experiencing. It is a non-threatening intervention of telling a story about another client—individual, couple, or family—with some similarity to the client's distress. It is a metaphorical description of key elements of the client's negative pattern with conjectured underlying emotions woven into the narrative. The story links the client's actions to the conjectured underlying emotions. The therapist often prepares the disquisition in advance rather than responding in session on the spur of the moment.

In the following example, the therapist is working with a remarried couple that has difficulties being unified in their approach to the children. Loyalty binds exist between the biological and stepparents. The therapist uses a disquisition to get them to consider their own stuck relationship in light of another couple.

> *"Sometimes couples get locked into a pattern that is difficult for them to understand. I have been thinking about a couple I know that gets stuck around holiday celebrations. They can even see it coming, but they just feel helpless once the issues get going. She has a close relationship to her family and wants to be part of her family's holiday gatherings. He sees this as her family's control over her. At any rate, he tends to challenge her desire to hang out with her family as a sign of her lack of commitment to their marriage. She resents his judgmental attitude and is angered by his critical comments about her family. He then backs off and becomes passive and sulks. She is furious at his behavior and sees him as overly demanding and immature. Funny thing is that they both want this 'family dance' out of their relationship. He wants reassurance that he is important to her, as family holidays tended to be painful times for him. She didn't get that he wanted reassurance and support, and he didn't see that she wanted to be there for him but couldn't because she felt too controlled. I wonder sometimes if this couple could identify with what it is like for you both when dealing with family expectations."*

Exercise 3.22. Practicing a Disquisition

Imagine you have a couple, Ted and Jed, who have begun to make changes. Jed, the more withdrawn partner, is re-engaging in the relationship and has been more forthcoming with his needs and hopes for the relationship. At the same time, Ted, the more anxious pursuer, is now getting what he said he wanted from Jed and now shifts between receiving this new attention and distrustful rejection of Jed's attempts. Ted concludes: "How do I know he is really sincere?" Compose a disquisition that

- Includes acknowledgment of Ted's difficulty in trusting Jed's new changes.
- Provides a description about how other clients have had a similar struggle.
- Describes a particular pursuer's mistrust of a more engaged withdrawer.
- Includes reference to the fears and distrust underlying this change.

____

____

____

____

____

Exercise 3.23. Selecting Empathic Conjectures

1. Cherise and Samuel have a long-standing pursuit/demand–withdraw/defend cycle with Cherise expressing chronic dissatisfaction with Samuel's "commitment" to her. The couple says this frequent fight dates back to Samuel's lack of support following the death of her father. Choose the best conjecture to help Cherise access the hurt and betrayal underlying her anger.
   a. "This anger you feel is often the result of an attachment injury you experienced with Samuel's lack of accessibility."
   b. "Your anger is a reactive emotion. Do you think you might really be grieving that he was not there for you?"
   c. "I hear your anger and frustration, and I wonder if it is a loud message to Samuel that your trust in him was shattered when he backed away at your father's death and that your heart is still breaking?"
   d. "I know you are angry at Samuel, but can you tell him what hurts you as well?"
2. Later Samuel is asked about his experience in hearing Cherise recount how abandoned she felt when he left her alone at her father's death bed. Samuel talks about his confusion, of not knowing how to respond to her feelings. He admits that it's sometimes safer if he just "takes it in" rather than trying to respond. Choose the empathic conjecture that would be most helpful to lead Samuel to the leading edge of his experience:
   a. "So, you see her emotions and back away because it is not safe. Is that it?"
   b. "It makes sense that you are uncertain how to respond to her emotions because her feelings are strong, and you have not done what she wanted in the past."
   c. "Can you ask her to tell you what she would like from you?"
   d. "So, it's confusing, and you hold back, almost like something bad will happen if you show your concern. It's scary to not know if your offer will be received or rejected?"
3. As treatment progresses Sam and Cherise have a clear sense of how their cycle is blocking them from having *a healing injuries conversation* about this event from years earlier. Sam is able to acknowledge that he does shrink in the face of Cherise's anger and tears, and Cherise is able to acknowledge that when Samuel shrinks, she does get angry and demanding—determined to get him to hear her pain, terrified she no longer matters to him. Choose the best conjecture to help expand Sam's openness to hearing the vulnerable depths of Cherise's breaking heart:
   a. "So, she sees you stone-faced, a stoic man, but inside, you're shrinking like a little boy, not knowing what to do, just afraid, afraid that she will not want what you have to give her? So, you hide from her, not knowing what to say or do, just hoping to disappear."

b. "So, she shows contempt, and you withdraw. You defend yourself, and she goes on the attack. That must be so difficult to brace yourself to listen to her side of the story!"
c. "It is so very difficult to hear—startling, almost—to discover that Cherise is still shattered over the moment you walked away when her father was dying. I wonder if it is also amazing to hear that her anger at you is not about despising you but about how important you are to her and how much she needed you and still needs you today?"
d. "How does she know the difference between your fear and your indifference? How can she know when you are ready to listen to how you broke her heart?"

Catching Bullets

Catching bullets is an intervention used in the face of an aggressive remark where the therapist deftly reframes the "bullet" with an empathic conjecture before the stinging impact penetrates the other's skin and triggers a reactive self-protective move of distancing or firing back. This intervention evolved in response to delicate moments when one person risks to disclose some newly distilled, vulnerable experience and the partner reacts with accusations and disbelief. Consider the withdrawer who takes the courageous step of acknowledging a core fear of being a failure in their partner's eyes and their pursuing partner scoffs in disbelief and fires back with an attack. One of the EFT therapist's greatest resources in these moments is being able to predict that a new experience or disclosure can be very disorienting or seemingly unbelievable, particularly when this experience has not been previously been shared.

There are three common bullets faced in working with individuals, couples, and families. First, a common bullet moment seen when vulnerability is shared between couples or families, often in the powerful change events of Stage 2. This bullet response results when one partner shares and the receiving partner is so disoriented at this new expression that he or she responds with an accusatory tone, mistrust, or minimization. A 12-year-old Micah makes a tearful, vulnerable disclosure, "It's like no one understands, and they just all want me to go away!" Dad jumps in to say, "If we wanted you to go away, we would have told you! There is no reason to talk like that!" The therapist protects Micah from this hurtful comment and says to Micah's dad, "When Micah just took this big risk to tell you about his fear that you don't really want him in the family, you interrupted him pretty quickly to say he has no need to feel that. Sounds like it was so hard for you to hear that he does feel misunderstood and unwanted, and in your best attempt to reassure him, you actually discounted his feelings, yes?"

Second, sarcastic or unkind accusations toward a family member in early stages of therapy are also moments of aggression that an EFT therapist will seek to contain by *catching the bullet*. In an early session, Lilly says, "I feel all alone in this relationship." Ben retorts, "The problem is she is just like her entire family—so difficult, always sending these stingers!" The therapist interrupts, reflects the present process, and conjectures to reframe. "Ben, it sounds like when Lilly says she feels alone, you feel the sting, and you fire back with accusations about her family. You don't know how to tell her that her saying she feels alone actually stings you—that it hurts you to hear she feels alone—that you are letting her down somehow. Do I get it?"

A third bullet can be when an individual makes a derogatory remark about self or hears, in their imagination, an accusation from an imagined other in a therapist-choreographed encounter. Todd, who struggles with bouts of depression and self-judgement, says, "I don't deserve better anyway. My life's been easy. Many others have it worse." To catch the aggression, the therapist begins with reflecting present process, "Slow down, please, Todd. You were telling me how heavy all this news has been—disappointed to have been moved to a new department at work, frightened to hear your sister has been diagnosed with cancer, and shocked at your brother's decision to move to a new country—and suddenly you downplay the struggle and move to concluding you don't deserve better! Without noticing, perhaps, you turn against yourself, when you don't know who is there to recognize and care for you and the enormous losses you are facing?"

To contain aggressions toward self or another, the EFT therapist catches a bullet by reflecting present process and reframing the reactive response then conjecturing about the reaction as a disorientation or disbelief and at times adds a positive attachment intention.

Exercise 3.24. Catching Bullets Through Reflections and Reframes

How can you catch the following bullets by reflecting what just happened and reframing to normalize the reaction in an attachment frame?

1. Catch the bullet Claudia sends to her mother: A 70-year-old mother says to her adult daughter, "I am beginning to get now, Claudia, what a burden I placed on you as a child when your dad died. You were only a child, and you needed a mother, but I wasn't there for you." Her daughter interrupts her, "I don't want to hear it! Your recognition is coming a little too late, don't you see? It's like you just expect me to say it's all okay, and it is not!"

   ____

   ____

   ____

   ____

2. Catch the bullet Mary sends to Darnell: Mary starts to talk about a painful event, and Darnell shrugs his shoulders. Her voice gets suddenly shrill as she says, "If only Darnell would stop giving me silence and a cold shoulder whenever I want to talk about what happened, maybe we'd have a chance, but he's useless actually as a partner. Living with him is worse than being a single parent!"

   ____

   ____

   ____

   ____

Task 3. Restructuring Interactions

The third task in EFT involves using newly reprocessed emotional experience to restructure patterns of interaction. EFT assumes that change does not come simply from new emotional experience but rather from the new contact and interactions that arise from that new emotional experience. "If deepening engagement with core emotional vulnerabilities, especially with fears, unmet longings, sadness and loss, and shame or fears about the self, is the first key element of the change process . . . , the second element is that new facets of experience are explicitly rendered into action or enacted by the client. They are owned and expressed and in an interpersonal context" (p. 28, Johnson, 2019).

For this reason, it is extremely important that the EFT therapist be comfortable and proficient in using restructuring interventions. Interventions aimed at restructuring interactions and interventions used for reprocessing emotional experience are always intertwined. However, for the sake of clarity, three basic interventions used in EFT to restructure interactions are presented separately here:

1. Tracking and reflecting patterns of interactions.
2. Framing and reframing problems in terms of repetitive patterns or attachment responses.
3. Restructuring interactions by choreographing new events that modify patterns of engaging and interacting with emotion, with self and with others. The shaping of encounters between attachment figures in couple and family sessions or in EFIT, with a therapist, with imagined others, or between parts of self is the focus of this section.

Tracking and Reflecting Interaction

The EFT therapist starts *where people are* by tracking and reflecting the client's present pattern of engaging. Through this process, the therapist pieces together reoccurring sequences, of triggers and action tendencies, making them explicit, and helping clients to take ownership for what triggers them to react and what their typical behavioral reactions are when they perceive a threatening cue.

As the therapist tracks and reflects clients' patterns over time, the ways in which partners and family members pulls for a particular response from the other becomes tangible and clear. With individuals, it becomes clear how they are stuck in cyclic patterns of interpersonal interactions, triggering internal emotional responses and internal responses, in turn pulling for repetitive interpersonal reactions.

The identification of these patterns provides a meta-perspective for clients, helping them to stand outside themselves and view their own interactions. Tracking and reflecting also provides an opportunity for clients to expand their sense of the interconnection between inner experience and interpersonal interactions. They begin to see how the real problem is not themselves or another person but the repetitive pattern that is keeping them stuck.

Tracking and reflecting interaction is akin to and intertwined with reflecting emotional experience, although tracking interventions focus most explicitly on the behavioral aspects of emotion. As with reflecting emotional experience, the therapist's collaboration with the client and immersion in the client's experience make the intervention powerful and give it meaning. Through tracking and reflecting, the therapist eventually constructs a frame for understanding the client's distress in the context of the repetitive cycle of triggers and responses. Through tracking and reflecting interactive patterns, the therapist accesses first reactive emotions and then underlying core emotional experience (Table 3.4).

Table 3.4
Tracking Interactions

Therapist Focus	Possible Responses
Recent incidents	"So, you had a fight last night, and when he said, 'I'm so frustrated with your ignoring me,' you were initially shocked and then reacted with a series of complaints about how he has ignored you for years."
Recurring patterns	"When you are not getting along with your daughter and are feeling distant, that is when you begin to question her and she gets very annoyed at you for the questions, is that it?"
In-session moments of interaction	"Help me understand what just happened here. You were telling me that others' jabs tear you up on the inside, and you suddenly folded your arms and said, 'Really, it's silly really. I'm just overreacting.'"
Attachment: significant moments of interaction	Greetings, partings, and moments of needing comfort, support, reassurance, physical touch, or intimate contact have particular attachment significance. These moments are likely to trigger clients' sense of attachment security and to evoke positive or negative cycles of interaction. For example: • "I walk in the door, and when you don't look up, I feel you couldn't care less." (greeting) • "I was afraid and then pissed when you didn't call." (wanting contact) • "I was overwhelmed and confused and needed someone to talk to." (needing reassurance) • "After mom died, it felt so good to have him close to me." (needing support) • "When we don't make love, I start to build a wall." (wanting connection) • "I wish when you left in the morning, you would say good-bye." (parting)

Exercise 3.25. Tracking and Reflecting the Unfolding of Emotional Experience

This exercise is designed to help you learn to track and reflect interaction. Notice that the excerpt contains both a recent event and an in-session moment. You will see that the therapist's reflections of Nick's interactions and experience are filled in. Your task is to fill in the blanks reflecting Nora's interactions and experience:

Nick: Yeah, I'll tell you how this goes between us. Last night was a good example. I came home. I walk in the door, and she doesn't look up. She ignores me." (To wife) "Yeah, and then you were pissed off because I wasn't all cheerful.

Nora: (wife jumps in) You don't really get this at all. When you came home, I was working with your son trying to help him with his homework. You didn't offer to help. You went straight to your office. I can't ever count on you. I used to get up and give you a kiss, but you seem to walk right past me, and I don't see you for the rest of the night, so I quit. You are hardly a part of my life anymore. Why don't you make the family a priority in your life? (Nora gives Nick a stern look.)

Nick: Of course I went to my office because you give me that attitude every day. Who wouldn't leave and go be alone?" (Nick looks down and away.) "If I try to come in and help, you just get angry, and we start fighting. It doesn't matter what I do. I can't get it right with you.

Therapist: Wait a minute. Let's slow this down. Let me get what's going on here. This sounds important to me.

1. Reflect the danger cue for Nick:

Therapist: When Nora didn't look up when you walked through the door, a danger bell rang for you, yes?

Reflect the danger cue for Nora:

Therapist: ____

2. Reflect Nick's simple actions:

Therapist: Nick, You're saying you walk in, you walk past Nora, you go to your office.

Reflect Nora's simple actions:

Therapist: ____

3. Reflect Nick's perceptions of Nora's actions:

Therapist: Nick, you see her as ignoring you, that she doesn't care, that she is pissed off, It seems to you that it doesn't matter what you do, you can't get it right.

Reflect Nora's perceptions of Nick's actions:

Therapist: ____

4. Reflect how Nick's perceptions cue his actions:

Therapist: It seems to you that she is mad and that it doesn't matter what you do—that no matter what you do it is wrong, so you distance yourself.

Reflect how Nora's perceptions cue her actions:

Therapist: ____

5. Reflect Nick's reactive emotion evoked by the interaction:

Therapist: You perceive that she is not interested in you, and so you put up your guard and get defensive.

Reflect Nora's reactive emotion evoked by the interaction:

Therapist: ____

6. Reflect Nick's core underlying emotion:

Therapist: You experience her as not interested, and you feel hurt, lonely, and rejected.

Reflect Nora's core underlying emotion:

Therapist: ____

Reframing

After the intervention of reflection and tracking, reframing is the second intervention we are exploring in Task 3. The basic reframe in EFT involves tying couple and family distress and individuals' presenting problems to the basic stuck patterns of interaction or engagement (with others and with emotional experience). The EFT therapist reframes each client's behavior in the context of their typical pattern or interactive cycle. The cycle of interaction is then labeled as the *enemy* or the problem, shifting the focus away from a specific person's personal deficiencies. This reframe externalizes the problem, essentially saying, "The real problem is not you, or your partner, son or daughter, parent, and so on. The pattern in which you are caught is the real enemy here." The cycle is framed as the enemy preventing couples and families from having safe, responsive connections. It is also framed as the enemy holding individuals in self-protective prisons of depression, anxiety, isolation, and other emotional distress.

This reframe provides a non-pathologizing context for clients to become curious about this imprisoning pattern and motivates then to work together to reshape this imprisoning cycle into one of safety and secure connection. The reframe of secure attachment—the antidote to presenting problems and distress—is a pattern where significant others are safe and responsive and each person feels lovable, valued, and competent.

In this section on the intervention of reframing, you will have opportunity to explore two types of reframes. The first is framing the cycle, not a person, as the problem. This is a de-pathologizing, non-blaming reframe. The second is finding hints of secure attachment possibilities within clients' stories of distress and thus painting a picture of secure attachment while also validating their current distress. That is, planting seeds of secure attachment in early sessions.

Reframing the Problem as the Cycle

Negative interaction patterns cause clients to experience attachment insecurities and distress and, in turn, to react in negative ways, causing more distress in an endless, vicious cycle of negative behavior and attachment distress. By reframing *the cycle* or distressing internal and interpersonal patterns of interaction in terms of attachment fears and insecurity and as preventing safe, responsive contact, the therapist reframes the distress not only as a struggle against the enemy of the negative cycle but also as a struggle for secure attachment.

The most commonly used reframes in EFT are that anger and criticism are framed as attachment protest for a response rather than as random aggression; withdrawal and defense are framed as fear of rejection rather than indifference or uncaring; and the *problem* is framed not as an individual and his or her *flaws* but as distressing patterns of interaction—ways to cope with attachment insecurity.

Example 1: An EFT therapist reframes the distress between a mother and 14-year-old son as a problem not being the teenager or the mom but the explicit problematic cycle in which they are caught:

> *"We've been talking here about this cycle in which the two of you are caught. Mom, you experience Carl as not being available to talk and as shutting down. You get afraid that you will lose him if you don't do something. So, you push him to talk, but he just gets more silent. And, Carl, you experience Mom as pushy and angry,*

and you try to defend yourself the only way you know how, which is by shutting down and pulling away. Of course, your shutting down just gets Mom to try even harder to get you to talk. The more you try to protect yourself by shutting down, the more she pushes. And, Mom, the more Carl shuts down, the more you get afraid of losing him, and the more you push him to talk. The two of you are caught in this never-ending vicious circle that leaves both of you feeling frustrated and distant."

Example 2: Reframing a partner's withdrawal in a couple relationship as "protecting the relationship and the partner"

Therapist: "You withdraw when you are confronted by her anger because it's hard to bear the feelings that you've done it wrong. And you know that fighting back is not an option. Fighting back is to risk a massive meltdown, to risk getting out of control, and to risk hurting her, and that's not an option. So, you withdraw to protect yourself, Julie, and the relationship. Is that right?"

Example 3: Reframing a partner's criticism and pursuing as "fighting for connection"

The angry, critical behavior of a pursuing spouse can be difficult to understand, manage, and frame for a beginning couple therapist. However, when viewed from an attachment perspective, these behaviors are adaptive and make sense. In attachment terms, critical pursuing behavior is understood as attachment protest, a reaction to the unavailability of the other, and an attempt to regain responsive contact and to pull the other close by fighting for the relationship.

Exercise 3.26. Reframing Critical Pursuit as "Urgency for a Response"

Selma, who lost her first husband to police violence, is fraught with distress over her husband John's quietness. She swings between raging at John and going silent for days. She knows he is a kind man, but she is terrified he has lost his love for her. John says maybe she has a mental illness because she acts so bizarre!

Please create a de-pathologizing reframe for her critical pursuit as urgently seeking a response in the context of their cycle:

____

____

____

Exercise 3.27. Reframing Isolation as Seeking Protection

Latonya struggles with depression and social isolation. She lives alone and just celebrated six months of sobriety. She says the isolation is getting to be too much; however, even though she says she wants friends, she refuses to reach out to anyone. "People only hurt me and let me down. I'm not taking any more chances! I know it sounds stupid to say I want friends, when I refuse to let anyone in."

Please create a de-pathologizing reframe for her avoidance and isolation in the context of her story:

____

The previous example, reframes the problem of self-isolation as "seeking protection." Although this behavior is not a solution, the reframe takes the focus away from naming Letonya as the problem. It validates her pattern of isolating as her best protection in the present context. It also contains an example of finding hints of secure attachment possibilities within her story. This leads to the second type of reframe, discussed next: Finding hints of secure attachment within the distress.

Beginning EFT therapists often pay too little attention to creating a positive frame that both provides an image of secure attachment and implies the possibility of making that a reality. The therapist will "paint a picture" or imply the possibility of secure attachment. Some clients who are distressed have had a secure attachment earlier in the relationship and so already have an image to build on. Others have had few secure relationships and will need repeated exposure to images of secure attachment to make the frame meaningful for them.

EFT employs three methods to "imply possibilities" of safe attachment:

1. Validating the current distress pattern while implying the possibility of safe attachment:

   "You're not sure that you could find anyone in your life that feels safe to turn to in need?"

2. Highlighting exceptions to the problem that point toward safe attachment:

   "It seems that you were able to confide in her here today in a way you aren't usually able to do. Is that right? So, maybe you can do it. You just need more moments of feeling safe enough to take these risks."

3. Implying possibilities by giving them an image of safe attachment:

   "So, if you were able to go to your mom for support and to share with her when you were feeling overwhelmed like this, that would be different? It would be like being in a foreign country?"

Example: Painting a Picture of Safe Attachment in Couple Therapy

Therapist: I think what you are both telling me is that in a way, this fight was about wanting to come home to a safe haven where both of you could have a moment to connect and feel supported by the other. Marcus, you walked in the door tired and discouraged about the bad day at work and wanting to see a kind, accepting smile on Linda's face, wanting a moment to connect and to feel that someone was on your side. But instead, you bumped up against Linda being irritated and unavailable, and you felt hurt and got defensive. And, Linda, you were feeling swamped and depleted, struggling all day with the children, and you were 'drowning,' wanting someone to throw you a life raft. Instead of feeling that you are together in the boat battling the storm together, you feel alone. Is that it? Am I getting it? And I think what we are working on here and what is hard to imagine is that sometimes the relationship could be a resource or a safe haven where you could turn to each other for a moment of contact or support. That when one of you falls out of the boat the other can help pull you back in. And if both fall out, you can work together to save yourselves. I think that is what you both are fighting for but are having trouble creating.

Exercise 3.28. Painting a Picture of Safe Attachment in EFFT

Fifteen-year-old Ahmaud is getting into shoplifting troubles and getting hurt by his friends. He wants nothing to do with his mother's attempts to help him. Please create a reframe for the distressed cycle between Ahmaud and his mother that paints a picture of possible secure attachment.

____

____

____

Restructuring Interactions by Shaping Encounters

This is the third intervention for Task 3, restructuring, that you have the opportunity to explore. The restructuring intervention is not a simple micro-intervention like the other interventions we have reviewed in this chapter. Traditionally called enactments in couple therapy, the restructuring intervention is also known as engaged *encounters* across all modalities of therapy. These interpersonal encounters are specific dialogues shaped in a predictable manner by the therapist. This manner involves four basic elements: (a) engaging the client to distill their experience and shape a coherent message; (2) helping the discloser and the receiver of the message to anticipate the disclosure; (3) making a direct request for the disclosure; and (4) finally, helping the disclosing client to maintain focus and remain engaged when they exit or become distracted.

The encounters are shaped between attachment figures in couple and family therapy. In EFIT, the encounters are imagined dialogues with a significant other, between parts of self, or an encounter with the therapist. Recent EFT literature (Brubacher, 2018; Johnson, 2019, 2020) describes encounters to be a substantial part of the EFT macro-intervention known as the EFT Tango. The Tango, a simple way to conceptualize the repetitive flow of EFT interventions, is presented at the end of this chapter with opportunity for you to practice with the case of a transgender couple, Jade and Beau. That case example provides a walk through the process of restructuring in an early session.

The elements of choreographing or shaping of encounters for Task 3 restructuring can be remembered with the acronym SHAPE:

Simplify (distil) the message.

Heighten present moment engagement with repetition.

Anticipate contact.

Present disclosure to relevant other. (Direct the client to disclose.)

Engage. (Keep the client engaged in the process with refocusing, redirecting, repeating, and *slicing the risk thinner.*)

Encounters can be shaped for the following purposes (Johnson, 2020):

- Enacting present positions and typical action tendencies, so they can be directly experienced and expanded
- Turning new emotional experience into new ways of interacting
- Highlighting new or rarely occurring responses
- Choreographing change events

Encounters are focused and choreographed, allowing the client little room for failure. When clients cannot follow the directives, the difficult moment is processed not as a failure or resistance but as an opportunity to further explore and process their experience in the moment. The therapist will "slice the risk thinner" into a manageable, congruent message that the client can express. At times the manageable disclosure might be a simple as, in EFFT, "Can you turn and tell your dad, then, 'I am just not ready to tell you how much I am hurting from what you did'?" Or in couple therapy, to partner, "Can you tell her then, 'It's too hard, I'm just not ready to tell you how freaked out I get over all the time you spend on Twitter.'" Or in EFIT, to an image of a parent who committed suicide, "It is too difficult to tell you that your death feels like a slap in the face—too hard to tell you when I know you were in such pain."

Throughout the course of therapy, the therapist will create numerous encounters. These create "bite-size" amounts of interaction, allowing clients to "digest" small moments of engaging in new ways with experience and with others. By creating many small corrective emotional experiences through encounters, the therapist gradually moves the process one step closer to shaping more secure bonding interactions. The following case of Beau and Jade in EFCT illustrates how all interventions combine towards shaping, processing, and integrating encounters with the macro-intervention of the EFT Tango.

BRINGING IT ALL TOGETHER WITH THE EFT TANGO

The micro-interventions of EFT explored throughout this chapter comprise the macro-intervention of EFT—the EFT Tango. The EFT Tango, known as "the heart of EFT intervention" (Johnson, p. 54, 2019) is a succinct depiction of how all the EFT micro-interventions lead up to creating corrective emotional experiences that are shaped in Tango Move 3, processed in Tango Move 4, and consolidated in Tango Move 5. The EFT Tango is a dynamic metaphor for the five essential "moves" that are used repeatedly though the entire EFT process and demonstrated through the remaining chapters of this book. To use the five moves of the EFT Tango macro-intervention, an EFT therapist (1) reflects the present-moment process, (2) assembles the elements of emotion in that process and deepens the core emotion, (3) shapes interpersonal encounters to disclose newly discovered experience and to restructure the *dynamic*, (4) processes and expands the impact of sharing and receiving the disclosure, and (5) integrates and consolidates the corrective emotional experience. These five moves are used repeatedly across sessions, with different degrees of intensity and pacing, depending on the stage of change. From Stage 1, stabilization/de-escalation, through Stage 2 restructuring to Stage 3 consolidation, the five moves of the Tango can be seen. Repetition and reflection intensify the power and the function of every micro-intervention in the EFT Tango Moves.

Exploring an early session of EFT couple therapy gives an overview of the five moves of the EFT Tango as they utilize the micro-interventions described earlier. Jade and Beau, a transgender couple, both using they/them pronouns, begin therapy, caught in their typical distressed interaction. Jade, an anxious pursuer, complains that Beau is never available—always too busy trying to impress others. Jade protests, "I can never get Beau's attention in the most dire moments of need—like at the party last night. Once again I was alone and couldn't get you to even look at me." Beau, in exasperation, pleads, "Can't you see how hard I am trying to show you that you are important—to make you happy?" and then suddenly flips into frustration that Jade never remembers or gives them credit for anything!

Next you can interact with the therapist moving through the five moves of the of EFT Tango with Jade, who pushes for Beau's response, and Beau, who withdraws and defends against Jade's demands. After you fill in your chosen responses, you can compare them with the options offered at the end of the chapter. This isn't about right and wrong; rather, it is about exploring and applying EFT interventions. Take note of how your answers are creatively different from the suggested responses.

Tango Move 1—Reflecting the Present Process

Empathic Attunement

Before finding words to reflect the present process between Jade and Beau, the therapist empathically attunes to Jade's story and complaints of being alone and Beau's failing efforts to please Jade. The therapist also attunes to the rapid interactional responses each partner makes to one another.

The therapist tunes into her own body to get a felt sense of Jade's exasperation and loneliness; then the therapist tunes into her own body to get a felt sense of Beau's frustration with numerous failed attempts to make Jade happy; and finally, she senses in her own body the push-pull-push dynamic between them. After having a felt sense of the present moment struggle, the therapist uses a combination of empathic reflections and tracking interventions to mirror back to Jade and Beau their present moment process.

[Note: If, instead of Jade and Beau, the client was an individual without a relevant *other* physically present in the room, the therapist would also seek to attune to the client's story of distress, which is invariably relational at its core.]

Empathic Reflections and Tracking

To empathically reflect and accurately track the current distressed pattern between Jade and Beau, the therapist uses the simple formula of *The more . . . the more* with action words that describe the actions each is taking in the present moment and empathic reflection of the most poignant, alive apparent emotion. "It seems the two of you have slipped back into your familiar pattern. In this moment, Jade, the more you complain and get exasperated with Beau (Jade's action tendency), the more, Beau, you explain yourself and then flip into angry responses. Then, Jade, the more Beau explains (Beau's action tendency), the more you complain, and round and round it goes with both of you feeling frustrated, alone, and unappreciated (empathic reflection of their emotional experience).

Exercise 3.29. Tango Move 1—Reflection of the Present Process

Please summarize the pattern between Jade and Beau and their emotional experience of this pattern. This attachment framing of their problem is de-pathologizing and hopeful.

The pattern: ____

The emotional experience: ________________________________

Tango Move 2—Assembling and Deepening Emotional Experience

Affect assembly is an active process by which the therapist assembles the elements of emotion first for one partner and then the other. In Stage 1, the emotional experience of each partner is assembled. You can begin with either the withdrawer or pursuer. "The relationship to emotion changes as a result of identifying the different elements of emotion"

(Johnson, 2019, p. 2). Because the therapist knows that people calm down and have more access to adaptive action tendencies when elements of emotion are assembled, she is in no rush to deepen emotion in this early session. She wants most of all to help Jade and Beau discover and more actively engage with the emotion that is driving their part of the negative cycle.

In EFT Tango Move 2, the therapists uses validation and evocative responses and questions to assemble emotion. Additionally, some redirecting and empathic conjectures are used. To savor and deepen the new emotional experience that is accessed in this process, the therapist will, in the latter part of Tango Move 2, use heightening and perhaps conjecture.

The therapist begins with Jade to validate how their feelings, meanings, and action tendencies are legitimate and understandable in the context of their negative stuck pattern with Beau. In this validation process, the therapist is targeting specific elements of emotion. In the transcript in Exercise 3.30, please fill in the blanks to indicate which element of emotion has just been identified. One blank may also indicate the core underlying attachment emotion.

Exercise 3.30. Identifying Elements of Emotion in Tango Move 2 Assembly

Identify in each blank which element of emotion has just been illustrated (That is, cue, bodily arousal, meaning made, action tendency or core emotion).

"It makes sense, Jade, that the more Beau tells you that you don't notice how much they are already doing __________, the more you push to say ______________. "None of that counts when I just want you to notice me! You even see me! You just don't care!" ______________. Your voice chokes as you say those words ______________. The more alone and invisible you feel, ____________________ the more you push Beau to show up ____________________.

Exercise 3.31. Validation in Tango Move 2 to Link Elements of Emotion

Create a validation linking Beau's danger cue (Jade's action tendency to complain) to their action tendency, attachment meanings or reactive emotion.

____

____

____

Evocative Questions and Responses

Now, the therapist wants to add more specificity and engagement to Jade and Beau's affect assembly. To do this, the therapist can use evocative responses and questions to focus on the emerging, unclear edges of experience. By accessing and expanding the key elements of emotional experience: cue/initial perception of danger or safety, bodily response, meaning making, and action impulse, the therapist can assemble the pieces into a coherent whole. After the emerging edges are distilled into more coherence, the therapist will heighten, savor, and linger in the depth of newly accessed emotional experience.

All evocative questions are to be followed by reflections to savor, link, and heighten emerging experience. To assemble Beau's emotional experience, the therapist first of all **reflects and validates** their obvious frustration. "It must be frustrating, indeed—when what you hear when Jade says they were alone and couldn't get you to look at them (cue) is that you can never satisfy them—can never make them happy (meaning)!"

Exercise 3.32. Using Evocative Questions to Assemble and Link Elements of Emotion

Begin by replaying the cue and then evoke Beau's bodily response, the meaning they make of Jade's action, and the automatic action impulse: "You hear Jade say (cue) that they couldn't even get you to look at them last night, and a danger bell rings, "Oh, oh, this isn't good!" (immediate sense of attachment threat). How can you evoke:

1. Bodily response: ______________________________
2. Meaning making: ______________________________
3. How can you put it all together into a coherent whole along with Beau's action impulse?

   ____

   ____

Beau confirms, "That is what happens—Jade complains, and I immediately hear I can never make them happy—can never satisfy them, and it's so frustrating!"

Redirect and Refocus

In Tango Move 2, there are times a client exits or minimizes and the therapist redirects and refocuses to triggering moments to return to exploring, assembling, and deepening.

To evoke Beau's underlying core emotion just before his explanations, pleas, and reactive emotions, the therapist redirects back to Beau's bodily arousal, and validates the difficulty, "Can we go back to the moment of the hurt in your stiffened back? You hurt inside (bodily arousal) and your start to feel angry that Jade doesn't seem to see how important they are to you? (meaning). This sounds like a very difficult moment! (Beau: Very!) Will Jade ever see—will I ever make Jade happy? That must be dreadful, to fear you cannot make Jade happy or satisfied with you? Your body startles (arousal) and what happens inside?" (evocative question to elicit core attachment fear).

Beau: Dread. Dread—my stomach drops—dread I can never make it with Jade—like I have already lost the game.

Heightening With RISSSC

This example of refocusing also had the impact of heightening as the therapist repeated in a soft, slow, low voice how very frightful Beau's emotional experience is. EFT therapists heighten emotional depth by using repetition; images; a simple, soft, slow voice; and the client's words. They stay with, linger, and intensify newly emerging emotional experience.

Exercise 3.33. Heightening in Tango Move 2 With RISSSC

How could you heighten Beau's dread with repetition of their bodily felt sense linked to the attachment meanings in the dread?

Empathic Conjecture

Conjectures are empathic reflections just slightly ahead of what the client has expressed. They are informed by immersing in the client's attachment story and hearing the implied messages on the leading edge of what they are able to put into words. Conjectures are consistently offered with tentativeness and an invitation to be corrected (e.g., "Does that fit for you?").

Exercise 3.34. Deepening in Tango Move 2 With Empathic Conjecture

How might you respond to Beau's dread of never being able to make Jade happy with a conjecture that could deepen into their core fear in the context of continuing to try to please Jade and then giving up in frustration?

At this point, before assembling Jade's emotion in EFT Tango Move 2, the therapist will likely choose to shape an encounter (EFT Tango Move 3) for Beau to share this newly coherent emotional experience with Jade. After processing that encounter (Tango Move 4), the therapist will return to an EFT Tango Move 2 to assemble Jade's emotional experience.

EFT Tango Move 3—Choreographing Engaged Encounters

Catching bullets and *seeding attachment* are variations of reframing and conjecture also used in Tango Move 3. Restructuring is the kind of change that happens later in therapy; however, the interventions used in the restructuring task are relevant throughout therapy as illustrated in this early session with Jade and Beau.

Exercise 3.35. Shaping the Message for an Encounter

The therapist chooses to shape an encounter for Beau to more deeply experience this newly formulated core fear linked to their typical action tendency while disclosing it to Jade. How could you shape an encounter for Beau to share with Jade how they do in fact fire back with explanations and frustrated pleas for Jade to appreciate how hard they are trying and that under that frustration is an uneasy sense of dread and fear that they will just never make it with Jade?

Exercise 3.36. Anticipating the Encounter

Next, the therapist checks whether Jade is ready to receive a disclosure from Beau. How might you check with Jade if they are ready to hear this, repeating specifically the core of what you are asking Beau to share? Repetition of the distilled message heightens awareness and emotional engagement.

____

____

____

Empathic Reflection and Validation to Repair Alliance Rupture. If Jade replies with, "I guess, but it won't change much, will it? In fact—don't bother. I already heard Beau and I don't get why you want Beau to tell me. I don't want to hear any justification for their explanations and pathetic pleas!" there appears to be a threat to the therapeutic alliance. Jade seems not to be finding the process to be relevant to their concerns. This calls for some therapist transparency, empathy, and unconditional acceptance.

Therapist: Of course, you do not want any justification for Beau's explanations and pleas. You have been living in this lonely spot for so long and—feeling left all alone. I get that. When Beau acknowledges that they don't tell you about their fear but instead give fiery explanations, it brings pain for you, and you feel irritated about how long you've been stuck in this pattern. You are right—asking Beau to tell you about the dread inside just before the explanations is not likely to change much yet. For now, I am inviting Beau to let you know that they are aware of how they automatically push aside this dread of failing you and get quickly caught up in giving explanations and pleas that are so painful to you.

Refocus the Receiving Partner. Refocusing Jade, the therapist says, "I'd like Beau to have a chance to tell you themself. Are you okay if they share with you just now?" Jade nods acceptance and turns to Beau.

Exercise 3.37. Refocusing the Experiencing Partner and Directing the Encounter

How could the therapist refocus Beau on the link between the underlying dread in their stomach and their automatic action impulse to fire back with explanations and pleas, and then invite them to share with Jade (choreograph an encounter)? (Hint: Go back to the sinking stomach.)

____

____

____

Beau does the encounter with Jade: "I do—it's true—I don't tell you about my sinking stomach. I live in dread I could lose you if I cannot make you happy, and then I get frustrated with you. I explain and defend myself and beg you to give me credit and actually blame you!"

Tango Move 4—Processing the Encounter

Exercise 3.38. Catching a Bullet While Processing an Encounter

Jade gets triggered into their negative cycle: "Well, I'm tired of your angry explanations, and I don't care about your stomach!"

How could the therapist gently validate Jade's interruption, block the aggression, and reframe it as disorientation?

____

____

____

To process Beau's emotional experience of the encounter, the therapist contains Jade and asks Beau an evocative question.

Therapist: Jade, let's hear what it was like for Beau to so bravely turn to you and look you in the eyes and admit that they don't share this fear but come after you with fiery explanation. What was it like Beau to look right in Jade's eyes and share this with them?

Beau: Oddly—a relief. I wish I could share this fear more. I'm tired of getting so frustrated with Jade. They deserve better. I don't tell Jade that my stomach knots in dread of their unhappiness.

Therapist: Ahhh, big relief to be so open and honest with Jade about this core fear that drives you to get frustrated and defensive! (heightening, tracking, to process)

Exercise 3.39. Evocative Question to Elicit Jade's Inner Experience—Processing the Encounter

Repeating the core of what Beau shared, how can you invite Jade to reflect on what it was like to receive this message from Beau?

____

____

Jade: Honestly, I was shocked. I had no idea Beau could admit they fire back in defense. No idea when Beau is firing back and pleading with me that they have any dread or fear—certainly not any fears of losing me! No idea they even care! This is a weight off my shoulders, really.

Tango Move 5—Integrating and Validating

After processing (Move 4) and integrating (Move 5) this encounter, the therapist will assemble and deepen Jade's experience in the pattern (Move 2) and shape an encounter for Jade to disclose to Beau a clearly distilled message of their experience (Move 3). After processing each encounter with each partner with Move 4—"What was it like to share?" and "What was it like to receive?"—the therapist will do a Tango Move 5 to integrate and validate what Beau and Jade have just done. Thus, there may be several Move 5 integrations within the session. At the end of the session, there will be a clear Tango Move 5. In that summary validation, the therapist will emphasize, in this early session, that even though Beau and Jade haven't yet changed their automatic pattern, it is a significant shift for them to have identified together how they typically get caught and to have named the underlying fears that drive this pattern.

The Tango Moves are not always done in a linear fashion, though Tango Move 2 does help to prepare clients for Tango Move 3 encounters, and the impact of Tango Move 3 encounters is maximized and heightened through Tango Move 4 processing. There are frequently multiple flows between Moves 3 and 4. Once an EFT therapist is familiar with the EFT micro-interventions and the macro-moves of the EFT Tango, they can improvise with creativity.

Exercise 3.40. Summary Statement to Integrate the Work of the Session

How could you summarize the work of this session, helping the couple to celebrate the experience they had and to leave the session with some coherence? Assuming Jade had also acknowledged in their encounter with Beau that, "It is true, when you don't respond to my pushes and pleas for you to be more involved with me, I do push harder and louder and do get very critical of you! I am not ready to tell you how afraid I am that you just don't care about me. I am still convinced most of the time that you don't care enough to hear me!" How could you validate and integrate the specific significance of this session as the couple took ownership for the pattern they are caught in and some of the underlying emotion propelling this cycle?

____

____

____

____

Exercise 3.41. Review of EFT Tango Moves

The EFT Tango is a macro-intervention combining all the micro-interventions. Next are questions to help you review and verify that you are clear about the focus of each move.

Select the response that best describes what an EFT therapist does in each move of the Tango.

1. In Move 1 of EFT Tango, Mirroring Present Process, the therapist:
    a. Provides clients with clear insight into a de-pathologized view of their problem.
    b. Reflects present process, particularly the triggers and behavioral responses in clients' typical pattern of engagement.

c. Empathically reflects and tracks the impact of past traumas and family of origin incidents.

d. Deepens clients' core emotional experiences driving negative coping patterns.

2. In Move 2 of EFT Tango, Affect Assembly and Deepening, the therapist:

   a. Reflects and mirrors how the core attachment fear that is driving ineffective patterns of emotion regulation and relational processes.

   b. Intersperses many evocative questions and validating reflections to help clients to choose new ways of interacting.

   c. Assembles the elements of emotion, with evocative questions as a path into deepening present moment experience of the core, underlying attachment fear.

   d. Heightens all elements of emotion except for bodily arousal which is reserved for Tango Move 4 processing.

3. Move 3 of EFT Tango, Choreographing Engaged Encounters:

   Choose the one item below that is **NOT** an accurate statement about Tango Move 3.

   a. Tango Move 3 is the heart of reshaping interactions because in this move, the therapist typically speaks for the client, and the level of risk is at its lowest.

   b. Tango Move 3 can be an encounter between attachment figures in couple and family therapy and in EFIT, with an imagined other not physically present in the room, with the therapist or between parts of self.

   c. Tango Move 3 includes shaping the message to disclose, anticipating the disclosure, directing and the disclosure, and refocusing and redirecting when required.

   d. Shaping an encounter follows reflection of present process and assembling and deepening emotion so the client is sufficiently emotionally engaged with their experience for the encounter to have an impact.

4. Move 4 of EFT Tango, Processing the Encounter:

   a. All moves of the Tango culminate in Tango Move 4 when clients are helped to shape an encounter that turns new emotional experience into new interactions.

   b. Emotional engagement is not important while processing an encounter.

   c. Catching bullets, evocative questions, and validation are all micro-interventions used in Tango Move 4.

   d. Tango Move 4, processing an encounter, is only necessary if the encounter does not go well.

5. Move 5 of EFT Tango, Integrating and Summarizing:

   a. Tango Move 5 is never done more than one time per session. It is a clear summary at the end of each session.

   b. Tango Move 5 summarizes, validates, and integrates the work in each session and helps to create safety and security with the celebration and coherence it provides.

   c. The primary purpose of Tango Move 5 summary is to help a more withdrawn, intellectual client recognize that there is value in explanations.

   d. Tango Move 5 is the one Move that is reserved primarily for couple therapy. It is rarely used in EFIT and EFFT.

ANSWERS AND SUGGESTED RESPONSES

Exercise 3.1. Attunement with the Attachment Perspective.

Hugo may be fearing rejection/judgement. His view of other is that his boss is out to hurt him. (unsafe other) He has a positive view of self (competent).

Exercise 3.2. Stance of Empathic Attunement.

Answer: All but C. illustrate a stance of empathic attunement. The therapist failed to attune by wanting to help Bob see Marie's point of view rather than attuning to Bob's experience, to Marie's experience, and to their relational experience of getting caught in a self-reinforcing feedback loop.

Exercise 3.3. Stance of Acceptance.

Answer: Only B. illustrates a stance of acceptance and respect for the client's present moment experiencing. A focuses on a diagnosis and not the person. C conveys a lack of acceptance for the way the client is regulating her emotion and is more about the therapist's need to remove distractions. D conveys judgement and makes assumptions without joining first with the person to learn about her experience.

Exercise 3.4. Therapist Genuineness.

Answer: D. While illustrating some therapist honesty, D. is lacking in terms of genuine therapist engagement with the client's longing for tools to get to a better place. It is disrespectful and nonempathic.

Exercise 3.5. Therapist Self-Disclosure/Transparency.

Answer: E. All of the responses are examples of therapist self-disclosure.

Exercise 3.6. Continuous Alliance Monitoring.

A. is the only response in which the therapist acknowledges in a genuine, open manner what they have just done that may have been a misunderstanding and that uses empathic, evocative responses to invite open dialogue.

Exercise 3.7. Emotions Common to Human Experience

1. Anger	a) to fight, attack, defend
2. Joy	b) to move toward, to engage, connect
3. Sadness	c) to seek comfort and nurturance
4. Fear/anxiety	d) to fight, flee, seek protection
5. Shame/disgust	e) to disappear, to hide, to retreat
6. Surprise/curiosity	f) to move toward, to explore

Exercise 3.8. Identifying Basic Emotions

1. Sadness/despair, 2. Shame/disgust, 3. Shame/disgust, 4. Joy/elation, 5. Fear/anxiety, 6. Anger/rage

Exercise 3.9. Linking Interpersonal Triggers, Action Tendencies, and Experienced Emotion

1. fear of being hurt/rejected.
2. his son's lack of response/his son won't talk to him.
3. to shut down in despair or to attack.

Exercise 3.10. Distinguishing Core and Reactive Emotion

1. anger/rage; surface/reactive
2. pain shifts to curiosity; immediate/core
3. fear; immediate/core
4. numb; surface/reactive

Exercise 3.11. Attuning to Core Emotions and Longings Underlying Reactivity

1. Reactive emotion: numb; possible underlying emotion: shame, fear of rejection.
2. Reactive: anger; possible underlying emotion: desperation, loneliness, fear of abandonment.
3. Reactive: annoyance, numb, helpless; possible underlying emotion: fear of rejection, judgement.
4. Reactive: No reactivity here. This is a congruent expression; core emotion: Fear of rejection, frozen, trapped

Exercise 3.12. Focusing on Core Emotion

1. **D.**
2. **C.**
3. **B.**

Exercise 3.13. The Role of Assembling Emotion in Shaping Experience

1. **C.**
2. **B.**
3. **A.**

Exercise 3.14. Tracking and Assembling Elements of Emotion

1. **Hurt:** the complexity of sadness/despair, anger, and fear of loss.

2. **Cue:** He refuses to comfort her.

   Initial Perception: Danger.

   Bodily Arousal: Body stiffens, face flushes, wrings hands.

   Meaning Made: I am on my own. He doesn't care.

   Action Tendency: Turns away, sighs.

   Assembly: *When Jack says he doesn't want to comfort you (the cue), your back stiffens, and you begin to wring your hands. His comment must be so difficult to hear—perhaps to you it says he doesn't care—that you are on your own in this relationship, and so you simply turn away—as if there is no hope of mattering to him. Is that it?*

3. Anger. A validation: "Of course you are angry if Jane is critical of you, and you are hurting from her recent affairs."

   The attachment threat is that Jane turns away to other affair partners, and when Marcy pushes for a response, Jane calls her demanding. The threat to Marcy is that Jane is abandoning her.

4. Cue: Jane's criticism and labeling her as "difficult and demanding."

   Basic Perception/Initial appraisal of Safety or Danger: Danger

   Bodily Arousal: Becomes still and tightens up.

   Meaning Making: I am being attacked. Jane is scapegoating me. I am flawed, and it's my fault.

   Action Tendency or Impulse: Attacks in self-protection

Exercise 3.15. Reflecting Surface Emotions in the Context of the Distressed Cycle

1. Reactive Emotion: Anger

   Brief reflection of reactive emotion in context of the cycle: "You're saying at some point in this, he gets angry and raises his voice toward you, pushing for an answer. But you don't have one, which sounds really upsetting and frustrating. In turn, you get angry with him and get right back into his face, too, with your own anger. Is that how the cycle goes?

2. Reactive Emotion: Numbness, nonchalance

   Brief reflection of reactive emotion in context of the cycle: You hear Lara's accusations, and you take it to mean she just doesn't care about you. To cope with how much it could hurt, you shrug it off and act like it doesn't bother you a bit.

3. Brief reflection of reactive emotion in context of the cycle: You hear Jake's irritable voice. Inside you get tense, and you fear you will not measure up to his demands. The harder you try to please him, the more frustrated he gets. This continues for a while, until you go cold, and shut down and walk off alone.

4. C.

Exercise 3.16. Practicing Validation

a. "It makes sense that you wonder what is going on and worry when you don't know where he is, and of course a call from him would make a difference at those times!"

b. "Yes, that is tough. You are working so hard to earn her trust, and it makes sense that you see her request for a phone call as a sign that trust is not building in the relationship."
c. "You are so afraid of where this is leading. You fear you've already lost Sara. You'd hoped if you just tried harder, you'd get her to trust you again, but you are terrified that you've ruined your relationship beyond repair!"
d. "Right, Sara, you cannot simply turn on the trust, and when you hear Leo's fear, you are doubtful, and you back away. And Leo, you hear her pulling back and doubting, and if she is going for safety, you are, too. You sense her pulling away, and you pull back, too—it's too risky, fearing there is little hope for you to regain her trust. She fears and pulls back, and you see this, and you pull back too."
e. "So, when conflicts come up, you see things he could do differently. But when he responds defensively, you try to let him know what his 'mistakes' are and how to he can improve. You learned with your family how to make your point with sharp words, and when you run into clashes with your son and want so desperately to help him, you find that the more defensive he gets, the louder you get, until he walks away from you."

Exercise 3.17. Evocative Responses that Expand a Client's Experience

1. "So, what is happening for you as you talk about this? It's like your face is full of emotion."
2. "So, you're angry, but there also tears—and what do these tears say?"
3. "What happens for you Jane when you see that look on Stephanie's face?"
4. "And Stephanie, what is happening for you when you hear Jane talk about this fight?"

Exercise 3.18. Forming Evocative Responses

1. "So, this feeling of sickness, is it more like fear, or hurt—maybe something else?"
2. "What happens inside of you when you are so exhausted from this argument that you have to lay down?"
3. "Sheri, what's it like for you to hear Paul talk about leaving?"
4. "So, you could count on your grandfather's support and care. What do you think he would say to you now about these fears in your relationship with Karen?"

Exercise 3.19. Images or Metaphors to Heighten

1. "So, it is like he locks you out. Closes the door, and you don't have the key."
2. "It's like you have lost your voice in this relationship. You speak, but he does not hear."
3. "It's frustrating and maddening to try so hard but not get through. You seem to end up in the same place you started from."
4. "So, you found something that you thought you lost. Like it might never come back, and it's almost like it means even more to you because it seemed like it was gone."

Exercise 3.20. Heightening Client Experiences

1. **C.**
2. **B.**
3. **C.**

Exercise 3.21. Heightening by Reflecting and Tracking

1. "So, when you pull away you're afraid that you won't be loved, that you are not good enough, not worthy, you will be rejected. That Joe will say, 'You just don't measure up.'"
2. "That's amazing. Describing this safety and security brings tears to your eyes. It's been such a long time since you felt this—like cool water after days wandering in the desert."
3. "Lucinda, it's like you hide your fears of disappointing your son—You hide behind this wall of positivity and kindness—trying to meet every one of his demands, when inside you fear you are not the mother he wants."
4. "It's like work is your castle. You feel strong and competent, and when Chris comes around and those feelings of insecurity grow, not feeling good enough, wondering if he really loves you as you are, you run. Run for safety."

Exercise 3.22. Practicing a Disquisition

"It's hard for you, Ted, to see this change and believe it. It's what you have been hoping for, but it's somehow hard to believe it's real. I know for some of the couples I have worked with, this is one of the toughest steps. It's like a person takes all these risks coming to therapy and opening up, and then they find there are even more risks, like believing that your partner has changed, that the words someone has wanted to hear are really true. And it is also hard for some people because they are still angry with all the hurt of the past, and this change does not wipe it all away. I've experienced this distrust with other couples – mistrusting the change and fearing that there is now an expectation that, "Since my partner has changed, I'm supposed to change, too." It's difficult, and it's scary for many partners to know what to do with all this change. I am not sure what it's like for you, because your situation may be different?"

Exercise 3.23. Selecting Empathic Conjectures

1. **C.**
2. **D.**
3. **C.**

Exercise 3.24. Catching Bullets

1. Claudia, when you mother begins to talk about how much she let you down as a child and begins to show some remorse and empathy for how hard that was for you, it's almost like you step in quickly to stop her. I imagine it is hard to

listen to her when it triggers deep pain and fear that she wants you to forgive her immediately? That just feels too hard to do at this point, am I getting it?

2. Mary, it sounds like when Darnell shrugged his shoulders, just as you began to talk about that painful event, you got that frantic sense again that you can't find him when you need him. You get so desperate for him to respond to you and be with you, that you turn the volume up to get him on board with you, is that it?

TASK 3. RESTRUCTURING INTERACTIONS

Exercise 3.25. Tracking and Reflecting the Unfolding of Emotional Experience

1. "When Nick came went straight to his office and didn't offer to help with your son's homework, a danger bell went off in you, yes?"
2. "Nora, you're saying you don't kiss him, you don't think there is any way to connect with him, so you give up."
3. "Nora, you see that he walks by without saying anything and your sense is that he isn't involved, and you get angry because it feels like you can't count on him."
4. "Nora, you feel that Nick isn't there for you—that you are alone and unimportant to him, so you've stopped reaching out. You give him some harsh looks, but mostly you pull away."
5. "So, Nora, you are saying, 'I don't see you, can't count on you. I'm alone. You are gone. And you sink in despair and resentment?"
6. Nora, underneath you are feeling all alone. You feel almost a panic that you've lost Nick—that you are no longer important to him, and you sink in fear and sadness at this loss, yes?"

Exercise 3.26. Reframing Critical Pursuit as "Urgency for a Response"

"You have these 'sore places' from the tragic, unjust loss of your first husband. You want to be able to trust again but it's so hard. When John is quiet, you can't bear the longing and being uncertain about whether you're important to him, so you get angry and fight to get a response, or you go silent to protect yourself."

Exercise 3.27. Reframing Isolation as Seeking Protection

You keep to yourself for now (implies it may not be forever, but validates it makes sense in the moment) because you don't know anyone just now who is safe to reach out to, at this time. Keeping to yourself seems like the safest way to live just now. You have been hurt by so many other people that you are afraid to trust anyone! I also hear that you do long to find some friends that you could potentially trust. You hope eventually to be able to distinguish hurtful others from some potentially safe others.

Exercise 3.28. Painting a Picture of Safe Attachment in EFFT

Therapist begins talking to the mother: It is difficult to picture a family where you trust Ahmed to make wise decisions, to come to you when he needs you and to also make some decisions on his own. And Ahmed, it is hard to picture a family where you feel it is safe to come and ask your mom for support when your friends are harassing you and letting you down.

Exercise 3.29. Tango Move 1—Reflection of the Present Process

The pattern: Jade complains about Beau's distance from them and pushes to get Beau's attention; Beau pleads to have their efforts noticed and flips into frustration for not getting credit.

The emotional experience: Both are apparently feeling frustrated, unheard, unappreciated, and alone.

Exercise 3.30. Identifying Elements of Emotion in Tango Move 2 Assembly

cue/trigger, action tendency, meanings, bodily arousal, core attachment emotion, action tendency

Exercise 3.31. Validation in Tango Move 2 to Link Elements of Emotion

It makes sense Beau that the more unhappy Jade is about not being able to find you when they need you, the more you hear you are failing to get their approval and the more frustrated you get and lash out at Jade for being unhappy with you.

Exercise 3.32. Using Evocative Questions to Assemble and Link Elements of Emotion

1. "Where in your body do you get that 'Oh-oh sense'?"
2. After Beau responds, the therapist asks, "What does that stiffened back (or knotted gut or whatever bodily arousal Beau identified) say?"
3. You hear Jade say they couldn't even get you to look at them last night (cue), a danger bell rings, "Oh, oh, this isn't good!" (immediate sense of attachment threat) You startle, and your back stiffens (bodily arousal), and inside you say to yourself, "See—I can never satisfy Jade—cannot make then happy no matter how hard I try!" (meaning making), and then you get frustrated and begin to explain that you already do a lot and you plead with Jade to give you some credit (action impulse).

Exercise 3.33. Heightening in Tango Move 2 With RISSSC

"Your stomach drops with dread—deep inside your stomach, before you get frustrated or fire back, is that heavy dread that you cannot make it with Jade—fear that maybe you will never make Jade happy! (This is the typical withdrawer's attachment fear of rejection.)

Exercise 3.34. Deepening in Tango Move 2 With Empathic Conjecture

"It sounds like you live in fear—that you are on guard for Jade's rejection, dissatisfaction? You don't talk about it—instead you try and try to please Jade and then fire back when what you do is not enough. I imagine your fear of failing to make Jade happy could be a fear that if Jade he is not happy you could lose this most important person? Is that it? Like that sickening slur from your drunken father who called you too lazy for anyone to love?"

Exercise 3.35. Shaping the Message for an Encounter

T: Can you turn to Jade and let Jade see this—Can you tell them, "It's true I do fire back at you with explanations and frustrated pleas—when inside my stomach is sinking with dread that I can never make you happy—never be someone you are happy with"?

Exercise 3.36. Anticipating the Encounter

T: Jade—are you willing to listen to Beau share with you about their explanations and pleas being code for this dread on the inside that they can never make you happy?

Exercise 3.37. Refocusing the Experiencing Partner and Directing the Encounter

Can you go back to that sinking stomach feeling, Beau? (B: Sure can!) And can you turn and tell Jade that inside when your stomach is sinking with dread that you can never be someone that they are happy with, that you don't share that—instead you fire back with explanations and pleas?

Exercise 3.38. Catching a Bullet While Processing an Encounter

T: Yes, Jade, of course you are so tired of these explanations that you almost want to shut Beau down, yes? It's very difficult to believe Beau's fear of losing you, under all their pleas and explanations, yes?

Exercise 3.39. Evocative Question to Elicit Jade's Inner Experience—Processing the Encounter

T: Jade, how was it to hear Beau acknowledge that indeed under this fear of losing you if they don't make you happy, that they do fire up at you in defense and explanations? What happened inside for you?

Exercise 3.40. Summary Statement to Integrate the Work of the Session

You have done amazing work together today, guys! Together you have been able to make sense of the pattern you get caught in over and over again—leaving you, Jade, feeling alone and afraid that Beau just doesn't care or hear you. And leaving you, Beau, quaking in fear that Jade is fed up with you and is about to tur away from you! Jade, you were able to let Beau know that under your loud protests and critical anger, you are really just trying to get a response. And Beau, you were able to let Jade know that when you shrug or fire up in defense, you are really terrified you have already lost Jade! Together you created a clear picture of your cycle: The more Jade pushes for response, the more Beau hears discontent, and the more Beau disappears or fires up in defense. The more Beau disappears and defends, the more Jade pushes and demands, leaving you both alone and in fear.

Exercise 3.41. Review of EFT Tango Moves

1. **B**
2. **C**
3. **A**
4. **C**
5. **B**

SECTION II

EFT AND THE COUPLE TREATMENT PROCESS

4

STAGE 1: ALLIANCE, ASSESSMENT, AND CYCLES

This chapter reviews the first tasks undertaken by the EFT therapist in joining with a couple and assessing their relationship, which encompasses the initial steps of the EFT process. The focus of the EFT therapist is on gaining an understanding of each client's emotional experience of their partner and of their relationship. As the intake session progresses, the therapist tracks and delineates the negative interactive cycle that traps and disconnects the couple. The therapist then reflects the cycle, validates the emotions stirred up by the cycle, and frames it as the source of the couple's distress and deprivation. EFT therapists assume that therapy starts from the first meeting and that assessment is an ongoing process throughout the therapy process. The initial focus of the EFT therapist can be summarized in the following two steps.

EFT STEPS: Stage 1, De-escalation and Relationship Stabilization

1. Create an alliance and delineate conflict issues in the core attachment struggle.
2. Identify the negative interactional cycle where these issues are expressed.

A good first EFT session consists of a compelling and intimate conversation between a warm, empathic therapist and a couple who may begin as nervous or even skeptical. As the session progresses, the couple usually begin to feel safe enough to take the risk of sharing private fears, doubts, and hurts. If things go well, the therapist can help them discover that their negative reactions to each other, while understandable given their individual experiences, trap them in a compelling cycle that leads to conflict and distance. The couple leaves the session feeling understood and hopeful that they have found somebody who can help their relationship.

OVERVIEW OF EFT ASSESSMENT (STEPS 1 AND 2)

To an observer watching an EFT initial assessment session, the therapist's work may seem effortless. However, the therapist is very clear about what needs to be accomplished and how it will be done.

- The therapist's first objective is to connect with both partners, building an alliance with the couple in which each partner feels safe, accepted, and understood

DOI: 10.4324/9781003039457-6

by the therapist. The therapist is empathically attuned to the clients and takes a collaborative, accepting, and genuine stance with the couple.

- Using the therapeutic skills of reflection, validation, evocative responding, and some reframing, the therapist listens to their story, trying to understand how their relationship evolved and why they sought out therapy at this time.
- The therapist also assesses the clients' background and attachment history and begins to form hypotheses regarding vulnerabilities and attachment issues underlying each partner's position in the relationship. The therapist looks for blocks to secure attachment and emotional engagement within and between partners.
- As the couple's story unfolds, the therapist begins to enter the experience of each partner, discovering how each constructs his or her experience of this relationship. The therapist watches for specific focus points or areas of difficulty and intervenes as they occur.
- The therapist tracks and discovers with the couple the typical and recurring sequences of interaction that perpetuate their distress (i.e., the cycle, dance, or pattern). This is done with curiosity and acceptance of their perspectives.
- The therapist also assesses the couple's responsiveness to each other and to the EFT interventions by asking them to interact or by touching on core primary emotions. The therapist also notes the strengths and positive elements in the relationship.
- As the session continues, the therapist assesses the nature of the problem and the relationship, including its suitability for couple therapy in general and for EFT in particular. This includes understanding the goals and agenda of each partner to ascertain whether these goals are feasible and compatible not only in terms of the partners' individual agendas but also with the therapist's own ethical considerations and expertise.
- The therapist then creates a therapeutic agreement between the couple and the therapist, a consensus of therapeutic goals and how therapy will be conducted.

We now introduce you to a couple, named Inez and Fernando. Excerpts of their therapy transcripts are used throughout this book to illustrate how their therapist, Jane, navigates the steps and stages of the EFT treatment process.

EFT SNAPSHOT: INEZ AND FERNANDO

Jane enters the waiting room to warmly greet her clients, Inez and Fernando. They are a heterosexual couple who share in their background a Spanish heritage with ancestors who emigrated to North America generations ago. Jane brings them into the office, where chairs are placed so that the couple can easily face each other and the therapist. The EFT therapist sits with the clients and not behind a desk. This way the couple can begin to feel the collaborative nature of the session, and the therapist can easily observe the clients' body language.

Inez is short and plump with salt-and-pepper, stylishly cut hair. When she smiles, dimples appear. Fernando is tall, tanned, and quite striking looking, with an abundance of white hair and brown eyes. Jane learns that the two are in their late 50s, and both are retired. For Fernando, retiring was a difficult process. Vice president of a high-tech company, he was offered a buyout package three years earlier and believed he had been forced out of the company that he had spent much of his working life building. Since retiring, he had embarked on several ambitious projects around the house but spent the majority of the time on the computer. "Not playing games," he added hastily, "but important research for the political party." Fernando previously had a long relationship with a psychiatrist, who helped him through considerable anxiety related to his work relationships and performance. He had also recently been struggling with symptoms of depression, including weight gain, sleeplessness, irritability, and lack of energy and motivation. Inez stayed out of the workforce to raise their three children. Approximately two years earlier, she was diagnosed with depression but had recently dropped out of treatment and stopped her antidepressant medication. She also currently experienced depressive symptoms, including weight gain, difficulty sleeping, and lack of motivation to do much at home. She was, however, involved in many activities outside the home, including art classes and volunteer work at a local food bank.

The couple reported that they had tried couple therapy two years earlier. Inez liked the counselor, but Fernando, who felt blamed by her, ended their sessions. Their children had all left home and were well on their way to establishing their own lives. Their sons were both married and had good jobs, and their daughter was finishing university.

The couple were prompted to try therapy for a second time because they were not getting along with each other. "In fact," said Fernando, "I can hardly bear it, the way she talks to me. She treats me so badly I feel just awful, and I just won't take it anymore." Jane asked if they could help her to understand what happened at home that resulted in Inez treating him so. Inez merely shrugged and said that she had difficulty getting herself motivated to do much around the house.

The following transcript begins after this basic information is gathered and as the therapist begins to track and understand the negative interactive cycle. You will see that the therapist interventions focus on three tasks:

1. Exploring what happens between partners, including asking questions that invite partners to describe how they relate during times of conflict. As she listens, the EFT therapist also tentatively reflects to the couple their present process, the cues partners send, and how they respond to each other in session. As the session progresses, the therapist periodically summarizes the cycle, tracking and ordering what has been learned about the negative dance between them thus far.
2. Exploring what happens within each partner to discover how they view and experience the relationship. The therapist enters the inner world of each partner, reflecting their unique perspectives, personal struggles, and feelings throughout the session. The therapist's interventions enable both partners to feel heard, understood, and accepted. Partners begin to listen to the distress each feels in the relationship.
3. Instilling hope by highlighting the couple's strengths and introducing attachment reframes when there is an opportunity to reflect partners' positive intentions or desire for connection.

The therapist begins by revisiting a recent situation as an example of the negative cycle

Inez: Look at this morning, for example. We were getting ready to come here to see you. He's throwing things round the kitchen and yelling at the dog—he kicked her, actually.

Fernando: And you come along and attack me!

Inez: I didn't. I just asked what's wrong. Maxie hadn't done anything wrong, and you kicked her.

Fernando: I didn't kick her; I pushed her out of the way with my foot. I was worried we'd be late for our appointment.

Therapist: Sounds like you get a bit worried and tense. Is that it, Fernando? (Reflecting the "worry") (tracking Fernando's emotional experience)

Fernando: Yes, I get anxious inside, and then she's in my face, you know? She wants to know exactly what's going on.

Therapist: And what's that like for you? (Goal here is to understand his experience and get a sense of the cycle.)

Fernando: I just want her to back off. Back off!

Therapist: You want her to give you some space? (reflecting; mild reframe)

Fernando: Yes.

In the following excerpt the therapist is Reflecting process with a "between focus":

Therapist: So, what happens then? (tracking cycle)

Inez: He snaps at me. (Inez looks sad; she looks down at her fingers.)

Therapist: That's hard for you, eh, Inez? (empathic reflection)

Inez: (tightens her mouth) It's always been that way. I just do my thing. I should be used to it by now.

Therapist: So, you kind of suck it up, is that right? (tracking cycle)

Fernando: No, it's not! She lays right into me. My heart goes thump, thump in my chest. I feel attacked and disrespected. It hurts. Boy, I see a side in her that I don't like to see! When she gets angry, I see an ugly woman inside. Hatred! It consumes her face. Over the last five years, she has been enraged at me.

Therapist: So, let me get this . . . a situation comes up where you feel anxious, Fernando, and you get . . . tense and edgy, and Inez, you approach him to find out what's up. That's when you try to get her to . . . to leave you alone, Fernando? And sounds like you get a bit . . . short with her, and from your perspective, that's when she gets really mad? (therapist stays with process; attempts to begin to describe cycle)

Fernando: She attacks me!

Therapist: And then you get all upset on the inside, and what do you do then? (Tracking cycle.)

Fernando: I get out of there. I go off to the computer.

Therapist: So, you go off on your own then? (Tracking cycle.)

Fernando: Yes, that's my only option.

Next the therapist Reflects, a "within focus" on Inez before reflecting the cycle again, filling in the picture more and more of what happens between them:

Therapist: That feels like that's the only thing you can do. Get out of there and go off to the computer. And so, Inez, what's that like for you? (Tracking cycle)

Inez: (sighs heavily) What else is new? What else is new? I'm on my own.

Therapist: When he leaves, then you feel like you're on your own? (Reflection of Inez's experience)

Inez: (looks down at her fingers, which are tightly woven together) That's how it always is.

Therapist: You feel on your own a lot, Inez? (Empathic question)

Inez: (nods, keeps looking down at her fingers)

Therapist: Sounds like that's hard for you, Inez, yes? Makes you feel real mad sometimes? (Empathic reflection; empathic conjecture based on Inez's body language)

Inez: (nods again and sighs)

Therapist: That's a heavy sigh, Inez. Sounds like this is really hard. Hard for you to talk about? (Reflects nonverbal; empathic question.)

Inez: (small voice) Yes. (long pause follows)

Therapist: So, it sounds to me like you are both left feeling really low after one of these things. (Both partners nod glumly.) It seems like there's a sort of pattern here that you are both getting stuck in, yes? I'm not sure exactly what triggers it, but it seems to get going when you see him scowling and uptight, is that right, Inez? That's when you go to him and try to get him to tell you what's up? To let you know what's wrong? (Attempt to delineate cycle)

Inez: (nods) Yes, I want to settle him down.

Therapist: You want to settle him down. It makes you feel uncomfortable when he . . . (Reflection; attempt to explore experience)

Inez: There's no need for it. It's ugly! Why be like that? Why not be nice to people?

Therapist: Right, for you it's difficult . . . (Attempt to enter Inez's experience)

Inez: It hurts me. It hurts me to see him in a horrible mood. Why? Why all the time?

Therapist: (softly) It hurts you when he's in a mood? (Empathic reflection, evocative responding)

Inez: (begins to tear) I feel like he hates me. He hates me, hates the dog—he hates us all.

Therapist: That must be really painful for you. To get that feeling. To feel like he hates you, Inez. (Empathic reflection, based on her tears; reflecting with a "within focus")

Inez: (nods; reaches for a Kleenex) That's when I yell at him.

Therapist: Aha I get it, hmmm . . . no wonder, if you get the feeling he hates you, yes I can understand you 'attack' him. (Validation also acceptance)

Inez: I blow up like a puffer fish. And I yell at him.

Therapist: A puffer fish! Like you get twice as big? (Reflection)

Inez: And four times as angry.

Therapist: And for you, Fernando, that's when you feel that you need to get away? (Tracking cycle)

Fernando: Well, that's ridiculous! Of course, I don't hate her. What a stupid thing to say. I just need for her to cut me some slack.

Therapist: So off you go to your computer? (Tracking cycle)

Fernando: Well, it's safe there.

Therapist: So, yes, it seems there's this pattern you get into here . . . this sort of bickering pattern where, Fernando, you get tense; Inez tries to settle you down; and you feel crowded. So, you try to get her to "back off." And, Inez, that's where you get hurt, get that awful feeling he hates you. And that's where you puff up and turn up the volume, and, Fernando, here's where you get hurt, disrespected . . . and you withdraw to the safety of the computer. Is this how it is? (Again, attempts to delineate cycle)

Inez: Yes. Anything can start it off.

Therapist: So, what happens next? (Tracking)

Inez: We each do our own thing. He's on the computer all day.

Fernando: And you do your painting all day. Or you're never there.

Therapist: Sounds like it's very lonely. How do you get close again? (Empathic conjecture; tracking)

Inez and Fernando: We don't.

Fernando: That's why we're here.

Therapist: You're here because you don't like the pattern and because you'd like to get close? (Reflection and reframe that emphasizes attachment needs)

Fernando: (nods)

Inez: (shrugs, looking down at her fingers)

Therapist: I see you shrugging, Inez. Does that fit for you? (Reflection of nonverbal communication; clarifying)

Inez: I tried for years for us to get close, and now I'm tired.

Therapist: (low, soft voice) You've been trying to be close to Fernando for a long time, and now you are tired. But you're here, Inez, so perhaps there's a part of you that is still hoping?

In this transcript, the therapist listened empathically to Fernando and Inez, trying to help each partner feel understood and accepted. As she listened to their story, she began to track and describe the sequences of interaction that perpetuate the couple's distress. She also began to enter the experience of the partners in an effort to find out how each constructed her or his experience of their relationship. The therapist flows organically between reflecting the within experience of each partner and the process that occurs between them, representing Move 1 of the EFT Tango. Jane learned that Fernando becomes anxious inside, and this generates a need for space. He then snaps at Inez, and then he feels attacked when she reacts to his snapping. Inez feels hurt and rebuffed by his snapping and responds by puffing up in anger. The couple then withdraw from each other and appear to have no way of regaining the closeness.

In a first EFT session, the therapist picks up on the emotions inherent in their story, acknowledging and validating them as you saw earlier. It is often the reactive emotions stirred by the negative cycle (e.g., anxiety, anger, discouragement) that we first encounter, and then softer hurts and fears peak through as the couple feel safer. The therapist's goal here is to meet her clients where they are at emotionally in order to build a therapeutic alliance of attachment security.

CREATING A THERAPEUTIC ALLIANCE—A SAFE HAVEN IN THERAPY

Creating a therapeutic alliance is the therapist's prime objective in the initial stage of therapy. If clients feel safe, supported, understood, and accepted by their therapist and confident in her skills, then couple sessions can provide a safe haven where partners can risk exploring both their relationship and their own primary attachment-related emotions.

Thus, the EFT therapist deliberately sets out to create a collaborative alliance with the couple, and, throughout the therapy process, continually monitors this alliance to ensure it remains intact. If the therapist believes the alliance is in any way threatened or ruptured, she will take active steps to repair it. Repair of a ruptured alliance is fully addressed in a later chapter.

Therapists can promote the therapeutic alliance by obvious actions like being on time for appointments and sitting with clients rather than behind a desk. In order to foster the alliance, the EFT therapist also takes a therapeutic stance that involves being empathically attuned. Being empathically attuned allows the therapist to be genuine and accepting of what the clients say. These aspects of the therapeutic stance are discussed next.

Empathic Attunement

Simply put, empathic attunement is the therapist's ability to tune into the client. As the client describes his or her experience, the therapist metaphorically allows herself to step across into the client's world. By doing this and by using her imagination, her personal experience, and/or her present feelings, the therapist can connect with the client's experience. The therapist can hear, for example, how a wife berates her husband for the long hours he works and the weeks he spends away on business and "feel into" her attachment experience of loneliness even before the client can voice this herself.

Empathic attunement permits the therapist to "be with" the client in a way that engenders a sense of "feeling connectedness, of being in attunement with another. It feels like an unbroken line" (Stern, 1985; p. 157). An empathically attuned therapist creates with the client a shared experience whereby the therapist mirrors and echoes the client. By tracking and attuning to emotion, the therapist signals to the client, by use of verbal and nonverbal responses, the important messages provided in Table 4.1.

Table 4.1
Therapist Response and Impact

Nonverbal: Therapist Does	Verbal: Therapist Says	Impact on Client
Makes eye contact, nods, leans forward, has an open posture	I hear you; I am with you. Says "hmm" and "aha" to indicate attention.	Reassured: "My feelings actually make sense to this person."
Echoes or mirrors the client's affect. The therapist looks concerned when the client is sad and laughs when the client laughs.	I hear you; I am with you. Joins with the client using the client's words and images.	Comforted: The client can maintain a working distance from the emotion and not become overwhelmed.
Offers a tissue when the client weeps	I support you.	Safer: Reduced need to defend against difficult emotions as they are accessed.
Open and receptive stance	I am not judging you.	Open: Explores his or her own experience more deeply.

Example: Empathic Attunement

Let's take another look at Jane's session with Fernando and Inez.

Fernando: I just want her to back off. Back off!

Therapist: You want her to give you some space?

Fernando: Yes.

Therapist: So, what happens then?

Inez: He snaps at me. (Inez looks sad; she looks down at her fingers.)

Therapist: That's hard for you, eh, Inez?

Inez: (tightens her mouth) It's always been that way. I just do my thing. I should be used to it by now.

This is an example of Jane being empathically attuned to Inez. Jane puts together the harshness of Fernando's tone as he says, "Back off" and the sad look on Inez's face as well as the tightening of her mouth as Inez looks down at her fingers. If Jane's partner snapped at her, it would certainly be painful for her. It might also make her angry. Jane's response to Inez stems from her awareness of all these factors and her ability to step across into Inez's world to connect with her experience.

In this small excerpt, the therapist might equally well have stayed "in tune with" Fernando's experience and explored his need to have his wife "back off."

Exercise 4.1. Attuning Empathically

Imagine that Jane caught a glimpse of Fernando's eyes widening in panic just a split second before his response of flash anger. Using your own life experiences, imagine the kinds of fears Fernando might have about a loved one seeing his vulnerability. See if you can come up with a response to Fernando that would be empathically attuned to his window of tolerance.

____

____

____

Acceptance

The therapeutic stance of acceptance means the therapist does not judge the way a client responds but rather understands responses in light of the client's experience. Notice that the previous example is also an example of the therapist's simply accepting Fernando's need for space rather than frowning on the response. The therapist might then move into exploring and understanding his need for space. In the following example, the therapist accepts—and even validates—an angry response from Inez by understanding her response in the context of her experience.

Inez: (nods; reaches for a tissue) That's when I yell at him.

Therapist: Aha, I get it, hmmm . . . no wonder, if you get the feeling he hates you, yes, I can understand you "attacking" him.

Exercise 4.2. Extending Acceptance

As the therapist tracks the cycle, she says to Fernando:

Therapist: So, you go off on your own, then?

Fernando: Yes, that is my only option.

Write a therapist response that best demonstrates acceptance:

____

____

____

Genuineness

As the therapist steps into the client's world, she is genuine in her reactions to what she hears from the clients. She is available for a real human encounter with the clients. When clients perceive the therapist as accessible, engaged, and responsive in a very genuine way, they are more able to relax into the therapeutic alliance and trust the therapeutic process. The EFT therapist will try to answer frankly and honestly within her own comfort zone any questions the clients may ask her, including about her own life. If a client is confrontational with the therapist, the therapist will endeavor to understand the interaction between them, including her own part in what led to this response. Here, the therapist mistakenly refers to the couple's oldest child as Sarah. Fernando curtly reminds her that Sarah is their youngest child.

Fernando: (sharply to therapist) Were you not listening?

Therapist: Sorry, Fernando, yes, I was confused there.

At the end of the session, Fernando turns to Jane and asks her if she ever fights with her husband.

Exercise 4.3. Expressing Genuineness

Reflect for a moment about your own internal reaction to Fernando's question. What concerns do you have about how to respond to this question? Let yourself be curious about what concerns or fears Fernando might have that are reflected in his question. Write a response that strikes a balance between therapeutic genuineness and offering reassurance.

____

____

____

Exercise 4.4. Reviewing Alliance Formation

1. The prime objective of Steps 1 and 2 is
   a. To identify the negative interactive cycle. ____
   b. To discover the attachment style of each partner. ____
   c. To create a therapeutic alliance with each partner. ____
   d. To take a relationship history. ____
2. Which of the following is not necessary to develop the therapeutic alliance?
   a. Making eye contact ____
   b. Mirroring and echoing the client ____
   c. Accurate empathic reflections ____
   d. Going over time in the sessions ____

Exercise 4.5. Practicing Empathic Attunement

Now consider the case of Gerald and Barbara, who have the following exchange in their initial session:

Gerald: We seem to be getting on just fine, and then suddenly we're not. Barbara launches into a tirade. It comes right out of the blue! She ambushes me! Before we know where we are, she's telling me she wants a divorce. Me—I'm like a turtle. I withdraw into my shell where no one can hurt me. . . . (a tear begins to trickle down his cheek) We haven't even had a hug in years.

Barbara: We aren't getting on fine! You come home every night and switch on the TV, and there you stay for the night. You never even see me. I don't exist for you. That's why we never hug. I'm too busy sucking up my anger. I suck it up and suck it up, and then I can't take it anymore—I blow!

1. Which response is not an example of empathic attunement to Gerald?
   a. "It sounds like it's all very confusing for you. One minute things are fine, and the next minute there's the threat of divorce." ____
   b. "So how do you get out of the shell?" ____
   c. "Right! You withdraw into your shell, where it's safe." ____
   d. "It seems like it's safe in that shell but terribly lonely." ____
2. Which response is not an example of empathic attunement to Barbara?
   a. "That must be painful, to feel like you don't even exist for him." ____
   b. "You're feeling continually so far away from him that hugs are out of the question." ____
   c. "Can you talk about your anger with him?" ____
   d. "I can understand why you blow now and then if you're always sucking up your anger." ____
3. Try to step across into Gerald's world. What do you guess is his experience? Pick the answer that best captures his probable experience.
   a. Angry, irritated, and distant ____
   b. Lonely, puzzled, sad, and possibly angry ____
   c. Attacked, defensive, and angry ____
   d. Stonewalling and blaming ____
4. Now try to step across into Barbara's world. What is her experience? Pick the answer that best captures her probable experience.
   a. Angry, irritated, and disengaged ____
   b. Lonely, puzzled, sad, and possibly angry ____
   c. Attacked, defensive, and angry ____
   d. Angry, hurt, and rejected ____
5. Write your own empathic response that signals to Gerald that you have understood him.

____

____

____

6. Write your own empathic response that signals to Barbara that you also understand her.

____

____

____

THERAPY SKILLS USED IN ASSESSMENT

In this section, the EFT skills most frequently used are described and exercises are provided for practice. The skills we will discuss include reflection, validation, reframing, and "catching the bullet."

Reflection

Beginning EFT therapists are often surprised at how much reflection is used in EFT, particularly in the early stages of the process. Reflection of internal and interpersonal responses is the predominant micro-intervention in the first move of the Tango, creating focus in the session. It helps the partners tune into their emotional world (within) and begin to notice how their behaviors pull each other into negative interactions (between). As in other therapeutic approaches, the clients' words are reflected, especially in the beginning of the session. Reflection of content signifies to the client that the therapist is listening and grasping what they are trying to convey. It also helps clarify the therapist's own understanding of the content presented.

In the initial session of EFT, the therapist also reflects the client's experience, surface or reactive emotions, and core (primary) emotions. (In some cases, especially in first sessions, core primary emotions can only be guessed at. Some clients may not be aware of their core emotions or may not be ready to acknowledge them). The therapist may also reflect incongruence between a client's verbal and nonverbal communication to bring clarity to mixed signals being sent. Finally, the therapist may reflect and comment on interactions between partners (e.g., a significant look is exchanged, or one partner may reach to comfort the other).

Reflecting Client's Experience

Reflecting a client's experience slows the pace of the session and helps the therapist to keep the focus on the clients' experience of their relationship. Such reflections can open a gateway to exploring and deepening the experience. A good reflection can better organize and anchor the client's experience so that he or she can tune in on a deeper level. For example, Fernando describes the process whereby he lost his job and finishes his description with the following exchange:

Fernando: Finally, I had no choice, and I accepted a buyout package. But it was rough—I was one of the main founders of that company.

Therapist: Sounds like retirement was an extremely painful experience for you, Fernando.

Fernando: (looks pained and upset) Yes, yes, it was a hard time. I felt so pushed out, like I was no longer any use.

This led the therapist into further exploring his experience around losing his job and asking if he had shared these feelings with Inez. The question links an individual experience of loss (within) to the relational experience of confiding (between), assessing how much partners use each other as a resource for support.

Exercise 4.6. Reflecting Client Experience

Now using the following example,

Emily: Charles was having a crisis at work when I had my surgery, and he wasn't there for me at all.

Write a therapist response that simply reflects Emily's experience

____.

Reflecting Nonverbal Communication

The therapist should also notice and reflect clients' nonverbal communication. These may include signs of strong affect (e.g., weeping, reaching for tissues, eyes becoming red, looking down at hands, flushing, clenching fists) or of efforts to dispel feelings (e.g., swallowing hard, looking away, biting lips). Alternatively, one client may give the other a hostile look, or roll her or his eyes, or reach to comfort the other. The therapist may choose to note these nonverbals internally, or depending on the therapist's sense of the developing alliance and of the client's willingness to respond, she may choose to reflect them to the client. Now consider the following exchange between Fernando and Inez:

Inez: (sighs heavily) What else is new? What else is new? I'm on my own.

Therapist: When he leaves, then you feel like you're on your own?

In this example, the therapist reflected Inez's experience (e.g., saying I am on my own, when he leaves). She might equally well have reflected Inez's nonverbal communication as follows:

Inez: (sighs heavily) What else is new? What else is new? I'm on my own.

Therapist: You give a heavy sigh there, Inez, as you say, "I'm on my own."

Exercise 4.7. Reflecting Nonverbal Experience

Review the following example of a therapist reflecting Emily's experience.

Therapist: That must have been a difficult time for you.

Emily: (long pause; Emily tears, and then reaches for a tissue)

Now write a therapist response below that best illustrates reflecting nonverbal communication:

____

Reflecting Incongruence in Verbal and Nonverbal Communication

Reflecting incongruence between what is said verbally and what is said nonverbally can be done very respectfully and gently.

Therapist: Yes, Fernando, I hear you say that this doesn't bother you when it happens, but I also see tears when I look into your eyes, and that gives me the impression that at one level, you might get quite upset by this?

Exercise 4.8. Reflecting Incongruence

Write a response that reflects the incongruence between what Charles says and what the therapist observes and then invites the possibility of underlying pain or hurt when: Charles grins as he says: *Yes, she's been mad at me for a long time.*

Validation

Validation is used extensively in EFT assessment. The therapist's goal is to affirm the client's experience, to convey to each partner that his or her emotions and responses are legitimate and understandable in the context of their experience. The experience of being validated is profound for many clients who have not been explicitly validated throughout their lives in their most important relationships. It helps clients feel deeply understood and thus helps to build safety in the therapeutic alliance. Equally important, when the clients feel validated, they can risk saying more about their experience. Further, validation helps clients to feel entitled to their feelings, and as their feelings and responses are validated and normalized by an emotionally attuned therapist, clients are better able to regulate feelings of shame and self-judgment.

Validating the Client's Experience

The therapist may use validation to respond to a client's description of past experience or their present here-and-now experience in the session. This includes reactive (or surface) emotion, which usually involves either anger or denial of any feelings. The therapist always places emotions in the context of the client's experience (the cycle and attachment significance) and validates it.

Sonia: Trouble is, he won't speak to me for days after we fight.

Therapist: And what's that like for you?

Sonia: I feel . . . it makes me feel desperate, afraid. It's like I feel, well—that's it, you know? It's over.

Therapist: So, after one of these fights, then, for you, it's like you lose him. And you feel desperate, afraid that he's gone forever? (empathic reflection)

Sonia: (begins to cry) Yes, I feel certain he won't ever speak to me again. I must be such a baby to get so scared.

Therapist: Well, I can easily understand how afraid you get. He's very precious to you, right? (affirms and legitimizes her experience; places it in an attachment context)

Exercise 4.9. Validation

Write a validation statement for Julia's experience when she says:

Julia: Things are so tense when he comes home from work. The kids stop playing—God! Even the dog hides under the chesterfield sometimes! He's just really grumpy, and anything sets him off. It makes me feel very nervous.

Now feel into the emotion in Julia's words and then write a therapist response that best validates Julia's experience.

The therapist takes care that her validation of one client does not invalidate or alienate the other. This is especially so when the couple appeal to the therapist for her perspective on their story. (At these times, it is far safer to comment on their process than on the content they are describing.) See the following example with Jack and Frank.

Jack: Take this morning. He was beating an egg, and he spilt it on the counter. He just went for me . . . screaming, yelling, like, anyone would think I spilled the damn egg, not him! I felt completely attacked and beaten up.

Frank: What did I yell? What did I yell? I yelled that an egg only costs 10 cents and it's not worth YOU starting World War III over it like you usually do. There's your answer!

Therapist: So, I get from your perspective, Jack, it feels like he gets on the offensive easily, and you feel beaten up on, and that's really hard for you. And on your side, Frank, I can also get there is history between you both that leaves you feeling the best defense is a good offense.

Exercise 4.10. Validation With Care

Now consider your new couple are very angry with each other as they discuss their finances. Marjorie is adamant that she should take over the budget and pay the bills so she can have some role in the family finances. Brian insists he's doing a good job and she needs to back off.

Brian: I'm doing it fine! You're out of line! You're always trying to get in there and correct me and do it better. It's infuriating!

Marjorie: Well, then, we're at an impasse. I'm sick of not being part of this. We're not a partnership, and I'm not going to let myself be treated like that anymore.

Imagine the message each partner is getting in this argument and use it to validate each of their positions.

Reframing

A strong foundation in attachment theory enables the EFT therapist to see her clients' longings that are veiled by the negative behaviors in their cycle. As with any intervention, EFT therapists tailor their reframes to fit their clients' sensibilities, self-awareness, and stage in therapy, including their alliance with the therapist. Thus, in initial sessions, reframes may be just one step beyond their own words. As therapy moves along, the therapist uses her understanding of the intrapsychic issues that the partners are struggling with (e.g., fear of conflict, a need to protect the self from the other, a longing for closeness) to craft reframes that touch more deeply on their core attachment needs. Refer to Chapter 3 for common examples of reframes for withdrawing and pursuing behaviors. Now consider how the EFT therapist might reframe Angela's response.

Angela: Too right. I'm angry. He spent last weekend fishing with his buddies and then stayed at the bar three nights last week. Once again, I'm on my own. Anyone would give him hell when he got home.

Two possible attachment reframes:

Therapist: Right. For you it's about wanting time with him, and giving him hell is about letting him know you want to be important to him, too.

Therapist: Right. When you don't get enough time with him, you protest loudly because you really miss him and feel incredibly lonely.

The following examples illustrate how the EFT therapist might respond to a partner's defensive avoidance:

Frances: I don't know what Ingrid wants. I just hear that everything I try to do for her is not enough. She complains constantly, and there's nothing I can do to change it. So, yes, I do get irritated and would rather walk out of the room than stay there, making things worse.

Possible attachment reframes:

Therapist: It upsets you to get the message that what you do for Ingrid isn't enough, so you try to shut down and exit the conversation rather than getting into an argument.

Therapist: I see that you are always getting the message that you are disappointing to Ingrid. It hurts so much that you just have to protect yourself from that pain and fear of making things worse.

Exercise 4.11. Reframing and Attachment Themes

Now feel into the attachment longings inherent in Kevin's statement listed next. Write two reframes, one that is lighter for early Stage 1 and a second reframe that taps into more core attachment experiences for deeper into Stage 1 work.

Kevin: We were at the meeting, and I was so proud to be with her. Her speech was awesome. And then at coffee time, she completely ignored me. I thought, "What am I? Chopped liver?" I was livid! Yes, I know I went for her on the way home.

____

____

Catching the Bullet

At the beginning of the initial session, the therapist may notice that spouses direct hurtful comments at the other. As the session progresses, the therapist gains some understanding of these comments and where they originate. She will interrupt such comments and bypass the aggression, focusing instead on the underlying pain. By "catching the bullet," the therapist takes the sting out of the comments and helps to create safety in the session. Consider the following example:

Husband: (angrily to wife) Why don't you just call your lawyer and get the divorce rolling—you're always threatening it anyway.

Therapist: I think what I am hearing from you right now is that it's too painful for you. It's so painful and difficult for you to hear her criticizing, that some part of you moves to shut her down and end it.

Exercise 4.12. Catch the Bullet

You are the therapist in a session in which a woman describes how her partner didn't understand her sadness following her third miscarriage. Her husband's response is swift and angry.

Husband: If I had a dollar for every time you weren't there for me, I'd be a rich man.

Reflect inside for a moment about your own response to this man's harsh reaction at the moment of his partner's vulnerability. Can you notice your internal responses (anger, impatience, confusion, protectiveness toward her) and also make room for curiosity about what might be behind his sharp reaction? Write a response that "catches the bullet" and speaks to the pain that most likely underlies this behavior.

____

____

____

Exercise 4.13. Assessing a Couple's Reactive Responses

As the initial session unfolds, you learn that Aaron's first wife Rachael was killed in an automobile accident. Aaron's relationship with his former mother-in-law, Ruth, is now the subject of many of Aaron and Sarah's fights. As the couple discuss Aaron's recent lunch engagement with Ruth, you hear the rage in Sarah's voice as she attacks her husband.

Aaron: This is all in the past. I only wanted to honor Rachael's mother for what we had together and what we all lost.

Sarah: You say it's in the past, but it isn't. Even last night you defended Ruth! You said, "Let's agree to disagree." Are you for her or for me?

Aaron: (weeping) My caring for Ruth is different. Actually, sometimes I don't even like her very much. But she's the mother of my first wife and the grandmother of my son. I just never wanted to ride roughshod over her feelings.

Sarah: There it is again! You care for her feelings—you ride over mine. Who is in your heart? Her or me?

1. What is Sarah's reactive (surface) emotion?
   a. Anger ____
   b. Loneliness ____
   c. Numb denial ____
   d. Fear ____
2. The therapist says: "Sounds like it's really hard for you, Sarah, that he maintains ties with Ruth?" This therapist response in an example of
   a. Reframing. ____
   b. Reflection. ____
   c. Catching the bullet. ____
   d. Validation. ____
3. The following exchange then occurs between the therapist and Sarah:

   Sarah: Yes, of course it's hard for me.

   Therapist: Can you help me to understand, Sarah, what it means for you when Aaron spends time with Ruth?

   In this exchange, the therapist is trying to
   a. Validate Sarah. ____
   b. Understand Sarah's experience. ____
   c. Reframe her anger. ____
   d. Catch the bullet. ____
4. Write a statement that validates each partner without invalidating the other.

   ____

   ____

   ____

KEY FOCUS POINTS IN THE ASSESSMENT PROCESS

As the couple's story unfolds, the EFT therapist is trying to understand each client's experience of their partner and of their relationship. How does each partner construct their reality in this relationship? How do they perceive themselves in relation to their partner? How do they process their experience of their partner? What does their partner's reaction or behavior mean to them? The therapist works to familiarize herself with the process within each partner and between the couple in front of her (Tango Move 1). She enters the experience of each partner: How does each construct their experience of this relationship and regulate their emotions? Inez feels that Fernando is often mean and snappy. This makes her angry, and she yells at him, at which point he withdraws to his computer. She believes that he dislikes—even hates—her: "Why else would someone treat me like this?" Jane, the therapist, asks Inez: "What's that like for you, Inez?" The question elicits the response that with Fernando, she feels "on her own." This is a glimpse into her experience of this relationship.

Here are some questions that help you to explore the client's experience:

- "So what's that like for you?"
- "How do you feel about that?"
- "What does that mean for you?"
- "What happens for you when . . . ?"
- "Can you help me to understand how it is for you when . . . ?"

The therapist reflects and acknowledges the emotional experience of each client. As the session progresses, the therapist begins to discover and differentiate surface or reactive emotions from more primary, core emotions. Reactive emotions are made explicit in the here and now and then placed in the context of the problematic pattern and validated (e.g., the anger and the attack from Inez as she feels pushed away and unimportant to her husband). Core emotions may or may not be discovered in the first session because often clients are not as aware of them at the beginning of therapy. It can take several sessions to fully assemble and deepen the emotions stirred up in the negative cycle. With Fernando and Inez, the therapist was able to see in the session when Inez did not acknowledge core emotion (perhaps sad, lonely, rejected, unimportant) but instead "puffed up" into anger, her reactive emotion.

How does the therapist know what to focus on and how and when to intervene? The EFT therapist watches for the following focus points that signal what to notice and when to intervene.

Focusing on the Impact of Strong Affect

As one partner tells his or her story, the narrative is interrupted by a strong emotional response. When a client is experiencing strong affect, the therapist sees signs such as crying, flushing red, biting one's lip, turning away, or perhaps clenching the fists. The client is usually unable to continue speaking. Consider this example:

> *Maria tells the therapist that if she tries to share problems and difficulties with Tony, he seems angry and withdraws from her. "I feel so . . . so. . . . " She stops speaking because she is flooded with strong emotion.*

The EFT therapist zooms in on this response, giving the message that it is safe and appropriate to share this experience in the session. The therapist says gently to Maria: "I can see this is hard to say, Maria. Take your time; it's okay." Maria reaches for a tissue, and the therapist helps her to talk about her hurt and her sadness.

Focusing on Limited Affect

Sometimes, as one partner tells his or her story, the lack of emotion is striking. Perhaps the client is describing a dramatic, traumatic, or clearly painful experience from a detached position that is not congruent with the content presented. For example, Pierre says things have been really difficult with Louise since their 2-year-old son died two years ago from a head injury following a fall. The therapist says to him, "This must have been so very hard for you both." Pierre shrugs and replies almost nonchalantly, "That's life; shit happens."

The therapist stays engaged with Pierre's response, reflecting with curiosity his lack of engagement in the personal experience being shared. Through these moments, the EFT therapist seeks to discover the significance of this minimal response, particularly in terms of the couple's engagement and how they view their relationship. The therapist says, "You say that lightly, Pierre. Perhaps that kind of helps you to keep the pain at bay?" Pierre swallows hard and nods. The therapist does not push Pierre further because they have not yet established a good alliance and instead moves into exploring if the couple have shared their mutual pain and given support to each other.

Focusing on Personal and Interactional Landmarks

Partners may recount experiences that they cannot forget or resolve. The stories open a door into the client's experience of the relationship and the client's sense of self in relation to the partner. The partner often may not really understand the significance of the story and may be exasperated that the other is still focusing on it. Consider Hélène's story of when recovering from surgery, she asked Serge to go to the corner store to buy her some bottled water before he went to work. Serge refused, saying that it would make him late for work. He reminded her that she could use the water filter. Serge could never understand why Hélène kept bringing up this incident.

The EFT therapist responds to Hélène: "It sounds like this was an important moment for you, Hélène. Can you help me to understand what this meant for you?" The therapist learns that this was the second incident during Hélène's recovery where she came to believe that she could not count on Serge when she really needed him. This stood in sharp contrast to the care she had lavished on Serge when he had broken his leg one year previously. From the bottled water incident, Hélène concluded that she wasn't important enough for Serge to go out of his way for her when she needed.

The therapist focuses on exploring this specific story and uncovers the meaning of the story from the client's perspective and whether their partner understands this experience. The therapist also validates the core or reactive emotions emerging through the process. For Hélène, this meant that she wasn't important enough for Serge to go out of his way for her when she needed him. Thus, this relatively small incident had a very important meaning for her. The therapist then asks Serge how he felt as he listened to his wife's story. The therapist validates the importance of the story for Hélène and explores how the couple's cycle became cemented around this incident.

In a similar way, specific interactions between a couple can signal typical positions that partner's take with one another. The interaction might indicate the availability for contact or support in the relationship (e.g., one partner cries, the other partner looks away) or the interaction might suggest a power or dominant position. In the case of Edith and Harry, a past interaction came to symbolize the couple's experience. Following the suicide of her brother three years earlier, Edith had become severely alcoholic. She had recently finished a recovery program, and in the initial session, she described her rapid and successful recovery with great pride. When the therapist asked Harry, her husband, what her drinking period had been like, Harry replied that it had indeed been very painful. Immediately Edith whirled around and glared at him, saying: "You didn't suffer!" Harry gulped and told the therapist that things were now going very well.

The EFT therapist responds by observing the interaction or making note of this moment that typifies the relationship. In this case, the therapist decided to explore it. First, she referred to the interaction: "I noticed that was a tricky moment for you both when Harry said your drinking was painful." Then the therapist made an empathic conjecture and asked Edith: "Tell me if I'm wrong, but my guess is it's incredibly hard for you to hear that he was hurt by your drinking." This led to Edith beginning to weep and talk about how difficult it was to hear his experience around her drinking.

As couples discuss their relationship, the therapist also observes comments or responses that seem to define power/control or closeness/distance as partners talk to each other, talk to the therapist, or tell stories about their relationship. The therapist is working to get a clear picture of each partner's position in their pattern, their partner's response to this role, and how each partner perceives and feels about such positions. In the following example, Alex complains:

> *"Well, I'd love to go back to Greece for a holiday, but I would never make a decision like that. The only kind of decision I'm allowed to make is when to change the kitty litter!" His wife replies: "That's fair. Why should we go somewhere I don't want to go, when I'm the one who earns most of the money?"*

The therapist says, "It feels like the only decision you can make is when to change the kitty litter?" Alex nods his head. Therapist asks then: "And how is that for you?" Alex pauses for a long time, then he bites his lips and shifts uncomfortably in his chair. Then the therapist says, "I see you biting your lip and looking uncomfortable, Alex, and I'm wondering what is happening for you." The process then moves into exploring the power dynamics of the relationship.

Focusing on Positive Interactions

The therapist notices how couples interact when there is opportunity for positive contact, as when one partner moves to physically comfort the other. In particular, it is noted how such gestures are received—is the partner open to receiving comfort, and, if not, how does this partner exit from contact? For example, as Tina begins to cry, her husband reaches over and takes her hand. Tina pulls her hand sharply away.

Exploring moments of positive contact, the therapist may note the tendency to move toward or move away from positive contact. These moments may provide opportunities to acknowledge efforts to comfort and receive comfort as examples of strengths in the relationship. In this case, the therapist might respond to Tina's reluctance by saying, "You're not feeling open to receiving comfort from him right now?" Had Tina accepted his comfort, the therapist might have said, "I notice you reached and took her hand there—that was to comfort her?" The husband nods. The therapist then says, "This is one of the good aspects of your relationship, then. You can comfort her, and you, Tina, can accept his comfort and care." In other moments, a partner may turn away from a positive more open moment of contact, and here the therapist might say: "I see you turning away as you hear her caring words, and I am wondering what is happening for you right now."

IDENTIFYING AND DELINEATING THE NEGATIVE INTERACTIVE CYCLE

The EFT therapist observes how partners react to each other as they get into conflict or areas of tension by tracking a couple's predictable actions. The therapist maps these interactional moves in sequence and frames for the couple a negative pattern of interaction or negative cycle. In EFT, all negative interactive cycles are seen in terms of separation protest and attachment insecurity. Cycles are understood as being a reflection of unmet attachment needs and fears about oneself and about trusting another in love.

Each partner's position in the cycle is their response to how they experience the relationship. For example, a wife may feel lonely and unimportant to her husband, who, feeling a sense of inadequacy, withdraws. This makes her angry, and she pursues for contact by criticizing and demanding. Her husband, who hears confirmation that he is inadequate, shuts down emotionally and withdraws further. Thus, a partner's position in the cycle not only reflects the person's experience but also creates it by evoking their partner's fears and keeping the cycle behaviors going back and forth. Often cycles have a closeness and a control dimension. Pursuing spouses can feel controlled by their withdrawing partner closing down or diverting conversations, whereas withdrawn partners typically feel controlled by their demanding spouses.

> *Patty often feels lonely and unloved in her relationship. Her husband, Peter, has some feelings of inadequacy and frequently withdraws. Patty's typical stance is to take a critical, angry position, saying to Peter: "You are never there for me. I can't count on you because you are only interested in yourself." For Peter, this is confirmation of his feelings of inadequacy. He defends himself angrily before withdrawing further.*

Fortunately, there are only a limited number of basic interactional patterns, cycles, and positions that ensnare distressed couples. Therapists become adept at identifying and empathically exploring these patterns, as they are, in large part, the plot of the couple's distressing attachment drama. Over time, distressed couples become caught in a "dance" of repetitive interactional patterns. Each partner cues or triggers the other in what becomes a cyclical pattern of negative interactions. Partners may have their own ways of describing cycles, and if they do, the therapist uses the clients' own words. By doing so, the couple tap into their own felt sense of their relationship, and together with their therapist's help, create the story of their negative cycle. For example, a spouse might say, "He shuts me out, so I just try to bash the door down" or "I just build a wall—and then she pushes and pushes." It is not enough for the therapist to identify the negative cycle for herself, nor for partners to gain a cognitive understanding of their patterns. Rather, we empathically explore and reflect, so the couple come to experience their negative interactions as the cycle "in action."

The Basic Negative Cycles and Interactional Positions

Pattern: Pursue/Withdraw

The most common cycle is a demanding spouse interacting with a withdrawing or avoidant partner. In this pattern, the distancing or "stonewalling" position is in a shutdown, protective mode that often cues panic or aggression in the other partner as in "I will make you respond to me." Most other patterns can be seen as variants of the basic pursue/withdraw pattern. When trying to identify the couple's negative pattern, keep in mind that the positions are "default" options: They are what the partners do when they feel threatened or vulnerable. A common mistake of beginning EFT therapists is to be confused by a withdrawing husband who pursues for sex but who generally takes a withdrawn position, especially when confronted, rejected, or vulnerable. This cycle has been described by different clinicians in a variety of ways including demand/distance, criticize/stonewall, and complain/placate. In heterosexual couples, there can be a tendency to associate these positions with gender difference (e.g., the woman more often in the position of pursuer and the man more in the position of withdrawer). However, we have certainly encountered couples that break these stereotypes, so the EFT therapist needs to be open and curious to discover the dance of each couple through a bottom-up process of exploration. A male pursuer will tend to appear different from a female pursuer because of the possible coercive element to male pursuit. The therapist needs to take note of this, particularly when assessing for abuse. We also find that gender fluid and same sex couples most typically present in pursue/withdraw patterns.

Pattern: Withdraw/Withdraw

Sometimes the therapist will observe couples whose interactions appear to be a withdraw/withdraw pattern. In this pattern, both partners are reluctant to engage emotionally for fear of driving their partner away. They tend to be conflict averse, and in the face of conflict, both withdraw further. This may be the couple's basic pattern; however, it is more likely that a pursue/withdraw pattern underlies it. The withdraw/withdraw cycle frequently evolves from a pursue/withdraw pattern, in which the pursuer gave up reaching for their partner. The withdrawal of a "burnt-out" pursuer may involve an explicit refusal to engage unless the partner changes and sometimes represents the beginning of grieving and detaching from the relationship. In other cases of withdraw/withdraw patterns, the pursuer may be a "soft" pursuer who is hard to recognize because he or she does not show the overwhelming anxious energy seen in many pursuers and because he or she gives up the pursuit rather easily. These cycles are difficult for a couple to maintain over time.

Pattern: Attack/Attack

Therapists often observe attack/attack sequences and escalations in couple interactions. Most often these escalations are deviations in an otherwise pursue/withdraw pattern in which the withdrawer turns, erupts into anger, and fights when provoked. After the fight, the withdrawer usually reverts back to the withdrawn position until sufficiently provoked again.

Pattern: Reactive Pursue/Withdraw Cycle

These cycles evolve over time from insecure patterns that have been in existence long term. For example, over decades, a pursuing wife gradually gives up trying to get close to her husband and begins to limit her investment in the relationship. Her distancing, work-obsessed spouse does not notice. The children leave home, an important transition, and then the wife announces she is leaving. The couple come into therapy with a reactive cycle, in which the husband is frantically pursuing his wife in order to prevent a separation and the wife is cautious and withdrawn, refusing to commit herself to the relationship. This cycle is, of course, the reversal of their original pattern in which she pursued and he withdrew. In the case of a reactive cycle, the therapist works with the cycle presented in the session, but the fact that the pattern is recent and evolved from a far different long-term cycle provides an important part of the client's history and must be kept in mind by the therapist. Fernando and Inez are an example of a reactive cycle.

Pattern: Complex Cycles

These cycles are multi-move cycles that are typically high in reactivity and often occur in trauma-survivor couples in which anxiety and avoidance are high, resulting in more complicated sequences of steps. In one example, Doreen, who is a trauma survivor, angrily demands her partner, Jocelyne's, attention. Jocelyne comes forward to try to please and attend to Doreen, who rejects her overtures and tells her to "get away." Jocelyne becomes confused and anxious about Doreen's well-being, which prompts her to badger Doreen with questions until Doreen storms out. They then experience a cooling-off period during which neither partner talks about what happened, until they slowly begin to warm up toward each other. In another example of a complex cycle, the husband makes coercive demands for compliance and attention. The wife withdraws, the husband then escalates his demands, and the wife attacks in self-defense. Both partners then withdraw, and the wife becomes depressed for a period of three days or so. In turn, the husband reinitiates with a softer pursuit, and the wife slowly responds then a brief period of loving sexuality ensues. Then the cycle repeats.

Identifying the Cycle

When does the therapist begin to track and identify the cycle the couple typically engage in that leads to their distress? It depends on the therapist's own judgment as well as the couple's eagerness to get to the heart of their problems. Ideally, from the first session, the therapist will explore how each partner experiences the relationship and begin to notice and reflect sequences of emotion and behavior patterns. The therapist will also ask about background information to provide context for the conflict or difficulty the couple is experiencing and illuminate the strengths of their relationship.

Therapists working with distressed couples frequently notice that both partners complain about and criticize the other; both may even escalate to verbally attacking or to withdrawing or stonewalling (Gottman, 1994). When identifying the negative interactive cycle, the EFT therapist is looking for the overall predominant pattern that most typifies the couple's interaction. The couple will fall into this pattern when they are vulnerable or the relationship bond feels tenuous. In EFT, negative interaction cycles are seen in terms of separation protest and attachment insecurity. Cycles are understood as being a reflection of unmet attachment needs and fears about oneself and about trusting another in love.

The cycle can be identified by exploring what happens between them when they fight. The therapist may ask them to relay a specific recent example that is prototypical of their arguments. Watching a couple's interaction in session will also give clues to the predictable moves that partners use when experiencing distress. The therapist may also ask about the couple's relationship history, gathering details on defining moments or key stressors they faced and how they coped. The therapeutic task is to track the couple's interactions around closeness and distance.

The therapist will ask the couple to describe their interaction by asking leading questions. The following questions can be used to elicit the information you need:

- "What do you each do when things are stressful in your relationship?"
- "What do you do when you see 'the look' on your partner's face?"
- "What happens when you have a fight?"
- "Pretend that I am a fly on the wall of your kitchen; tell me, what would I see if the two of you were having a fight."
- "Play me the video. . . . "

- "What do you do then?" "So, what happens next?" "How does it end?" "How do you reconnect after an argument?"
- "Did your arguments always follow this pattern, or did it used to be different?
- "When do the two of you feel close?"
- "How do decisions get made in your relationship?"
- "Who is more likely to initiate conversations about your relationship?"
- "How do you each 'take care of' your relationship?"

These questions help to focus the discussion around delineating the cycle. As the pattern emerges, the therapist describes the position that each partner relies on in times of vulnerability, when attachment needs are activated. The cycle is identified as the predictable behaviors that make up a couple's default position when they feel threatened or vulnerable.

The therapist listens for statements that describe the behaviors (the moves) that each partner displays in their cycle as well as the emotion-laden statements (the music) that each partner may use to describe his or her relationship. If you are having trouble deciding on your clients' positions, listen for who takes care of the relationship by keeping it close (closing the gap, initiating conversations or pushing for contact) and who takes care of the relationship by avoiding conflict (minimizing or shutting down a conversation, creating space). Clients often use descriptive phrases or metaphors describing their own position in the relationship (e.g., "Me, I'm like a turtle. I climb into my shell, where it's safe."). A list of statements common to withdrawing and pursuing partners is provided in Table 4.2.

Table 4.2
Perceptions of Withdrawing and Pursing Partners

Withdrawing partners often say . . .	**Pursuing partners often say . . .**
"You never come near me or touch me."	"My heart is breaking." "I am going to die."
"I never get it right or satisfy him."	"He is never there. He is always at work."
"I don't bother—what's the point?"	"You never look at me when I talk to you. You just watch TV."
"I am amazed that you can take something so small and blow it out of proportion."	"There are birthdays that are forgotten or Mother's Day when nobody gives me a card."
"I don't know what I feel. I'm lost."	"I do it by myself and just take care of things on my own."
"You give me that look, and I'm paralyzed."	"I am way down on your list—after your work, the kids, your family, and then maybe me."
"She never initiates sex—it's always up to me."	"You're not there—no one has ever been there."
"I can never get it right or to your standards. It's like you have a scorecard, and I always come up short. That's all I hear, anyway, is what I do wrong, never what is going right."	"You won't listen. You never listen. It doesn't matter how long I talk or how many examples I give to you or how hard I try—I can never get through to you."
"I feel like you've got me dangling from the end of a rope that is going to fray at any minute, and it's going to be all over."	"It's like we are roommates or sisters. Any hope for passion or romance is futile—she just doesn't want it."
"I don't feel anything—nothing at all."	"Other couples seem to have lives that are full, and they enjoy each other. We don't have anything."

Delineating the Cycle

In delineating the couple's negative interaction pattern, the therapist outlines (a) the moves that each partner makes in the cycle (between process) and (b) the emotional music that primes these moves (within process). The therapist then links together the moves and the music, showing how they prime and maintain each other. The therapist also elaborates on how each partner suffers from being caught in this cycle. The therapist explicitly paints the cycle as the enemy that isolates the partners—the source of their pain and distress.

In the case of Fernando and Inez, we can understand their cycle by identifying the moves between and the music within.

- The Process Between: The moves Inez makes are (a) to "puff up and be angry" when she is hurt by Fernando and then (b) to withdraw to her painting or her outside activities. The moves that Fernando makes are (a) to be snappy and irritable when he is anxious, (b) to respond angrily to his wife's attack, and (c) to withdraw to his computer. In a later session, Fernando provides a metaphor for (b) and (c), as "I fire off a round, and I run for cover."
- The Process Within: The emotional music that primes the moves of Fernando and Inez. Fernando gets anxious around being on time and then feels "attacked" by his wife when she tries to "settle him down." This makes him feel disrespected, which results in anxiety, "makes his heart go thump in his chest." He then goes to the safety of his computer. Perhaps Fernando's moves are primed by feeling anxious or put down, not precious to his wife, or perhaps he feels he is failing in this relationship. Her attacks seem to confirm that she disrespects him, that he is not enough for her; if this is indeed his experience, then this would be hurtful or even scary (core emotion). The anger he shows when she attacks him is the reactive or surface emotion. Hypothesis: underlying attachment fear: "I am not adequate." Inez, on the other hand, feels hurt by her husband's way of interacting when he gets tense and upset, and because this is a long-standing pattern, she sees it as indicative that he dislikes—even hates—her. Understandably, this hurts her (core emotion) and makes her angry (reactive emotion). Hypothesis: underlying attachment fear: "I am not loved." Even "I am unlovable."
- Putting It Together: The therapist will then paint the picture for the couple and if necessary, explore and expand it until there is a good understanding of the pattern and the emotions that prime each partner's moves. The therapist may not achieve a complete understanding in the first session; however, the therapist will typically be able to draw out and observe the couple's behaviors, perceptions, and surface emotions. When the couple understand the complete cycle and the emotions that drive the cycle, they are ready to see the cycle as the enemy and begin de-escalating. A helpful homework activity mentioned in *Hold Me Tight* is for the couple to come up with a short-hand or nickname for their negative cycle (e.g., the tornado, the trap). This exercise helps partners take ownership over their cycle and gives them a shared language to notice and "call it" when it starts up between sessions—a powerful first step in breaking their negative dance.

Delineating the Cycle of Fernando and Inez

Fernando gets tense and edgy, and Inez tries to settle him down, causing him to feel distressed. He responds with anger, which reinforces for Inez the painful feeling that he dislikes or even hates her. Inez used to turn up the volume and get angry, but now she more often stays away and finds other things in her life to occupy her. Fernando withdraws to the safety of the computer. Each partner is then left feeling alone and unsupported, not important to the other. Neither partner reaches out to contact the other or to regain closeness. Instead, they each spend time apart, soothing themselves with other activities. The cycle has the couple trapped and leaves each partner feeling sad and alone. The predominant pattern for this couple in their early years was Inez pursuing and Fernando withdrawing. We still see elements of mild pursuit in Inez (moving toward to settle him), but this long-standing pattern has discouraged and disillusioned her, and thus we see her pursuit burning out. Interestingly, as the couple move into therapy, Fernando begins to pursue his wife. The cycle becomes a reactive pursue/withdraw cycle with Fernando pursuing Inez.

Exercise 4.14. Exploring Negative Cycles

Answer the following questions based on your observations of Wendy and Barry's relationship. Wendy states that Barry always seems to put other things ahead of her. She feels she is at the bottom of his list, which hurts. She fears that she is not very important to him and tries to talk to him, to get him to understand how unhappy she feels. Ultimately, the only time he turns to her, she says, is when he wants sex. This makes her angry, and she is critical of Barry, often escalating to shouting at him. Barry gets the message from Wendy that he is a disappointment to her. He feels he must be failing her. He feels insecure and inadequate, but he also becomes quite resentful of her criticism. He begins to avoid her, working long hours and often stopping at the bar on the way home. Sometimes he approaches Wendy for sex, but recently, she almost always refuses him.

1. The negative cycle of Wendy and Barry is
    a. Complex cycle. ____
    b. Attack/attack. ____
    c. Pursue/withdraw. ____
    d. Withdraw/withdraw. ____
2. Which of the following best describes their reactive pattern?
    a. Barry pursues, and Wendy withdraws. ____
    b. Barry attacks, and Wendy pursues. ____
    c. Wendy attacks, and Barry pursues. ____
    d. Wendy pursues, and Barry withdraws. ____
3. Wendy's reactive or surface emotion is
    a. Hurt. ____
    b. Fear. ____
    c. Anger. ____
    d. Shame. ____
4. Barry's reactive or surface emotion is
    a. Hurt. ____
    b. Fear. ____
    c. Anger. ____
    d. Blame. ____

Exercise 4.14a Putting Together the Emotions and Moves

Think of a couple you are working with who are in a basic Pursue/Withdraw cycle. Drawing on the aspects of their story that you have discovered thus far, write a description that pulls together the partners' cycle moves and their emotional music. Hints: (a) Try using **"when. . . then"** phrases, such as, When Partner A does _____, then Partner B feels _____ and does _____ (b) Conclude with **"the more . . . the more"** phrases, illustrating how the cycle feeds on itself, such as "**The more** Partner A distances and turns away, **the more** loud and angry Partner B becomes, and around and around it goes."

____

____

____

____

____

Taking a History of the Relationship

A key EFT assessment process goal is to hear and to understand the story of this couple. The therapist is essentially answering the questions: How did their relationship evolve, and why did they come for therapy at this time? The therapist wants to enter the world of each partner and understand how their relationship evolved to this point. Basic information is gathered organically, with questions and prompts like the following:

- How long have you been together? What attracted you to each other?
- Do you live together? Who else lives with you? How old are your children? What is your relationship with extended family?
- What was it like when things were good between you?
- When you fight or argue, do you feel as if you resolve issues? How do you make up? Who initiates closeness and sex? Have you been satisfied with your sexual relationship?
- What was your relationship like at the beginning? Were you once able to confide in each other? How and when did this change?
- Have there been significant stressors in your lives together? How have you handled them?
- What prompted you to come for therapy at this time? Whose idea was it to seek therapy? What changes would you each like to see happen?

Assessing a Couple's Sexual Relationship

Some couples present for therapy with a specific focus on improving their sexual intimacy, in which case the EFT therapist will begin to explore their sexual challenges and track how their negative cycle plays out in the bedroom. Therapists vary in their training and own comfort levels for working with sexual issues (e.g., desire discrepancies, vaginismus, erectile problems, premature ejaculation), and it is therefore important to only practice within your scope of expertise and seek consultation as needed. Additional assessment and consultation with other professionals who specialize in sexual health is advised in most cases.

The focus in Stage 1 of EFT will still be on the attachment themes that block the couple's intimacy. In long-term committed relationships, secure attachment enhances their ability to attune and respond to each other sexually, which in turn strengthens their relationship bond. For other couples, their sexual relationship will feel like a very sensitive conversation, and they need the therapist to choose their timing carefully while taking the lead in opening up this topic. A good place to start is to ask permission, "Would it be okay for us to talk a little about sexual intimacy in your relationship?" and then stay within your clients' window of tolerance. Even if it feels too sensitive for partners to talk about sex at the first invitation, the therapist has provided a door they can open further into the therapeutic process, once they are more comfortable.

A comprehensive sexual assessment includes conjoint and individual sessions that address questions about the partners' current sexual satisfaction and communication about their sexual needs, health factors, and medications that impact sexuality and their sexual history. The EFT therapist will also ask her clients what messages they received about sex as a young person, what stands out for them in the development of their sexual identity and orientation. What role did parents or other significant people play? How did parental figures respond to their emerging sexuality and/or coming out? Whether sex becomes a topic at the beginning or later in therapy, here are a few helpful questions to open up the conversation:

- How important is it for you that we address your sexual relationship in therapy?
- How satisfied are you in your sexual relationship now? Have there been changes in your sexual connection over time? What do you attribute those changes to?
- Are you able to talk about your sexual preferences or fantasies with each other?
- What happens when you try to talk about sex, physical intimacy, or affectionate touch?
- What characterizes your most gratifying sexual experiences with your partner?

See Appendix A for a full set of EFT Sexuality Assessment Questions compiled by Susan M. Johnson and Michael Moran to be used in conjoint and individual sessions.

Attachment Injuries

The EFT therapist also notices if there has been an attachment injury in the relationship. An attachment injury is a critical incident when one partner learns they cannot count on the other and often pulls away. Attachment injuries, their diagnosis, and their management, are discussed in Chapter 1. Attachment injuries may emerge in the couple's relationship history or may be identified through the process of treatment, often in Stage 2.

Assessing Current Attachment and the Broader Developmental Context

The EFT therapist's assessment begins with the couple relationship because it is most pertinent to the presenting issues. However, clients also have a need to tell their own personal stories, and the EFT therapist listens to each partner empathically. Learning about your clients' models of attachment and their strategies for regulating their emotions and maintaining connection enables the EFT therapist to better understand their expectations in close relationships, particularly concerning core existential questions, such as:

- "Am I lovable?" "Am I worthy of your attention and care?"
- "Will you cherish me?" and "Will you be there for me when I need you?"

The process goal here is to discover the clients' habitual attachment moves in close relationships that foster or block secure connection. Do they see their bonds with others as a secure resource to reach out to and seek support from in times of need? Or have they adapted to adverse life situations and insecure attachments by avoiding dependency or becoming anxiously preoccupied with the other's availability, or a mixture of both (Fraley & Waller, 1998)? Partners' attachment strategies can be assessed in three ways: (a) from the attachment history and background of each partner, (b) by understanding the interaction between partners, and (c) by using self-report questionnaires.

Assessing Attachment History and Background

The EFT therapist explores the attachment history and context of each client's upbringing. The assessment focus provides a rich understanding of the developmental world of each partner through learning about their family-of-origin, cultural context, and other formative influences. Differences in history and experience can impact a couple's negative cycle and amplify its effect. A key assessment goal is to explore their cultural background, religious influences, and social location as the setting for our clients' lived experiences of attachment. The therapist takes her time with this conversation and exercises cultural humility, noting internally any differences in background between partners. These themes are also explored in the individual sessions. The therapist asks each couple about their family of origin, key events, and major transitions, as well as previous significant adult relationships. Some possible questions include:

- What was your model of relationships like? Did your parents seem close? Were they openly affectionate? Did they fight? Did they resolve arguments and become close again? How did you experience any fights and arguments that occurred in the home?
- Did you have a secure relationship with a dependable parental figure? Who was available for comfort, confiding, and soothing? Do either of you have a history of loss or abuse? How did you cope with this at the time?
- What were your cultural, racial, or religious influences or experiences growing up? How do you identify with your background now?
- Were there major transitions, such as immigration, frequent relocations, or other significant adults, in the home? How did the family navigate these transitions?
- Have you experienced bullying, racialized trauma, or discrimination of any kind? If so, how was it handled by your family, school, organization, etc.?
- What stands out for you in terms of the development of your sexual orientation and gender identity? What role did family or others play?
- Have you felt safe to disclose how you identify in various aspects of your life to people who are important to you? How have they responded?
- How were emotions handled in your family? Were some emotions acceptable and others disallowed? Are there cultural influences that impact your expression of emotion?
- Have you experienced trauma or divorce in previous love relationships?
- To whom do you each turn for comfort and confiding now?

(For additional questions, see Appendix B.)

The therapist approaches these conversations as part of a process of safety and alliance building. She enters the clients' phenomenological world, honors their experiences, and captures a full picture of them. The therapist opens the door to these potentially sensitive areas, following the clients' pacing and lead in determining what is most meaningful for them. Couples experience this as an organic conversation that invites them to be curious and make connections about how their life experiences have helped shape them and their relationships. They also begin to explore differences in life experiences and culture. How they navigate these differences as a couple becomes part of their relationship story.

We use what we discover about our couple's history to explicitly validate how they learned to regulate their emotions: "No wonder you keep your worries bottled up inside. When you were little, it would have been dangerous to show your feelings. It makes so much sense to me that you close down emotionally and clam up in your arguments." In this example, we could also highlight places where experiences of discrimination reinforce the strategy of shutting down to avoid the fear of drawing unnecessary attention to oneself. See Guillory (2021) and Nightingale, Awosan, and Stavrianopoulos (2019) for examples relevant to African American heterosexual couples. In addition to providing validation for the client, it allows their partner to see behaviors in a new light and take them less personally. The depth of information we gather as we get to know our clients tell a story about the emotional tone of their upbringing, their sense of safety in the world, their losses and vulnerabilities, and how people were there for them or not. These experiences are intricately connected with attachment, and taken together, they profoundly shape our clients' expectations and how they respond in their close relationships. As therapy progresses, themes concerning family history, culture, race, and discrimination are revisited, and new elements emerge, illustrating the fluidity between assessment and therapy in EFT.

Assessing Partners' Interactions

Information regarding attachment strategies is also gathered by (a) observing the couple as they interact in the session and (b) asking how each typically responds to the other. Who seeks closeness? Do they seek support from each other? What does each partner do when the other is distressed? The EFT therapist listens for indices of secure attachment, heightened fear of abandonment, or avoidance of emotional closeness.

A client with secure attachments tends to

- Openly express positive and negative emotions.
- Give their partner the benefit of the doubt.
- Seek out their partner for support when distressed.
- Be available to comfort and support their partner when needed.

A client who draws on avoidant strategies tends to

- Avoid seeking support from their partner.
- Struggle to support their partner when anxious or needy.
- Withdraw precisely when needed by their partner.
- Dismiss or minimize threats and hurts to self.
- Intellectualize and restrict emotionality, focusing on problem solving or taking action.

A client with anxious attachment tends to

- Show an intense need for support and affection from partner.
- Catastrophize and amplify threats and personal hurts.
- Be vigilant and readily interpret partner's behaviors as a threat.
- Demand their partner's time and attention.
- Express emotions intensely.

A client with a mixture of fearful and avoidant strategies tends to

- Manage fears by avoiding intimacy and struggle with emotional and physical closeness.
- Hold in emotions and be reluctant to self-disclose.
- Have difficulty believing that their partners care about them.
- Avoid seeking support or when they do they withdraw when it is offered.
- Behave in a passive manner.
- Have experienced trauma or been violated in love relationships.

Exercise 4.15. Matching Attachment Strategies

Match the following attachment strategies to the following examples:

Attachment strategy:

A. Avoidant/dismissive attachment
B. Mixed anxious and avoidant attachment
C. Anxious/preoccupied attachment
D. Secure attachment

1. A woman asks her partner for support and comfort when she is laid off from her job. ____
2. Elise is extremely angry because Charles is late from work as he tries to meet an important deadline. ____
3. Peter looks out of the window as Shana tearfully describes her recent miscarriage. ____
4. As Jeff lights candles for their anniversary dinner, Lisa berates his efforts given he has only completed four of five tasks she asked him to do for her. ____

Self-Report Questionnaires

EFT therapists may also administer a self-report attachment style questionnaire such as the Experiences in Close Relationships Scale (Brennan, Clark, & Shaver, 1998). For a review of self-report adult attachment measures, see Ravitz, Maunder, Hunter, Sthankiya, and Lance (2010) and Mikulincer and Shaver (2016). Sandberg, Busby, Johnson, and Yoshida (2012) proposed a self-report assessment based on Johnson's (2008) partner questions reflecting an impression of accessibility, responsiveness, and emotional engagement. The BARE scale provides a brief reliable measure of core elements of attachment behaviors in adulthood. EFT outcome studies have commonly relied on the Dyadic Adjustment Scale (Spanier, 1976) as a general self-report assessment of relationship satisfaction. The Couple Satisfaction Index (Funk & Rogge, 2007) provides a robust assessment of relationship satisfaction in a brief format.

Individual Sessions

Following the first one or two meetings with the couple, the EFT therapist usually meets with each partner individually. This provides the therapist the opportunity to continue to foster the therapeutic alliance by listening and focusing on the individual's concerns and to obtain a history of previous adult relationships, including an understanding of how they ended.

Individual sessions enable the therapist to observe and interact with each client in a different context (i.e., without their partner). Clients can frequently be more candid about problems when the partner is not present, particularly about sexual intimacy or contraindications to therapy. The therapist can use individual sessions to explore information that is difficult to obtain in the presence of the partner. Here, for example, the therapist may ask about violence and other forms of abuse. Asking the individual whom she or he confides in can ease the therapist into asking about competing relationships, whether there is another partner or perhaps an online relationship.

The therapist also uses individual sessions to explore previous attachment relationships. Family of origin and background questions may be explored in further detail, and the therapist also asks about previous significant adult intimate relationships. The therapist will also assess for personal attachment traumas that may have an impact on the present relationship. This permits the therapist to further understand the client's model of intimate relationships and to discuss with the client the underlying feelings and attachment issues that might affect the present relationship.

Secrets and Individual Sessions in Couple Therapy

Conducting individual sessions leads to the question of secrets. Will an EFT therapist agree to keep information learned in an individual session from the partner? This issue is best addressed explicitly in the conjoint session and reiterated at the beginning of the individual session. The therapist may advise the client that although they have a right to individual privacy, holding secrets between the couple can interfere with the process of EFT, as well as their own goals for therapy. The therapist would encourage and support a partner to share secrets regarding, for example, ongoing affairs in a conjoint session, processing any fears and reservations about doing so first. Other information, for example, a past abortion never talked about or a brief affair that ended years ago, may not be considered necessary to bring into the current couple therapy process. If a client did tell the therapist that he or she was having an ongoing extramarital affair, and the client did not wish to share this information with the partner, then the EFT therapist would tell the client that she was unable to work with them because this secret would inevitably undermine the process of relationship change. The condition to at least place the other relationship on hold and be open about it in therapy is necessary to proceed with therapy.

CONTRAINDICATIONS TO EFT

Throughout the EFT process, the therapist is mindful of possible contraindications for couple treatment. There are five key areas in which individual factors may impact the viability of using EFT to treat couple distress. These areas include partners with different agendas, couples who are seeking separation, intimate partner violence, mental health issues, and the potential influence of untreated substance abuse. Therapist concerns in each area are listed next.

Different Agendas

It is not unusual for couples to present with differing agendas, and the EFT therapist needs to be able to clarify the impasse and present it clearly to the couple. For example, one partner may push for commitment to get married, while the second partner is ambivalent about committing because of unresolved issues in the relationship. Can the couple come to some common ground, for example, agreeing to put the question of marriage on hold until they can work on the relationship to see if they can resolve their issues? Are they both willing to engage in therapy under these terms? In another example, one partner's objective may be to persuade the other to be in an open relationship, while the other does not wish to do so. The EFT therapist will explore each partner's position and relational needs and support them in determining if they can work through this issue in a mutually satisfying way. Or alternatively, if their needs are fundamentally incompatible, the therapist will support them to go their separate ways. The goal here is to create a shift one way or another that helps them get beyond their impasse.

Separating Couples

When it is clear that one partner has emotionally left the relationship and the couple will be separating, EFT should not be offered. Occasionally, one spouse will initiate couple sessions in the hope of securing support for the other as she or he lets the partner know about the plan to move on. Partners may then be offered sessions to help them with pragmatic aspects to separation. The therapist may also work individually with the second partner or refer him or her for support or grief work with another therapist.

Intimate Partner Violence

The question of using conjoint treatment in couples when there is violence comes down to the type of violence exhibited in the relationship. Slootmaeckers and Migerode (2018, 2020) argue that EFT, with its goal of de-escalating destructive interaction patterns, has much to offer couples in which there is intermittent bidirectional aggression that arises out of frustrated and unmet attachment needs. This situational couple violence is distinguished from intimate terrorism, which involves unidirectional and pervasive use of power and control of one partner over another and is contraindicated for couple therapy. EFT involves encouraging partners to be vulnerable with each other; in highly abusive relationships (i.e., intimate terrorism), such vulnerability could be misused, putting the abused partner more at risk.

However, one abusive incident does not necessarily mean an abusive relationship, and, conversely, some relationships have no history of physical violence, but rampant verbal abuse is present in the form of threats, denigrating comments, and deliberate moves to hurt or intimidate the other. For example, a wife may confide in her individual session:

"He has never hit me . . . but I am afraid of him." The EFT therapist will listen for fear, and if one partner is afraid of abuse or reprisal from the other, the therapist will not proceed with EFT. Violent partners may be asked instead to participate in therapy or programs that foster exploration into the root of their triggers and at appropriate expression of the full range of their emotions, including anger.

An in-depth analysis and discussion of abusive relationships is outside the scope of our workbook. The reader is referred to several excellent sources (e.g., Bograd & Mederos, 1999; Slootmaeckers & Migerode, 2018, 2020). In addition, therapists may want to seek supervision or consultation when deciding how to proceed with abusive relationships.

Substance Abuse and Other Addictions

The EFT therapist views addictions through an attachment lens and focuses on the ways in which the substance or addictive activity (e.g., gaming, pornography, gambling) acts as an attachment substitute to distract, numb, and sooth deep emotional pain within the using partner. This de-pathologizing frame humanizes the using partner and orients the couple toward the creation of safety and security in their relationship. Thus, substance use or dependence does not necessarily preclude EFT, as long as couples can participate in sessions while sober. Early sessions will explore where the addictive behavior fits within the negative cycle and how the couple's emotions and behaviors organize around it. The therapist will explore how the addiction affects the relationship, as well as how the relationship impacts the addiction. An important goal in Stage 1 is for the using partner to acknowledge and take ownership over the addictive behavior to extricate the other partner of responsibility for their sobriety. Typically, the partner who is engaging in addictive behavior will also attend some form of individual recovery or group treatment for the addiction.

Depression and Other Mental Health Issues

It is not unusual for partners experiencing relationship distress to be depressed or anxious, and EFT can have a positive impact in alleviating symptoms of these disorders. However, if a partner has significant impairment and is untreated, the client may be referred for assessment and concurrent individual treatment. Depending on the therapist's expertise and scope of practice, the same is true for most other psychiatric disorders. For details on EFT couple treatment involving depression, see Denton, Wittenborn, and Golden (2012) and Wittenborn et al. (2019).

Creating a Therapeutic Agreement

The EFT therapist briefly describes how EFT is conducted and invites clients to ask questions or express fears or concerns. For example, the therapist may say:

> *"We find that distressed couples tend to get stuck in a pattern—we also call this a 'cycle' or 'dance'—that leaves them feeling unhappy, alone, angry or hurt, and far apart from each other. What I will do is to try to understand your pattern and also to understand the feelings that you each have within the relationship that are difficult to talk about. I will try to help you to understand each other and relate to each other in a deeper and more satisfying way."*

The couple are invited to ask questions (e.g., how long does therapy usually take?) and to express fears and concerns about the process, which are then addressed. Most EFT therapists predict therapy will take 8 to 20 sessions, longer if there are long-standing mental health issues, addictions, a childhood history of trauma, or attachment injuries within the current relationship.

Exercise 4.16. Assessing Contraindications

1. A client tells you her partner hit her during a recent fight. Write three questions you would ask to assess if you could continue with EFT.

   ____

   ____

   ____

2. In an individual session, your client tells you that his partner is drinking to excess, and he is worried that she may be alcoholic. You ask him if he has discussed his concerns with his partner.
   a. Your client says: "Yes, I have tried to talk about my concerns on several occasions, and it always leads to an argument." How does this statement inform your therapeutic goals in this session and your upcoming conjoint session? Write an intervention that reflects how you would explore this statement.

      ____

      ____

   b. Your client says: "No, it sits between us like an elephant in the room. There's no way I would bring it up." What is your therapeutic goal in this and the next conjoint session? Write an intervention that reflects how you would explore this statement.

      ____

      ____

Personal Reflections

Think of a couple you have worked with in the past in which there were "grey areas" concerning one of the contraindications mentioned earlier. Identify one or two things you would do differently now based on what you have learned in this chapter.

____

____

In working through contraindications, the couple therapist often faces ethical dilemmas that can become the source of considerable angst. To remind yourself you are not alone, write the names two colleagues or mentors you can trust to turn to for consultation and support.

____

____

Following the individual session and by the beginning of the second or third couple session, the EFT therapist will have developed a basic alliance with both partners and gained a sense of their histories and evolution of their relationship. The therapist will know whether the couple ever knew a happy, secure bond and will have a sense of the problematic cycle and how it impacts the emotional realities of each partner. The therapist will also have a sense of each partner's pain in this relationship as well as an understanding of how each attempts to deal with it. At this point the couple will also have the beginning of a sense of trust and ease with the therapist and a new perspective on their problem or cycle. Each partner will also have seen glimpses of the underlying emotions in their partner, and both will likely have some hope for the future of the relationship.

ANSWERS AND SUGGESTED RESPONSES

Exercise 4.1. Attuning Empathically

Suggested Response: A good response will acknowledge Fernando's discomfort of letting Inez in without overly interpreting, judging, or attempting to "correct" his behavior. Some possible examples are

- "Yes, I understand, there is something uncomfortable there about letting Inez into your space in those moments when you are anxious or on edge."
- "It's hard for you there, I notice; you need some breathing room. Can you say a little more about what happens there?"

Less desirable answers would be

- "Can you see, Fernando, how that leads to distance between you?"
- "Yes, but you sound rather harsh when you say, 'Back off.'"
- "If only you could tell her how anxious you get."

Exercise 4.2. Extending Acceptance

Suggested Response: Helpful phrasing can start with "It makes so much sense to me if you feel. . . then you would. . . " or "I really understand that. . . . "

Examples of responses that do not predominantly convey acceptance are

- "I can understand why you do that, Fernando, but do you think it is helpful?"
- "Inez, do you see how your attacking leaves him feeling like he has no choices?"

Exercise 4.3. Expressing Genuineness

Suggested Response: EFT therapists relate to their clients on a "human" level and in doing so normalize and universalize their struggles. A nice response to Fernando's question that balances transparency and reassurance could be: "Yes, of course, we fight sometimes; everybody does. We usually find a way to sort things out afterwards."

The following responses are less desirable as they may be alienating:

- "No, we are very happily married."

- "My personal life is not the issue here."
- "You have concerns about my relationship?"

Exercise 4.4. Reviewing Alliance Formation

1. **C.** Although all of the above are objectives in this stage of therapy, the prime objective is the creation of a therapeutic alliance.
2. **D.** Not known to be helpful in creating a therapeutic alliance.

Exercise 4.5. Practicing Empathic Attunement

1. **B.** Could be used when tracking the cycle, but it is not an example of empathic attunement.
2. **C.** Directing, not attuning
3. **B.** He seems not to understand why his wife launches into a tirade, he regrets the lack of hugs, and he withdraws to protect himself. He is tearful and probably anxious; he may possibly also be angry.
4. **D.** She is obviously angry and irritated. There is no indication that she is disengaged at this point. She may well feel hurt and rejected by Gerald.

Suggested Responses

5. A good response will include acknowledgment of some or all of the following: his confusion or lack of understanding of his wife's tirades, his loneliness and or sadness, and the move he makes to protect himself (i.e., creeping into a shell).
6. A good response will include acknowledgment of some or all of the following: how painful it would be to not feel seen or to feel she does not exist in her partner's eyes and given that experience, how understandable her anger is, perhaps even how hard it is to hold in her anger.

Exercise 4.6. Reflecting Client Experience

Suggested Response: A helpful therapist reflection here will simply feedback to Emily the experience of being left alone at a vulnerable time in her life: "You felt like he wasn't there for you at a key time when you needed him."

Less desirable answers would be

- "What was your surgery for?" This question misses her experience, although may be a piece of content that you could ask about at a different time.
- "I can imagine you must have been furious about that." This is overly interpretative.
- "So, you were both stressed out at the same time." This may be true, but it does not reflect the experience she was trying to convey.

Exercise 4.7. Reflecting Nonverbal Experience

Suggested Response: "You get tearful as you think of Charles not being there for you at that difficult time."

It is best to keep it simple and reflect what you see. The following responses are less desirable because they do not help Emily link her tears to her sense of not being able to lean on Charles when she needed him:

- "Take your time, Emily."
- "Perhaps you have never talked about this before?"
- "Let's move on to something that is easier to talk about."

Exercise 4.8. Reflecting Incongruence

Suggested Response: A good reflection acknowledges the two sides of what is being expressed (verbal and nonverbal) and gently invites the client to explore a deeper or more vulnerable experience, such as: "I notice you smile as you say that, Charles, but I wonder if there aren't some pretty painful feelings about her being mad at you."

The following responses are less desirable because they are confrontational or psychoeducational:

- "What's funny about her being mad at you?"
- "Sometimes, Charles, we smile when we have other feelings that we are not comfortable with sharing."
- "So, what do you do, Charles, to make her mad at you?"

Exercise 4.9. Validation

Suggested Response: A good intervention here picks up on Julia's experience of how tenuous their connection is to validate her feelings of anxiety: "Yes, if it seems to you like anything will set him off, I can understand how you would feel nervous, because he's so important to you."

The less desirable interventions below are misattuned to Julia's emotion and risk alienating her partner.

- "It sounds like the two of you fall into some kind of angry cycle at the end of the day."
- "Yes, Julia, I'm getting that he's very tightly wound, and that certainly isn't acceptable."
- "Yes, I can understand you must feel very angry with him."

Exercise 4.10. Validation With Care

Suggested Response: When the couple is in the heat of a contentious argument, the therapist wants to turn down the temperature by validating both of their perspectives, so each feel seen and heard: "So, for you, Brian, it feels like it's about her doing it better than you do, and I can understand that makes you mad. But for you, Marjorie, there's something here about not feeling included, not a partner, and I get that this is the part that's difficult for you, yes?"

The following less desirable interventions either miss the attachment themes entirely or only validate one side of the argument and thus the other partner will probably not respond well:

- "Yes, Brian, I understand it must be hard for you to get the message that you don't do it right. Can you see where he's coming from, Marjorie?"
- "So, Marjorie, this is about not feeling included and not a partner with him. That must be really painful to not feel included, yes? Can you let him know? Can you tell him how hard that is for you?"
- "Why don't you compromise . . . say, take it in turns?"

Exercise 4.11. Reframing and Attachment Themes

Example (early Stage 1 reframe): "Your anger was about your longing to be there at her side because she is so important to you, is that right?"

Example (later Stage 1 reframe): "But I imagine that you went for her because you felt really left out and abandoned, and that must have been very painful for you."

Exercise 4.12. Catch the Bullet

Suggested Response: A therapist response that exemplifies "catching the bullet" will jump in quickly to de-escalate the aggressiveness and keep the therapeutic process on track. Two suggested responses include

- "What I'm getting is that it's truly hard for you to hear her disappointment, so painful that somehow you move in to stop her."
- "What I'm hearing is that this is hard for you to respond to her tears right now because you have also had hurts in this relationship."

The following responses below are less desirable because they are confrontational and are likely to feed into the negative cycle:

- "Can you just listen to her, right now? She needs for you to understand this."
- "You sound really defensive as you say this to your wife."

Exercise 4.13. Assessing a Couple's Reactive Responses

1. **A**. Sarah is clearly very angry with Aaron.
2. **B**. The therapist simply reflects the difficulty she hears that Sarah has.
3. **B**. The therapist hopes to enter and understand her experience of Aaron's relationship with Ruth.
4. A good response will contain some or all of the following elements:

    - How she is anxious about her place in his life
    - Placing her anger in the context of her anxiety and importance to him
    - How torn he is in this situation
    - How painful this is for both of them

Exercise 4.14. Exploring Negative Cycles

1. C
2. D
3. C
4. C

Exercise 4.14a. Putting Together Emotions and Moves (Within and Between)

This exercise is about the therapist grasping the inner experience of each partner and the moves between them that spiral them into the negative cycle. You will describe and reflect the couple's cycle *to them* many times in Stage 1 to help them experience and internalize it. At a minimum, your cycle descriptions (to yourself and to the couple) should pull together their moves and reactive emotions. For example, one partner becomes angry and critical when triggered, and the other becomes frustrated and defensive in response.

As you move along in Stage 1, your cycle descriptions become richer and more elaborate, including more elements of the cycle. For example, one partner becomes critical when feeling hurt and not wanted and pushes for contact. The other partner then feels anxious and "in trouble" and becomes defensive in an effort explain and calm things down. Notice if the two sides of your description are even. Pursuing partners may provide more information than withdrawing partners initially. You may need to actively make room for withdrawing partners to draw out their experience, but this is important for creating a balanced alliance.

Exercise 4.15. Matching Attachment Strategies

1. D
2. C
3. A
4. B

Exercise 4.16. Assessing Contraindications

1. Questions that explore the history, intensity, and discern the nature of the violence (e.g., bidirectional/unidirectional, related to attachment distress/power and control, frequency, severity in terms of physical injuries) and fear of her partner will help determine the couple's suitability for EFT at the present time. Some sample questions include
   - Would it be okay for us to take some time together to talk about the circumstances around this incident and what exactly happened?
   - In the past, when angry, have either of you ever thrown things, slammed doors, pushed, slapped, grabbed, punched, or choked the other? Are you worried this may happen again?
   - Are you afraid of him? Has he made threats? Are you afraid he will act on his threats?
   - Does he try to control your contact with friends, family, or support systems?

2. **a. Suggested Response**: This client statement is an entry point into Tango Move 1 (reflecting process between and within). The therapeutic goal is to track and explore the cycle that organizes around the wife's drinking: "How do you express your concerns to your wife?" "What do you actually say? . . . And then what happens next?" tracking the play by play of the dance steps. Additionally, depending on the alliance, exploring what triggers the wife's drinking, "When do you find yourself drawn to drink? What's happening in your world?" quite naturally flows into her experience and provides a deeper understanding of what leads the wife to reach for alcohol.
2. **b. Suggested Response:** Here the client is exposing a block in expressing his concern to his wife. The therapeutic goal is to identify the fears underlying this block (e.g., fear of her anger, fear of making the relationship worse) so that he can work through them and with the support of the therapist, bring his fears and concerns about her drinking up in an upcoming conjoint session. Questions such as "What gets in the way of you sharing your concerns? What is your fear of what will happen if you do?" can open the door for further exploration.

5

STAGE 1: DE-ESCALATION AND STABILIZATION

As the emotionally focused therapist establishes a working alliance and makes explicit the negative interactional pattern that fuels the distress in a couple's relationship, a key focus for the therapist is engaging and ordering the emotional experiences that come to define this problem pattern. The reframing of the couple's problem as a negative pattern that is ordered emotionally and understood experientially leads to the de-escalation of this reactive process and couple's stabilization for the couple. This is the key change event of Stage 1 in EFCT.

Following the EFT change process, the focus of sessions is on accessing the unacknowledged emotions underlying interactional positions (e.g., pursuer, withdrawer) and reframing the problem in terms of underlying emotions and attachment needs. The cycle is framed as the source of each partner's emotional distress. Through this stage, the therapist remains focused on the EFT Tango through accessing present moment experience, ordering and deepening emotion, and engaging through encounters new experiences associated with the couple's pattern.

EFT SNAPSHOT: CYCLE DE-ESCALATION

After the initial sessions, Inez and Fernando began to see the cycle of negative interactions had taken over their relationship. Inez experienced Fernando as irritable, unhelpful, and withdrawn, while Fernando found her bossy and "in his face," and he pushed her away. Efforts to connect with one another seemed to lead to bickering, with Inez "puffing up" and shouting at him. Inez had shut down physically and spent more and more time away from the home. The couple settled into separate lives, and following his retirement, Fernando began to realize that his wife was not there for him anymore. They could describe their pattern but not distance from it because it often took hold of them in ways that left them losing hope for their future.

Inez had been feeling ill for three weeks. Her eyes were red and scratchy, and she had a cough and frequent headaches. She wondered if she was developing allergies and decided that she would shampoo the rug in the living room and completely dust the house. Fernando, who was beginning to understand that she was unhappy because he wasn't giving her more help with the household tasks, went to the store to rent the carpet shampoo machine and made a list of all jobs that needed to be accomplished that day. This was clear at the beginning of the couple's fifth session with Jane.

DOI: 10.4324/9781003039457-7

Inez: All I did was ask him when supper would be ready.

Fernando: Well, for God's sake! I hadn't had a moment all day. I was at everyone's beck and call. Inez—for God's sake, I'm trying.

Inez: All I did was ask when supper would be ready. You gave me "the look," and then you went for me. And you haven't spoken to me since.

Fernando: Well, look at the day I had. And I started out by helping you. I got the machine; I did the heavy work. . . .

Therapist: You said you're really trying, Fernando?

Fernando: Yes, I'm trying to stop this cycle. I'm doing things for her, trying to make things work better, but she nags, and I can't stand it.

The couple worked together on the carpet cleaning, when their daughter Angela arrived, and Fernando went off to his study to assist Angela with her taxes, leaving Inez to struggle with the carpet on her own. Inez silently worked alone, becoming more and more angry. Later that day Fernando was again called away by their son Chris, who was having car trouble and needed a ride. Soon after Fernando returned home, and an argument erupted between the partners. Jane catches up with the couple as their pattern takes full effect in session.

Therapist: That's a real hot button for you, Fernando, the nagging, the bossing—what happens for you when you feel she's bossing you?

Fernando: (sounds angry) It's total disrespect. I feel like she thinks I'm subservient . . . nothing.

Therapist: You feel like she thinks you're nothing? Yes, I can understand. That makes you feel angry. (validating secondary emotion)

Fernando: She doesn't value anything I do; it's like she sets the standards, I have to meet them. And I won't do it!

Therapist: So, what happens for you when you get that feeling, like she thinks you're nothing? (evocative response)

Fernando: That upsets me. So, I give out clear signals. Then I shoot and duck.

Therapist: You shoot and duck?

Fernando: Yes. I lash out and then isolate myself to stop getting hurt.

Therapist: So, what I'm getting is, when you feel "bossed" by Inez, you get a painful feeling like she's talking down to you, like she thinks you're nothing, and that really hurts you, yes? That's when you give out your signal to her—is that "the look"?

Fernando: (nods) Yes.

Therapist: So then when you yell and go off to the computer or down to your tool room—that's about protecting yourself from getting hurt?

Fernando: That's right. I get cranky. I get scarce.

Therapist: This is where the cycle takes over, yes? You get the feeling of being disrespected, and suddenly you are caught in your anger. You want to be close, to make her feel you're there for her, but then you get that feeling of disrespect that hurts you, so you "fire away," and then you withdraw to avoid further hurt? (tracking the cycle)

Jane focuses on Fernando's reactive responses, making sense of his experience in the context of the situation and in terms of his experience of their pattern. This begins the shift from talking about a problem to seeing a predictable pattern that organizes a specific moment of distress between the couple. Jane follows the impact of this reactivity on Inez in the present moment and begins to assemble her underlying pain in not knowing she mattered in this relationship and the sadness of being alone in all of this.

Fernando: Yes. It's like I put my armor on and disappear.

Therapist: You put on your armor so that you won't get hurt.

Inez: (angrily) Well, I'm the one that wasn't well yesterday. I needed your help, and you dropped everything and went off with Angela. To heck with me! I'm on my own! No wonder I yell at you.

Therapist: That's what happened for you yesterday, Inez. You got that feeling again, like you're on your own.

Inez: Yes! I don't count. I'm on my own, even in my own family.

Therapist: (RISSSC manner) That must be a very painful place to be, Inez. On your own in your own family.

Inez: (swallows and pauses) I've . . . I've been there for a long, long time. On my own. Even in my own home.

Therapist: (RISSSC manner) For a long time, you've felt unsupported and on your own, even in your own home. And that's been very hard, very painful? (heightening)

Inez: (looks down at her hands; tears well up in her eyes, and she sniffs) I feel unimportant, and I get resentful. (She straightens up.) I'm fed up with it. It makes me mad.

Therapist: Yes, I can understand that. I notice, Inez, as you said that, you looked really sad for a moment. I could feel the sadness, then you kinda sat up tall and said, "I'm fed up with it." Is that where the puffer fish comes in? You puff up and get mad?

Inez: (nods) That's right. I get angry. . . .

Therapist: But on the inside, there's all these tender feelings. . . .

Inez: (looks down at her entwined fingers, pauses, and nods again)

Therapist: It's hard for you to talk about the sadness on the inside? (Inez nods again) Mmm, so here's where the cycle kicks in, and you both are left far away from each other with all these emotions the other doesn't know about. (Fernando and Inez are now calmer, and Fernando reaches out to touch Inez's knee.)

Fernando: I'm sorry, Inez. I'm sorry I didn't tell you Angela was coming over. I clean forgot about it, to be honest with you.

OVERVIEW OF STABILIZATION

In this brief example, Jane focuses on the couples' pattern that disrupts their emotional balance and takes over their relationship. The therapist carefully tracks and punctuates the negative pattern, noting the impact of each partner's actions on the other. Essential to the EFT process is the attention given to each partner's emotional experience at different points of the cycle. The therapist works with each partner to assemble their experience and bring this into focus in the session. Surface emotions are acknowledged and understood, while underlying core emotions are evoked to frame a deeper awareness and felt understanding of the cycle. Note that the couple is able to refer to the cycle as external to their relationship, and the therapist emphasizes the negative impact of the cycle on the couple by highlighting the distance that occurs as a result. In the EFT process of change, the therapist furthers the process of stabilization by focusing on the following two steps.

EFT STEPS: Stage 1, De-escalation and Relationship Stabilization

3. Access the unacknowledged emotions underlying interactional positions.
4. Reframe the problem in terms of the negative, underlying emotions, and attachment needs.

The therapist promotes each partner's ability to tune in to the music of their dance by accessing their underlying emotions. Through exploring the core emotions that are often unspoken or simply unaware to each partner, the therapist ties these experiences into the couple's cycle, thus making explicit the underlying vulnerability that is woven into these interactions. As couples gain a deeper felt understanding of the reoccurring pattern, the cycle becomes predictable and understandable, and seen most clearly through the lens of attachment theory. Attachment provides an emotional logic to the couple's distress and resulting reactive pattern

Key Therapist Moves in Promoting Stabilization

Four key moves are associated with the therapist's work toward stabilization. These shifts result from the therapist focus on Steps 3 and 4 of the EFT process of change when increasing attention is given to the couple's pattern and the emotional experiences that inform its negative hold on the couple. These key moves include validating surface emotions, processing incongruence, assembling underlying emotion, and reframing patterns.

- Accepting and Validating Surface Emotion: As partners increasingly express their surface emotions, the therapist focuses on acknowledging and validating these reactive responses. At the same time, the therapist draws out the experience of the partners as they become more aware of their partner's reactive experiences. For example, while focusing on the numb experience of a withdrawn partner, the therapist explores the experience of his partner as he learns more about this numbing. He begins to see his partner as numb or "frozen" rather than distant and unfeeling.
- Processing Incongruence: A second shift includes the expression of intense or incongruent nonverbal behaviors as the couple moves further into their emotional experience. This may be seen when a partner responds with intense crying or displaying laughing in the face of a partner's blame. As the therapist encounters these nonverbal expressions, the therapy process slows and the therapist connects nonverbal cues with the client's verbalizing of their emotional experience (Tango Move 1). RISSSC manner (i.e. Repetition, Images, Simple, Soft, Slow, Client's words) is used to address intense and incongruous nonverbal responses and begin to deepen emotional awareness and engagement (Tango Move 2).
- Assembling Emotion: A third key move in the process is seen as partners encounter new primary emotional experience and their partners react to this experience by exiting the interaction or discounting the partner's new emotional experience. As the therapist evokes the underlying emotional experience of a partner, the other partner may react to this new awareness by dismissing the other's experience or may simply close off or shut down in response to this information. Therapists respond to this shift by redirecting the session back to exploring the emotional experience of both partners.
- Reframing Patterns: A final shift that is common in Steps 3 and 4 occurs when partners identify the specific pattern of interaction that defines their cycle and negatively impacts their relationship. Here the therapist actively focuses on each partner's position in the cycle and how this cycle functions to defeat even the couple's best attempts to connect. Processing the couples experience as a predictable pattern provides the couple an "emotional logic" for their distress.

Digging Deeper Into Negative Cycles and Interactional Positions

The EFT therapist tunes into statements that describe partner behaviors and attends to the emotion-laden themes they use to describe their experience. These themes often include metaphors or descriptive phrases the therapist can use as "emotional handles" in accessing and deepening experience. Common phrases used by withdrawing and pursuing partners were highlighted in Chapter 4 (see Table 4.1). The therapist uses these "handles" as an entry point to the underlying experience associated with these statements. In the Move 1 of the EFT Tango, the therapist turns to the present moment and invites a partner to make space to explore these emotionally laden experiences. The interpersonal positions of withdraw and pursue are associated with related emotional states. Table 5.1 includes a list of possible emotional experiences associated with a withdrawer or pursuer position.

Table 5.1
Common Underlying Emotions of the Withdrawers and Pursuers

Withdrawers often feel:	**Pursuers often feel:**
Rejected	Hurt
Inadequate	Alone
Afraid of failure	Not wanted
Overwhelmed	Invisible
Numb—frozen	Isolated
Afraid—scared	Not important
Not wanted or desired	Abandoned
Judged, criticized	Desperate
Shame	Disconnected
Empty	Deprived

As the therapist mirrors the present moment (Tango Move 1) with empathic reflection and validation, partners are often more aware and available to explore their underlying experience. A key focus in stabilization is the assembling and deepening of these core emotional experiences (Tango Move 2). This begins with the therapist attunement to the emotional handles that emerge in processing a couple's negative cycle. Jane's session with Inez and Fernando captures a key moment when the therapist shifts focus to Inez's emerging sadness.

Exercise 5.1. Affect Assembly and Deepening

Review the following excerpt from the Jane's session with Inez and Fernando and respond to the questions that follow.

Inez: (angrily) Well, I'm the one that wasn't well yesterday. I needed your help, and you dropped everything and went off with Angela. To heck with me! I'm on my own! No wonder I yell at you.

Therapist: That's what happened for you yesterday, Inez. You got that feeling again, like you're on your own.

Therapist: (RISSSC manner) That must be a very painful place to be, Inez. On your own in your own family.

Inez: (swallows and pauses) I've . . . I've been there for a long, long time. On my own. Even in my own home.

Therapist: (RISSSC manner) For a long time you've felt unsupported and on your own, even in your own home. And that's been very hard, very painful? (heightening)

Inez: (looks down at her hands; tears well up in her eyes, and she sniffs) I feel unimportant, and I get resentful. (She straightens up) I'm fed up with it. It makes me mad.

Therapist: Yes, I can understand that. I notice, Inez, as you said that you looked really sad for a moment. I could feel the sadness, then you kinda sat up tall and said, "I'm fed up with it." Is that where the puffer fish comes in? You puff up and get mad?

1. Emotional Handles. Identify a key phrase or experience you see the therapist focus on to direct Inez toward her underlying experience. ______________________.
2. Identify Inez's surface and core emotions.
   Surface: ______________________.
   Core/underlying: ______________________.
3. Identify examples of the different elements of emotion the therapist uses to assemble Inez's experience.
   Trigger: ______________________.
   Bodily response: ______________.
   Meaning: ______________________.
   Action: ______________________.

Personal Reflection

What stands out to you about the therapist 's focus in this example? What do you see is similar to your work in accessing a partner's underlying emotion?

____

____

____

4. If you were to refocus on Inez's underlying sadness, provide two responses that each focus on a different element of emotion and form a statement or question to Inez that would help begin to own this experience more deeply. (Review examples from Chapter 3 on working with emotion, e.g., empathic conjecture, evocative responding.)
   - ____
   - ____

Exercise 5.2. Exploring Underlying Emotions and Pursue and Withdraw Positions

Now imagine Lynn and Sean, who have a pursue and withdraw pattern in their relationship. The couples often fight over expectations about spending time together. Sean experiences Lynn's efforts to arrange joint activities as controlling and invasive, and Lynn finds Sean's routine insistence for personal time and solitude rejecting. Sean complains that she is dependent on him, and Lynn claims that he is selfish and only interested in himself, not their relationship.

1. How does Sean see Lynn as "the problem" in their relationship? Finish the following sentence using words that he might use. "Things would be better between us if she would just ____________."
2. What surface emotions or actions might you expect Lynn to express in reacting to a moment when Sean abruptly exits dinner for his "man cave"? ____________

   ____

3. Now match Lynn's surface emotion to a possible underlying emotion she might be experiencing, perhaps beyond her awareness. (Refer to Table 5.1 for ideas.)

   ____

4. Would you consider Lynn the pursuer or withdrawer in this interaction? ____________

After asking Sean to help her clean up after dinner, Sean rebuffs her request, muttering under is breath that he needs "a break," and then impatiently offers to clean up later.

5. Now consider how Lynn might see Sean as "the problem" in their relationship? Imagine how Lynne might finish the following sentence using words that she might use. "Things would be better between us if Sean would just ____________."
6. What surface emotion might you expect Sean to have in response? ____________
7. Now match this surface response to a possible underlying emotion Sean might be experiencing, perhaps out of his awareness. (See Table 5.1 for ideas.)

   ____

8. Is Sean in the pursuer or withdrawer position in this interaction? ____________
9. In session, Lynn's frustration grows as Sean defends his needs as "the introvert" in the relationship, and she interrupts with a piercing criticism of his "childish obsession with video games" and utter disappointment as a romantic partner. In tears, she shares: "I am so tired of feeling unwanted and alone in this relationship." (then choking on her words as she looks at him) "I used to feel like I meant something to you, like I was special, but now I feel terrible, especially when you have all these reasons for not wanting to be with me."

   Now label Lynn's responses from her appraisal to action.

   Trigger: Sean defending his need for distance.
   Initial perception: ____________
   Bodily arousal: ____________
   Meaning making: ____________
   Action tendency: ____________

   Create two evocative statements or questions to deepen her emotions in the moment focusing on her bodily arousal, meaning making, or action. Practice forming two statements.

   ____

   ____

   ____

The EFT therapist repeatedly frames the emotional experience underlying each partner's position in attachment-related terms. The use of attachment theory provides a powerful frame for understanding a "connecting purpose" or intention for the problematic interaction cycle. The negative cycles marked by patterns of blame/pursuit and withdrawal/distance can be understood in the context of a couple's search for connection and ways of managing disconnection. These patterns result in a reduction in responsiveness, accessibility, and a loss of felt security in the relationship. As this occurs, a couple's behavior in this cycle becomes automatic and compelling, bringing more attention to the impact of these behaviors and less to the underlying reasons for these actions.

Exercise 5.3. Finding a Connecting Purpose

Reflect back on Inez and Fernando's cycle. What would you hypothesize is a possible "connecting purpose" for Inez's anger?

1. Possible connecting purpose: ________________________________
2. Now create a statement that reflects this possible purpose to reframe the function of her anger in these moments of disconnection. Example: "I wonder if in those moments where you lash out, if part of you is saying I need to make this different to be seen, to protest the loss of connection I feel?"

 ____

 ____

 ____

The power of de-escalation is helping couples uncover the underlying intent of the responses that make up these powerful negative cycles; if only to help couples at this early stage to see that their cycle is evidence of a problematic attempt to connect.

EFT Interventions and Delineating Cycles

The following exercises illustrate a combination of macro- and micro-level EFT interventions. For additional examples of these interventions, please review Chapter 3.

Exercise 5.4. Identifying the Common Interventions Used in Stabilization

The five interventions used most often in cycle de-escalation are listed. Match each of the following interventions to the example that best illustrates the intervention.

a. Validation
b. Evocative responding
c. Heightening
d. Empathic conjecture
e. Reframing problem in cycle

1. "What's it like for you to be in this relationship, always waiting for the bomb to go off? ________
2. "So, when the conflict gets going, it's like you both lose your balance, you do what you do, he does what he does, and in the end you lose each other. It's like the pattern takes over and it's 'here we go again!'" ________
3. "So, for you, his silence is killing you. It makes sense that you need to do something to break through and find out what he is thinking. The silence leaves you fearing the worst." ________
4. "So, you feel cornered. Trapped. Like there is no place to go, no place to run. You want to hide." ________

5. "And when you get angry to get his attention, it's like part of you is mad, and the other part is sad hoping to connect to him." ________

Exercise 5.5. Exploring Interventions and Stabilization

Now we examine how these interventions are used to help a couple access and explore the emotions that underlie their problem pattern. Read the following transcript of a cycle de-escalation event and identify the intervention used by the therapist throughout the session. Select the intervention(s) from the list in Table 5.2 and enter the appropriate intervention in the space provided after each therapist's talk turn. Two spaces are provided when more than one intervention is used.

Table 5.2
EFT Interventions used to Engage and Process Emotional Experience

Engaging Experience	**Processing Experience**
Evocative responses/questions	Empathic reflection
Heightening	Validation
Empathic conjecture	Tracking interactions/patterns
Restructuring	Reframing/catching the bullet

EXAMPLE:

Ingrid: (high-pitched, frantic voice) I just found myself getting so angry and resentful over the weekend; all I could think about was what wasn't done and how she was away having a good time, and I was doing all of the work.

Therapist: That was hard being alone all weekend with the work, and it was frustrating that there you were doing it all alone.

Validation

Tango Move 1: In this section, the therapist focuses on mirroring the present process. Identify the interventions the therapist uses to walk through a reactive moment in Stage 1. Keep in mind some therapist statements may combine more than one intervention.

Ingrid: (high-pitched voice) I wasn't lonely—I enjoyed being on my own. But she has come to expect me to do all the work, and she can just sit back and that's not fair. I don't think she is going to change at all! All I see is more of the same—just more and more examples of things not changing. I don't know if she can really understand what I need or even cares.

Therapist: It must have been especially frustrating. Here you are doing all the work and feeling like it's just one more example of how things aren't changing. You are trying so hard, and it feels like Frances is not doing anything.

1. 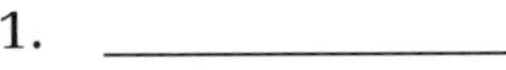

Ingrid: (irritated) I just keep thinking that this is the way it's going to be—I am supposed to do everything, and she doesn't do anything—she's lazy—she will do anything to avoid work. She's not changing—that's the way she wants it!

Therapist: That sounds like it is really frustrating and maybe even scary that maybe there was a part of you that was expecting, hoping that things will be different but then you are not seeing Frances change—and that begins to feel discouraging and hard to hold any hope.

2. ______________

Ingrid: I am not sure I am scared, but why should I change, and she not change at all? She should be changing first! I am the one that supported her in her work—I gave a lot! I gave time and have always been there. I don't see what she's giving. I can't give anymore!

Therapist: You gave a lot to help Frances. I would expect that you, like all of us when we join our lives with someone, had a lot of hopes of sharing your life with her and all kinds of dreams about building a future together with her, like working as a team.

3. ______________

Ingrid: (voice starts to calm) That's it. I don't feel like we are sharing. I am doing everything, and she just goes along for the ride.

Therapist: That is so hard because this is where the cycle takes over. You see yourself alone doing all the work, and Frances is not there. The resentment starts to build, and suddenly you are caught in your anger. You want to share with Frances, but you really don't expect she'll be there, so you up the ante so that she will respond—to which Frances withdraws, shuts down, and she is even more unavailable. Is that how it is?

4. ______________

Ingrid: (starting to tear) Yes, she is nowhere. I never know what is going on with her.

Tango Move 2: Therapist shifts to assemble affect and deepen underlying emotions. This slows the interaction to make space for more vulnerable underlying emotion.

Therapist: (RISSSC manner) That's very painful to you to have your partner but not be able to depend on her—that is a painful place.

5. ______________

Ingrid: I can't do everything. Frances just expects me to swallow it up and not say anything and just carry on like I always do.

Therapist: Hmm . . . so on one hand, you need to be with Frances and share with her. But on the other, it's like you are not supposed to speak or be able to say what you need, and actually the cycle gets in the way of that really happening, getting your needs met. Once it takes hold, you are off and running, and you end up nowhere but frustrated, distant, and alone. (Ingrid responds silently nodding while crying.) What's that like for you? It looks like it hurts a lot.

6. ______________ ______________ ______________

Ingrid: (calmer, softer) It seems like she doesn't want to help. It's just my feeling—maybe it's just a perception. (looking directly at Frances)

Frances: (irritably) That's not the way it is. I just came home. I wanted to relax. You can't expect me to start working the moment I open the door. I just felt like just walking out.

Tango Move 1: Therapist returns focus to Tango Move 1, mirroring the present process with Frances as she defensively responds to Frances' bid.

Therapist: It's hard for you to hear what Ingrid is saying, that she needs your help, needs to feel she can reach for you and get support. She gets scared when she can't, so she pushes. It hard to hear because you looked forward to seeing her, and when you got home, you saw her frustration, and you just wanted to get away?

7. ______________ ______________

Frances: I don't know what she expects. I was going to get around to it, but it doesn't matter what I do, it's wrong—so what's the use?

Therapist: This is a place that you go, Frances, when you are in the cycle, the place where you feel like there is no point. It seems like it doesn't matter what you do; it is wrong, that there is no point in trying. What's that like for you, Frances, when you are in this place? It sounds like an awful place for you.

8. ______________ ______________

Frances: I just want to get as far away as possible. There is no point sticking around. It really doesn't matter if I am around; I will only get it wrong.

Therapist: So, the cycle takes over, and when you see her frustration and disappointment, you just want to get as far away from that as possible, so you don't see it. It sounds like it really bothers you to see Ingrid's frustration, is that right?

9. ______________

Frances: Yeah. I feel kind of useless—to her anyway.

Tango Move 2: Therapist highlights Frances underlying experience, highlighting her feeling of "being useless." In Tango Move 2, the therapist works to access and expand Frances' emotions underlying her protest.

Therapist: (RISSSC manner) This is a really hard place for you, Frances, because when you see Ingrid's disappointment, it has a huge effect on you, and you end up feeling kind of useless, like you'll never get it right.

10. ______________

Frances: (starts to laugh, looking at Ingrid) That pretty well sums it up, right, Ingrid? I am pretty useless.

Therapist: So, you move away because Ingrid's disappointment with you is so hard to bear, not because you don't care, is that right?

11. ____________

Ingrid: You know I never said that. I just want you to help out more and see more of what I need.

Therapist: The cycle has a huge impact on both of you. It gets in the way of you, Ingrid, being able to get your needs met and has you feeling alone. And you, Frances, end up feeling bad about yourself and feeling like the only thing you can do is get away.

12. ____________

Frances: I might as well. It seems like it would be better that way. It's the only thing I can do.

Therapist: Better to get away than to be useless, like you are a deep disappointment or a failure in Ingrid's eyes. That's a painful place to be, yes?

13. ____________

Tango Move 3: Therapist organizes an engaged encounter focusing on Frances's experience of feeling "useless". Notice how the therapist heightens Frances' experience in setting up the encounter.

Therapist: I am wondering, Frances, if you could try to talk to Ingrid about this now. I know it is hard because when we feel like we're kind of useless . . . we do want to go away. We want to hide to protect ourselves. It's hard to stay visible. But could you try and tell Ingrid what it is like for you? How it feels inside?

14. ____________ ____________

Frances: (looking at Ingrid) I don't know how it feels. There are sometimes that I just feel such hate, and I just feel like leaving.

Ingrid: (in frustration) Well, if you feel hate, then we might as well just end it.

Tango Move 4: The therapist processes the experience of the couple as they attempt sharing the more vulnerable experience emerging in the session. The therapist keeps her emotional balance as both partners react and respond to the difficulty of engaging more vulnerable experiences together.

Therapist: It is very hard to talk about feeling kind of useless, especially in front of each other. It's easier lots of time to talk about hate—we feel bigger and stronger that way.

15. ____________ ____________

Frances: It's not that I hate her. There is such a feeling of hate. I am not sure if she even wants me. She would be better off without me.

Therapist: There is the overwhelming bad feeling that you can't please Ingrid, and you end up feeling that Ingrid doesn't want you.

16. ____________

Frances: (looking at Ingrid) You never touch me. I go to you for hugs and cuddling, and you never come to me.

Ingrid: That part of me has just shut down. I can't be close physically when there is nothing happening anywhere else.

Therapist: I know you need to protect yourself that way, Ingrid, but for you, Frances, it feels pretty painful not to be wanted or desired by your partner, and maybe you end up feeling that it is you, that maybe you are not worth much or even kind of useless in Ingrid's eyes?

17. ____________ ____________

Frances: (nodding, looking at Ingrid) Do you even love me?

Ingrid: I don't know how I feel these days. I feel like you are just making an excuse—an excuse for not doing anything.

Therapist: Frances, that takes a lot of strength and courage to ask how Ingrid feels, and it seems like this is a painful place for you, not to feel the love and wanting coming from Ingrid, and it seems like it is very hard, Ingrid, for you to hear and take in what Frances is saying now, maybe because it is too hard to believe that Frances actually cares about being connected to you. Now what I have heard you saying is that you do want her, you actually want more of her, more of her to depend on, to count on and not to feel so alone.

18. ____________ ____________ ____________

Ingrid: But I am not sure she wants to do it. Maybe she's just not capable. She's never had any successful relationships.

Therapist: It's hard to trust that she really wants to be there for you, that she really wants this relationship, this partnership, and that you are truly not alone.

19. ____________

Ingrid: I don't trust her. She has taught me not to trust her.

Therapist: It is so hard to even begin to trust her—you have been so disappointed in the past, that has really hurt, yes? I wonder if Frances has any idea how hurt you feel. I would expect that she doesn't know.

20. ____________ ____________

Ingrid: She doesn't want to know, and she just shuts me down.

Therapist: It's hard to think that she would even want to know how hurt you are, especially when the cycle takes over because all you see is Frances going away and not being there for you.

21. ______________ ______________

Ingrid: (starting to cry) I can't depend on her. She's not there. I feel so alone.

Therapist: What are you feeling, Frances? The look on your face looks like this bothers you to see Ingrid in such pain.

22. ______________

Frances: Well, it hurts. I don't want to see her so hurt.

Therapist: Can you tell her that?

23. ______________

Frances: I don't want you to feel so hurt. You've got to give me a chance. I am trying. I move away when I feel hopeless, like I'll never please you.

Ingrid: (looking intently at Frances) I don't know if you can.

Therapist: But Frances is here, and so are you, Ingrid, and you both are trying and struggling, the cycle pushes you apart and doesn't let you see each other, but I get a sense that you both want the same thing, to be close and be there for each other—yes?

24. ______________

Frances: I am trying. I will try.

Ingrid: We have to make time for each other. I don't want you to feel useless.

Tango Move 5: The therapist summarize the cycle reframe to consolidate a new experience of the couple's effort to face their distress and disconnection together through seeing their predictable pattern and the emotions that drive it.

Therapist: Time is important, but it seems like the cycle convinces you that you really aren't there for each other. But what you did tonight with Ingrid sharing a bit of her hurt and Frances seeing that and Frances being more verbal about where she is at—all this helps you, Ingrid, know more what is going on with her. I would expect it helps you to be able to see a bit of what is happening for her. That was great for both of you; you really worked hard tonight and took some risks, which isn't easy.

25. ______________ ______________

Reframing Interactional Patterns

The therapist can reframe the more anxious and preoccupied partner's pursuit and attacks as attempts to close the distance they experience and at the same time note the ways these reactions tend to drive away their partner, providing evidence to that partner that it is not safe to be close. The therapist can reframe the withdrawal of the more avoidant or ambivalent spouse as a response to help regulate the intensity of the emotional experience and calm down the relationship. Expression of emotion is then blunted, and positive and negative affect is reduced, which only tends to escalate the anxious pursuer's efforts to promote an emotional response to her or his concerns. The therapist's use of an attachment perspective provides a logical frame for the couple's cycle and its relationship to both their desire to connect and the negative experience that results when they cannot.

The therapist may use one of the following themes to reframe the partner's position in the negative interaction cycle. These include:

- "Fighting Against the Enemy": The therapist frames the cycle as the enemy who intrudes into the couple's relationship and takes over, keeping the couple from the closeness the couple seeks.
- "Fighting for the Connection": The therapist frames the cycle as a struggle to find a safe place in the relationship. Attachment needs are validated as the therapist paints a picture of the couple's cycle as a response to each partner's attempts to close the distance in their relationship. The therapist may use a separate frame for the pursuing partner and a different frame for the withdrawing partner.
- "Protecting the Relationship": The therapist frames the response of the withdrawing partner as an effort to protect the relationship from potentially damaging emotions or emotions that would overwhelm the relationship. The withdrawal is recognized as a protective response to a situation that may increasingly feel "out of control" emotionally.
- "Protesting the Loss of Connection": The therapist frames the response of the pursuing or attacking partner as a protest to the loss of connection and the perceived unavailability of the other. The intensity of the pursuit or attack becomes a way of getting the partner's attention or demanding a response. In attachment terms, any response is better than none. No response translates into the sense that one does not matter to the other and cannot impact the other. One is alone, and loss and isolation become tangible realities.

By the end of Steps 3 and 4, each partner will identify the habitual position that he or she takes in the relationship. Each will have also touched some of their inner world underlying this position and begun to understand their relationship in attachment terms. The negative cycle is framed as the enemy and block to partners connecting with each other in an intimate way.

Exercise 5.6. Identifying a Cycle Theme

Thinking back on Inez and Fernando's negative interactional cycle, respond to the following question.

1. Identify which theme best fits Fernando's surface emotional responses.
   a. Fighting against the enemy

b. Fighting for connection
c. Protecting the relationship
d. Protesting a loss of connection

2. How might you share this theme with Fernando and validate the connecting purpose of his reactive responses?

____

____

____

____

The EFT therapist facilitates a shift from the couple's focus on problems to a focus on the cycle of interaction by attending to the following actions. Through carefully tracking and reflecting the couple's problematic pattern of interaction, the therapist creates a non-blaming description of the couple's cycle. Using simple and straightforward descriptions, the therapist frames this pattern in the language of the clients. The therapist reflects the perception of the partners (e.g., "You see him as not really trying or even wanting to change") as well as the impact of each partner's actions on the other (e.g., "And when she does not respond, it is like she doesn't care or she's scary to you"). As the therapist maps the different moves in the couple's pattern, she clarifies the cycle by first working with one partner and then shifting to the other's experience. The cycle is framed as the enemy that takes over the couple's relationship, reducing the security of the relationship. Identifying the cycle helps the couple recognize the self-reinforcing pattern that provides a basis for engaging the primary emotions underlying this patterned behavior and placing it into an attachment frame. These interventions help the couple to externalize the problem so that the cycle becomes the focus rather than either partner. The couple experiences more safety in their relationship as a result. The process of cycle de-escalation is described in the following case illustration.

Stabilization: Exploring a Withdraw/Withdraw Cycle

Cycle de-escalation with a couple that is in a withdraw/withdraw cycle can look different from the more typical pursue/withdraw cycle. The quality of the interaction is different in that fights are less frequent and less intense; there may be less lovemaking, as there is an emotional disengagement. This relationship is characterized by conflict avoidance behaviors by both partners. The couple frequently have developed a reliance on recourses outside of the relationship to provide emotional sustenance, for example, children, friends, extended family, hobbies, and work. A variation on the withdraw/withdraw cycle is a "burnt-out pursuer," which can occur in long-term marriages in which one partner has been a pursuer but has given up that position and has come to rely on a more withdrawn stance as well. This type of withdraw/withdraw is flavored with feelings of resignation, defeat, and hopelessness.

Tracy and Adam, a couple in their early 30s, were married for ten years and did not have any children. They had successful careers in the same industry, which required a fair amount of travel. The presenting issue was that the couple had not had sexual relations since they had married, and this was now an issue because Tracy wanted to have children. In the first sessions, the therapist worked to establish an alliance with both partners and to alleviate some of the shame that they were both feeling about their problem by normalizing and placing the issue in the context of their cycle.

Tracy and Adam were caught in a withdraw/withdraw pattern as both had avoided addressing their lack of sexuality but continued to function well together as housemates and colleagues and within their family and social circle. They did not report any fights but that there might be some "tension" or silence between them that would wear off over time and after which they would be "good friends" again. At the point of therapy, Tracy was ambivalent about whether to stay in this relationship or pursue her goal of becoming a mother with another partner. Adam, for his part, wanted to save the marriage and was relieved that they were beginning to talk about their sex life, which had been so hard for them to talk about before.

Adam: I think things are going a lot better. We have been able to talk about this subject, which was so hard for us to talk about before. It is great that it's now out in the open, and we can do something about it.

Tracy: I agree. Just coming here was so hard to do. I didn't think I could do it and never expected that Adam would either. It's like we have finally taken the skeleton out of the closet.

Therapist: That was very difficult, and it took a lot of courage to talk to each other and me and admit out loud with a witness that this was a problem. It is a very hard thing to do for most people. (validation)

Adam: Well, I think it has helped a lot—we seem to be getting along better, talking more just about day-to-day stuff. Don't you think? (looking to Tracy)

Tracy: Yes, we are talking a bit more. We just couldn't do this before. We were just so busy with work. There were always more important things to attend to with our house and families. We did a lot in our time together, helping out my family, your mother, and all our traveling. We lead very busy lives.

Therapist: What's that like then to get this out in the open and to be able to talk more? How does that feel? (evocative responding)

Tracy: We have always got along fairly well. I know a lot of couples that all they do is fight. But that's not our style. We are very considerate of each other.

Adam: We are good friends, and we have a lot of friends. All my friends like Tracy, and the same goes for her friends. We never lack for things to do or people to hang out with. We keep busy.

Therapist: One thing that we have talked about so far is how the two of you were stuck in a cycle where you would avoid talking about things that were painful or where you thought the other person might get hurt and that a strategy that you both took was to kind of close your eyes and hope that it would go away. (framing the problem in terms of the cycle)

Tracy: But that is only part of our relationship. Sex isn't everything, and we have a lot of other things that are going well for us. We could never have got where we have if we had been arguing all the time.

Adam: I know I don't like an argument and just found it so easy to get along with Tracy. We enjoy a lot of things together and have a lot of the same interests.

Therapist: You have a lot of strengths as a couple and a bond that has kept you together for ten years, but I had also understood that you were at a crossroad in your relationship, that you needed to look at the lack of intimacy and how that was affecting you and how it was standing in the way of your future. Have I got that right or maybe I am off track? (refocusing; framing the problem in terms of the cycle)

Tracy: No, you're right. It's just so hard to talk about it. I would rather just go on and ignore it sometimes. I am afraid I am not up to it—there is a lot of other stress in my life. There is a lot going on at work right now.

Therapist: Maybe one thing the cycle has convinced you of is that it is hard to depend on your relationship to talk about things that are difficult. Yet they are things that are important to your relationship, the intimate things about sharing yourselves with each other. It's so tempting to rely on the old "let's sweep it under the carpet" and see if it will all go away. (reframing the problem in terms of the cycle)

Adam: I know I did that. I kept thinking that this is just going to get better, or I wouldn't think about it at all. It was too hard.

Therapist: It was hard to think that you were not making love to your wife and that this had gone on for a long time and it wasn't getting better? (empathic conjecture; mirroring the present process)

Adam: Yes. How could I do that? How could I let it go so long? I can't figure out what is wrong with me.

Therapist: Sounds like you end up feeling bad about yourself. (evocative reflection)

Adam: What else can I think? What other man would let this happen?

Therapist: It must be very hard then to think about or talk about when you end up feeling so bad about you. The feeling bad kept you stuck, stuck in the cycle. (evocative responding)

Adam: There was lots of time I just never thought about it at all.

Therapist: You had a way of putting it away in a compartment, so it didn't penetrate and you could protect yourself from feeling bad that way. (evocative responding)

Tracy: I wouldn't say that I ever saw him feeling bad. He sure didn't come off that way—we got along so well.

Therapist: It's kind of a mystery to you Tracy to hear about these feelings when the cycle blocked the two of you from really talking about your feelings. (validation)

Tracy: I never thought there was any point to talking about feelings. I knew it would just start an argument, and why rock the boat? There was so much going well for us.

Exercise 5.7. Mirroring the Present Process

1. How would you describe each partner's avoidance? Practice formulating an empathic reflection using: "when/then."

   Tracy:

   ____

   Adam:

   ____

2. Framing the couple's interaction as a cycle, provide a summary that connects the trigger to the action tendencies.

   ____

   ____

   ____

   ____

Exercise 5.8. Reframing a Partner's Avoidance

1. What is an attachment theme that describes Tracy's avoidance?

   ____

2. Form an empathic conjecture that points to the emotion underlying her action tendency to avoid "rocking the boat."

   ____

3. Now practice reframing Tracy's avoidance by summarizing her action and attachment them with her underlying emotion.

   ____

Now let's follow the therapist working with this pattern to move toward each partner's underlying emotion and the fear that maintains their cycle of avoidance.

Therapist: But to not have your husband hold you in his arms and for you to share with him your most special intimate self, how was that? It must have been hard, yes? (heightening, empathic conjecture)

Tracy: I got used to it. Actually, it started to feel kind of strange to do anything different— I mean who wants to kiss their brother? I am sorry, but that is how it came to feel.

Therapist: It sounds like that part of you, that special intimate part kind of got lost and that you have lost touch with those feelings in relation to Adam. How is that for you to hear that, Adam? (empathic conjecture)

Adam: (quiet and downcast) It's understandable. What else could you expect? It's been a long time.

Therapist: You look so sad when you say that, Adam. Is that how you feel? (empathic conjecture)

Adam: Well, it is hard to hear that your wife doesn't feel anything for you. I haven't lost that feeling.

Therapist: Can you look at Tracy and tell her that? (restructuring interaction, Tango Move 3)

Adam: You know I never stopped wanting you. I just didn't know how or what to do. After we stopped and then it seemed like you didn't want me, I didn't know how to get started again, and the longer it went on, the harder it got. I got so stuck there. I couldn't move.

Tracy: I find that hard to believe. You haven't made any attempts to be close to me, and I see how you look at other women—that certainly doesn't make me feel like you want me.

Therapist: That's hard to believe that Adam actually feels that way toward you, that he wants to be close and that he really desires you. It just gets so scary to face the fears that you "didn't want: him. (validation, Move 4, processing the interaction)

Tracy: It's hard to believe and also kind of weird feeling. It's hard to imagine that we could be any other way than the way we are. This just is the way we are, and I just wonder if maybe I should just be satisfied with what I have and look at all the positives in my life.

Therapist: Maybe it's even scary to imagine you in each other's arms. Maybe it seems awkward and weird and maybe even a little "abnormal" now. The cycle has prevented you both from looking at this and talking about this sooner, and the longer it went on, the harder it became for both of you. For you, Adam, it seemed to be a kind of frozen paralysis—that you didn't know what to do or how to approach Tracy. For you, Tracy, the cycle kind of froze your feelings of desire for Adam. The longer it went on, the more stuck you got, and the more distant the two of you became. It got to the point where it felt like you were more brother and sister than husband and wife. Is that how it feels? (validation, tracking the pattern)

The challenge to the therapist working with a couple in a withdraw/withdraw pattern is to block the couple's avoidance strategies without overwhelming them. The EFT therapist relies on a strong alliance that provides resources for safety and the security for the couple to begin to explore the more difficult emotions that are threatening to their sense of emotional balance. The therapist's confidence that this is a process that can lead to greater intimacy for the couple helps the couple to take greater risks in moving away from the cycle of withdraw/withdraw to a more engaged and responsive relationship.

Exercise 5.9. Following the Process of De-escalation

Bob and Sharon frequently argue about the couple's financial struggles. Both agreed that Sharon would manage the family finances. Bob is critical of Sharon's approach to handling the money and frequently challenges her decisions. Sharon experiences Bob as critical and hostile about finances but otherwise disengaged in their relationship. The therapist has helped the couple identify a common pattern in which Bob criticizes Sharon's financial decision making, and she responds with defensive silence and then later cross complains about his lack of commitment to the family. Bob then backs away further, and she escalates her efforts to get him to respond. He retaliates by blaming her for the family's financial problems, saying in the end that it is simply "All her fault, and she can't handle that."

In session, Sharon replayed a recent argument.

Sharon: I just get so frustrated that he asks me to pay a bill and then he is relentless in checking to see if I have paid it. It doesn't matter if I say I will pay it; he is after me till I pay it. But if I ask him for help around the house, I am "nagging" and "insensitive to the demands of his work." I am sick of him expecting me to do what he says and him not caring a bit about what I want or what I need. He can be a jerk sometimes.

Now as the therapist, follow the process of de-escalation. First reflect Sharon's secondary or surface emotion and then validate Sharon's present emotional experience.

1. As the therapist, write a statement using Sharon's comments that will reflect her surface emotions, including a statement validating her experience within the cycle. ________________

   ____

   ____

   As the therapist validates Sharon's anger, she notices Bob turning away and closing off from the conversation. He folds his arms and looks at the floor.
2. Now as the therapist, how would you bring Bob's emotional experience into the room?

   Form an evocative question that will help Bob connect his withdrawn posture to his emotional experience in the couple's cycle.

   ____

   ____

   ____

   Next, the therapist works to engage the underlying experience of each partner.
3. Using empathic reflection, how would you invite Bob and Sharon to connect the trigger to their reactive responses (i.e., surface emotions) in this interaction?

   ____

   ____

   ____

   Now imagine Sharon responds: "Yeah, I just want him to stop. To look at me. To see me, not the checkbook. Why can't he see it? He just doesn't get it. His money is more important than me."
4. What is her underlying core emotion? ________
5. Put into words how you would reflect her emotional experience focusing on Sharon's underlying emotion framing this reflection in the context of the cycle. Be sure to include an attachment theme for her self-protective actions.

____

____

____

Bob responds: "I just don't know what to do with all her anger. It is just too much, and she seems to take all this so personally. Frankly, it confuses me why she responds this way, and I don't know how to make it better or to convince her otherwise. I am so confused on how to make a difference in these moments."

6. What is Bob's underlying emotion? ______________
7. Put into words how you would reflect Bob's emotional experience focusing on his underlying emotion, framing this reflection in the context of the cycle.

____

____

____

Bob agrees and opens up further to his fear. As he talks, he shifts the conversation from his fear in the relationship to his fear that Sharon will make poor financial decisions and that he can't rely on her at this point.

8. What would you say to Bob to help him refocus on his fear and vulnerability?

____

____

____

9. What would you say to Sharon if she responded to Bob's vulnerability by dismissing his fear by saying: "Yes, we have missed a few payments, but we have never been in real financial trouble." What would you say to Sharon to help her refocus on her hurt?

____

____

____

Once the therapist refocuses the couple, the therapist returns to describe the couple's cycle and their positions in the cycle. Follow the therapist's framing of the cycle and then answer the questions that follow.

Therapist: So, when this argument gets going, Bob, you raise concern about how Sharon is handling the money, and she hears you being critical, like you don't trust her. And then, Sharon, you respond to his questions by telling him that things are okay and he need not worry. Bob, you hear her dismissing your concern and find ways to support your concern by bringing up past problems. Then Sharon feels attacked and responds by questioning whether you care more about her or the money. Bob, you then back away, not knowing how to respond to her anger, and, Sharon, you find yourself even more upset because he doesn't seem to care because he is not responding, and you use more anger and sharper words to get his attention. It's like you are fighting for your connection to Bob in these moments. This can lead Bob breaking his silence with another attack to push you away and Sharon you leave feeling like he has given up. He then withdraws again, leaving you alone. Do I have a sense of what happens in this cycle?

Bob: Yeah, that's it. I mean, I don't want it to go that way, but that is what happens.

Sharon: Sometimes it just feels out of control, like we end up in the same place no matter how hard we try to avoid it.

Therapist: So, this cycle, this dance you get caught in, pulls you both apart and leaves you confused, frustrated, and alone. And I get the sense that you both are looking for something else, some way to do this together, not alone, to not be divided by this cycle.

10. As the therapist in this moment, what would you do next. Choose the options that make sense to you. (mark all that apply—more than one answer is correct).
    a. Teach the couple about the relationship of negative affect to problem cycles. _____
    b. Refocus on Bob's intention and desire to not fall into the cycle. _____
    c. Validate Sharon's experience and focus on her sense of being "out of control." _____
    d. Invite the couple to process what it is like to see this experience together (e.g., making sense of their cycle), including the attachment motivations in the actions of each partner. _____
    e. Reflect and engage Sharon's sense of feeling out of control in these moments and the couple easily being divided by the power of the cycle. _____
    f. Focus on problem solving and financial decision making with the couple. _____

11. From and EFT perspective, which of the following is most likely true for this couple? (mark all that apply—more than one answer is correct).
    a. The couple's struggle to resolve financial difficulties is informed by the blocks to accessibility, responsiveness, and emotional engagement between the partners. _____
    b. The couple's emotional dissatisfaction and distress is best addressed by coaching problem-solving strategies related to finances. _____
    c. The lack of felt security in the relationship partners to rely on secondary attachment strategies (avoidance, anxious responding) to regain a sense of their emotional balance. _____
    d. Therapist assessment of patterns of power and coercion is essential in determining the appropriateness of conjoint treatment and assurance of the safety necessary to conduct EFT with this couple. _____

Exercise 5.10. Reviewing Cycle De-escalation

Select the best answer from options below.

1. The EFT therapist promotes cycle de-escalation by relating a couple's underlying emotions and attachment strategies to
   a. Surface emotions. _____
   b. Couple's presenting problem. ____
   c. Positions that each partner takes in the cycle. ____
   d. Automatic thoughts of each partner. ____
2. The process of accessing emotion in EFT includes
   a. Labeling feeling to help partners change their behavior. ____
   b. Venting emotions to diminish their effect in the relationship. ____
   c. Interpreting quality of emotional experience and possible splitting. ____
   d. Active engagement of emotional experience in the here and now. ____
3. Which of the following are signs of cycle de-escalation?
   a. Negative interactions are contained, and couples are able to exit cycles on their own. ____
   b. Partners are aware and understand the attachment issues that inform their and the partner's actions in the cycle. ____
   c. Couples are able to have conversations about vulnerable emotions and how they relate to their negative interactional pattern. ____
   d. Partners are more likely to have a more positive view of their partner recognizing the problem is the pattern rather than their partner. ____
   e. All of the above. ____

SUMMARY

In this chapter, we reviewed how the EFT therapist accesses unacknowledged emotions and fills in the picture of the couple's negative interactional pattern by accessing and expanding attachment-related emotions and needs. Processing these more vulnerable experiences in the context of the couple's predictable cycle begin to redefine the problem as the pattern that a couple can face together. New experiences of vulnerability also promise new opportunities for connection between partners. As partners are able to take greater risks together, new opportunities for closeness emerge; however, these moments often remain challenged by self-protective strategies that reinforce each partner's accessibility and responsiveness to emotion and vulnerability, particularly when it matters most.

ANSWERS AND SUGGESTED RESPONSES

Exercise 5.1. Affect Assembly and Deepening

1. **Suggested handles:** "on my own in my own home," "unimportant"

2. Surface: Anger, frustration, resentment

   Core: Hurt, sad, fear
3. Trigger: Fernando's leaving her alone

   Bodily Response: Tears, Looking away, swallows experience

   Meaning: "I am unimportant," I do not matter

   Action: "Puffs up and get mad." "Puffer fish."
4. **Suggested Responses**

   Meaning: As you say "I am alone in my own home," what happens in your heart? What's that like to be you in that moment?

   Bodily Response: Just now you swallowed hard as this sadness came up. Where does that sadness go? Where do you feel your sadness?

   Action: And when you feel unimportant and resentful what do you do?

Exercise 5.2. Exploring Underlying Emotions and Pursue and Withdraw Positions

1. **Suggested Response:** "Things would be better between us if she just let me do my own thing. She is always on me. There's just no space in this relationship. She is never happy even when I spend time with her."
2. **Suggested Responses:** Frustration, anger, alarm, despair
3. **Suggested Responses:** Hurt, alone, unwanted, abandoned, not important
4. **Answer:** Pursuer
5. **Suggested Response:** "Things would be better between us if Sean just see me and shows he cares. He is so preoccupied with his work and all the stress that comes with it, and then when he comes home, he disappears. That's all he cares about. It's like I don't exist in his world, and he is full of excuses for why he needs to be alone and not there for me."
6. **Suggested Responses:** Checks out, goes numb, avoids and goes silent, argues logically from an emotional distance.
7. **Suggested Responses:** Rejected, overwhelmed, afraid, shame, judged
8. **Answer:** Withdrawer
9. Lynn's emotional response

   Initial Perception: Alarm, desperation
   Bodily Arousal: Tears, choking back emotion
   Meaning: "I'm unwanted, not special, not precious or valuable
   Action: Critical attack

   Possible evocative statements or questions

   Bodily Arousal: "This is so difficult, so painful. As you choke back your tears, what happens inside of you in this moment? Where does the pain go?"

Meaning: "What's it like to say these words: 'I was special. I meant something to you. Now you don't want me.'" Action: "So you anger comes out full force in this moment, you need him to see this. This needs to matter? Am I getting what this is like for you?"

Exercise 5.3. Finding a Connecting

Purpose

1. **Suggested Response:** Inez is protesting Fernando's lack of responsiveness and dismissal of her needs. She is fighting to be seen and to know she matters in Fernando's world.
2. **Suggested Response:** Inez, your anger is like an alarm bell. It's an urgent call for Fernando to see what is happening between the two of you. It like the only way you can do something different when he is not seeing you and is going away? It's like you are fighting for connection in these moments that leave you alone and unwanted.

Exercise 5.4. Identifying the Common Interventions Used in Stabilization

1. **b**. Evocative Response/Question
2. **e**. Reframing problem in terms of the cycle
3. **a**. Validation
4. **c**. Heightening
5. **d**. Empathic conjecture

Exercise 5.5. Exploring Interventions and Stabilization: Ingrid and Frances

1. Evocative reflection/responding
2. Evocative reflection
3. Heightening
4. Reframing the problem as the cycle.
5. Evocative responding and tracking the cycle
6. Evocative reflection/responding
7. Tracking and validation
8. Tracking and evocative responding
9. Reframing in context of cycle
10. Empathic conjecture
11. Empathic conjecture
12. Reframing the problem in terms of the cycle
13. Restructuring with an enactment and validation
14. Reframing "catching the bullet" and validation
15. Empathic conjecture
16. Reframing and empathic conjecture

17. Tracking the cycle, empathic conjecture, validation
18. Empathic conjecture
19. Validation, empathic conjecture
20. Tracking and heightening
21. Evocative responding
22. Evocative question and empathic conjecture
23. Reframing the problem in the cycle
24. Reframing and empathic conjecture
25. Reframing and validation

Exercise 5.6. Identifying a Cycle Theme

1. **Suggested Response:** Different themes could apply in reframing Fernando's response to Inez's demanding responses. Fernando puts on his armor, shoots, and then ducks. He attacks and then avoids going away to protect himself in these moments from what he perceives as Inez's disrespect and disappointment in him. Inez becomes like a "puffer fish" when she feels abandoned or unwanted. Two themes appear most relevant in reframing this attack/attack interaction. First, the therapist could reframe their pattern as a fight for connection in which each lashes out when the response of the partner is hurtful. In similar ways, they are each fighting to be seen by the other (answer **B**). Alternatively, the therapist could also use the theme of fighting against the enemy or the cycle when the demands that they both feel in the relationship take over and this gets in the way of each of them finding the other with what they need most (answer **A**).
2. **Suggested Responses: B**. When the cycle takes over, you both find yourself caught in this struggle to be seen, both of you making efforts that don't seem to matter or count. You both fight to be seen when you feel unwanted or disrespected and want the other to know what is happening for you. It's like you are both fighting for something different, fighting to find your connection. **A**. When the demands go up in your relationship, you can easily find yourself on opposite sides with the cycle taking over. When, Fernando, you are hoping Inez sees your efforts to make things better and, Inez, you want Fernando to see you and the impact of the needs that can become overwhelming. You both are fighting against the cycle that leaves you alone and without the support of the person you need most.

Exercise 5.7. Mirroring the Present Process

1. **Suggested Response**

   Tracy: "When there is tension or a difficult conversation coming up with Adam, then you are more likely to ignore this or move to a different topic rather than getting into the difficulty and distress."

   Adam: "When things get difficult for both of you, like the issue of lovemaking, then you are more likely to go on assume that the tension will get better or maybe even go away."
2. **Suggested Response.** Both of you seem to appreciate that you can get along and stay away from conflict and arguing, which makes things seem more safe but not

more close. It's like this cycle of avoidance or escape that takes over in moments when there is a concern or trouble and then you each move away in your own directions trying to keep the peace but losing sight of the other and what really matters to both of you"

Exercise 5.8. Reframing a Partner's Avoidance

1. **Protecting the relationship.** Tracy moves away from conflict in the relationship, fearing that getting into a conversation about their feelings would lead to an argument. Instead, she would protect the relationship by not "rocking the boat" and sharing her disappointment and discouragement.
2. **Empathic conjecture.** In those moments, Tracy, it's almost like there is one part of you can see there is difficulty ahead; if we open the conversation to our emotions, this will "rock the boat," things will get difficult between us, so you turn away. And yet I wonder if there is also another part of you that really longs to go toward this challenge with Adam to somehow face the difficulty together but it's just so hard because there is so much at stake. Am I getting it?
3. **Reframing.** It makes sense Tracy that you turn away from this difficulty, avoid rocking the boat, to protect your relationship and turn away from the hard conversations and the fears that seem to have grown so big between both of you. This leaves you both stuck unable to move forward fearing to risk that which really matters.

Exercise 5.9. Following the Process of Cycle De-escalation

1. **Suggested Response:** "So you are frustrated, even angry, that Bob is after you about the bills, but he doesn't seem to see you, doesn't seem to hear your needs. And it makes sense that you would feel angry and hurt that he is not there for you, like the bills are more important than you. Is that it?"
2. **Suggested Response:** "Bob I wonder what is going on for you as you hear Sharon. It seems like you are pulling back, like this is too much, and you can't take it, or don't want to take this. So, you close off."
3. **Suggested Response:** "So, when these financial issues come up, Sharon, you hear Bob's concerns as an attack, and you get angry because there seems to be no way to please him. And, Bob, when she responds, you, too, see this as an attack, and you shut down and close off and stay out of her emotional reach."
4. Hurt
5. **Suggested Response:** "Bob's concern for the money comes across as criticism, and that makes you angry, but more than that, you feel alone, like he has chosen money over you, like you don't mean as much, like you do not matter, and that hurts?"
6. Helplessness/fear
7. **Suggested Response:** "So it's confusing, all this anger. You get lost in it all. You pull away. You are frustrated, lost, with nothing you can do. Like you feel helpless when this happens. Like things are out of control, leaving you vulnerable, and that is hard for you?"

8. **Suggested Response:** "What would it be like to tell her that it is hard for you to feel like things are out of control and that sometimes these financial issues leave you feeling vulnerable, and that is a hard place for you to be?"
9. **Suggested Response:** "And it is difficult to hear this; on the one hand, you hear him saying that it would be different if you handled the money better, but at another level, it's not about the money and how you handle it. It's about you, and that hurts? It's hard for him to trust you, and that hurts."
10. **B, C, D, and E**. Each of these responses focuses on the process of the couples' relationship. The EFT therapist is a process consultant and organizes the experience of the couple to provide a different experience of the relationship, one that moves from a focus on threat to one enabling a focus on vulnerability.
11. **A, C, and D**. Items A and C point to the pivotal role of felt security in couples' ability to share mutual influence in negotiating family tasks, including financial decision making. Bob and Sharon's negative interactional pattern confounds their ability to face the fears each share about the uncertainties of the financial situation. Financial decisions can be a source of power and coercion in a couple's relations, and the couple therapist must continue assess possible contraindication for conjoint treatment.

Exercise 5.10. Reviewing Cycle De-escalation

1. **C**. The EFT therapist makes explicit the ways in which underlying emotions and attachment strategies inform the predictable positions partners take in negative interactional cycles.
2. **D**. The EFT therapist assembles affect and deepens experience through the active engagement of emotional experience in the present moment. The macro-interventions of the EFT Tango highlight the process of working through emotional experience both within and between partners.
3. **E**. All of these descriptions serve as markers or evidence of de-escalation for couples in the EFT process.

6

STAGE 2: WITHDRAWER RE-ENGAGEMENT

In this chapter, we focus on withdrawer re-engagement, which is the first of two change events that define the process of restructuring attachment bonds in Stage 2 of emotionally focused therapy (EFT). Withdrawer re-engagement results when a previously withdrawn partner shares their attachment needs and wants from an emotionally engaged relational position. This partner experiences and asserts a newly discovered, often intense desire for a safe and secure connection with the other partner. In Stage 2, the therapist skillfully relies on the use of new emotional experience and expression to change interactional positions and restructure attachment bonds. Following the EFT Tango, these change events underscore the power and importance of engaged encounters (Move 3) and processing the impact of these moments (Move 4). Still at the heart of Stage 2 works is the assembly and deepening of emotion (Move 2) with a more explicit focus on each partner's attachment related needs. Each "partner now speaks from a position of increased efficacy, where he defines the relationship for himself, rather than reacting to the other's definitions" (Johnson, 2020, p. 171). As partners share more and more of their experiences in an emotionally accessible manner, these moments of sharing become the bonding moments necessary to restructure their bond, the goal of Stage 2.

EFT SNAPSHOT: WITHDRAWER ENGAGEMENT

Inez, the withdrawer, and Fernando had some close times following the last session, and as the therapist had suggested, discussed key elements of the previous session. They also began having a date night each week and reported increased closeness. At the beginning of their next session, Fernando reported that he was feeling "frustrated" with the therapy process. Note how the therapist draws attention to Inez's experience in the present moment and uses this to assemble her experience that then leads to a more engage emotional encounter. This represents a step in the withdrawer's move to greater re-engagement.

Fernando: I thought we were doing really well, getting better—you know, closer. Happier. But I don't know anymore. We're on a retirement budget, and these sessions are a stretch for us.

Therapist: Sounds like you're feeling discouraged, Fernando?

Fernando: Well, I just wonder if we've come as far as we can.

DOI: 10.4324/9781003039457-8

Therapist: Hmm. You sound a little disappointed.

Fernando: Well, actually, I don't want to sound angry with Inez. (directs an anxious look at Inez, who is looking down at her fingers) But quite frankly, it seems to me like (turns to Inez)—do you really have any desire for us to get close?

Inez: What do you mean?

Fernando: Well, you know. . . . You've been avoiding me again.

Inez: (continues to study her fingers) I've just been busy.

Fernando: (Fernando angrily takes the cushion behind him and drops it on the floor.) Fine then! You've been busy, and I think it's time we stopped coming for the sessions.

Therapist: This is what it can go like between you guys, isn't it? This is kind of like the cycle starting up right here and now. It's like you're reaching for Inez, right, Fernando? And when she doesn't respond you get frustrated, mad, but inside you feel. . . . (Therapist waits for Fernando to complete his sentence.)

Fernando: Like she disrespects me. Yes—and mad.

Therapist: So, Inez, you're quiet today. Where are you? What's happening for you?

Inez: It's been rough for me. Yes, I guess I've been feeling depressed and sad.

Therapist: You've been depressed and sad?

Inez: Well, my mother's visit is always hard.

Fernando: She's really a difficult woman.

Inez: She even follows me round the kitchen telling me I stir the sauce wrong or I'm putting too much flour in the gravy.

Therapist: So, having your Mom here's been really hard for you.

Inez: Yes, but then Fernando's been difficult, too. Snappy. Angry. And dealing with both. . . .

Therapist: (RISSSC manner) Ah, so you've had lots of messages to let you know you're not worth much, you don't count?

Inez: (nods tearfully)

Therapist: (RISSSC manner; uses Inez's words from previous sessions) Back to that really, really painful place where you don't count. You're not enough. No one cares. (Inez nods, weeping) So, Inez, what do you need when you get to that place, that painful place where you feel so small and defective?

Inez: I need for Fernando to be on my side. To stop taking his anger out on me. I am not a defective person. I work hard and I do a good job. I make good gravy, too!

Therapist: Right. You need for Fernando to see your value and treat you like you count. Can you let Fernando know now what you need from him?

Inez: (turns to Fernando) I want you to support me. When I'm feeling crummy and small, I want you on my side.

Therapist: You'd like for him to be beside you, not on the other side. So, what would you like from him?

Inez: I want you to come and support me when I'm upset and not get angry right away. Come and give me a hug and tell me you think I count. Like you did in here last week. (Fernando leans forward, looks emotional)

Therapist: That was good for you? Here in the session when he said that you're incredibly important to him?

Inez: (nods, weeping) It meant a lot to me.

Fernando: I guess I get anxious when you get quiet and withdrawn. I'm so busy worrying about me; I forget you need me there for you. (Fernando moves to sit beside her and puts his arms around his wife.)

DEEPENING EXPERIENCE AND DEFINING ATTACHMENT NEEDS

The EFT therapist prepares the way to withdrawer re-engagement through deepening core emotions and exploring underlying attachment-related needs often more clearly seen in relationship to one's view of self or view of other. Much of the work initially in Stage 2 requires a concerted focus on the underlying emotions that inform the more avoidant attachment strategies more common to withdrawing partners.

EFT STEPS: Stage 2, Restructuring Bonds

5. Access implicit needs, fears, models of self.
6. Promote acceptance by other; expand the dance.
7. Structured reach and respond, express attachment needs, create bonding interactions.

For each partner, the processing of emotional experience in Step 5 and the ensuing interactional events in Step 6 ready the partners for the further expansion and sharing of attachment fears, longings, and wants in Step 7. Requests for connection are made in Step 7 from an emerging, empowered, and accessible position that pulls for the other partner to engage in the same attachment-related process. Previous processing through Step 5 with the withdrawing partner naturally evolves into a heightened awareness and expression of needs and wants in Step 7. When one truly experiences a sense of thirst, for example, such awareness leads to a clear expression of need and desire for water. The formulation and expression of needs occur within the context of each person's interactional position in the relationship. As the attachment-related affect is engaged and expanded, new meanings organized by emotion emerge into awareness.

Statements made by the withdrawing partner in Step 5, for example, summarized as "I feel small and inept with you, and live in fear of you really seeing this and leaving me, so I go numb, defend, and withdraw" evolve and crystallize in Step 7 as "I am exhausted from all of this defending and numbing out. I want to feel special to you. I want you to hold off on the criticism and quit threatening to leave me. I'm not going to leave, and I don't want to feel small in this relationship anymore." The partner is now emotionally engaged and speaking from a position of increased efficacy, defining the relationship for himself rather than reacting to his partner's definitions. He has integrated attachment-related affect and subsequent newly emerging meaning into a new position that is emotionally accessible and responsive rather than distant and inaccessible.

As the withdrawing partner moves through Step 7, they are able to stay engaged with their immediate emotional experience and clearly ask for what they need to feel safe and connected in the relationship. These requests naturally stem from each partner's views of self and other. One spouse, for example, may share that "I am afraid that you can't love someone as disgusting as me. Who could?" Such a statement suggests a negative view of self as unlovable or deficient. Another spouse may state, "I don't think you really love me. I am not sure you ever have." Such a statement may revolve more around this partner's view of other. The EFT therapist should develop a sensitive ear to the nuances of attachment-related fears emanating from views of self and other when working through Step 7. The therapist does this by staying emotionally engaged to the immediate in-session experiencing of each partner from an open and curious stance.

The type of expression promoted in this step represents a new interactional stance that is much more equal and affiliative. These requests have the quality of *a new and authentic attempt at emotional engagement*. Emotional processing creates a different context and atmosphere than, say, negotiating behavioral contracts, seeking solutions, or gaining insight into family of origin. Requests are not made as demands on the other, nor are they stated in the context of blaming the other. Requests in Step 7 emerge from new positions that arise out of a new integration of emotional experience. When a more blaming partner makes an accusation, an engaged withdrawer is now able to steadfastly hold on to a new stance without resorting to the previous negative cycle of defending and withdrawing. For example, a withdrawer may state, "Yes, I temporarily resorted to my past behavior once this week. I've learned to react that way, unfortunately. But that was temporary, and I don't want you to take that as evidence that I am not trying or that I don't care and get so angry that I can't get close to you. I am working hard over here, and often I am doing things differently in ways that we both recognize and like, ways that bring us together. I need you to trust me in this."

In Step 7, partners are able to share specific requests in a manner that pulls the other partner toward them and maximizes the possibility that the other will be able to respond with accessibility and comfort. In short, *the attachment signals are clear*. The very nature of the requests tends to affirm the other partner's sense of being the prized one, the irreplaceable one, which has a powerful, immediate effect. From an attachment perspective, these interactions are extremely confirming and compelling. Common sentiments from the listening spouse, for example, after the engaging withdrawer shares attachment needs and wants, are often similar to: "I had no idea that I mattered this much to you. You really do need me. Wow, I am not alone in this after all." Here, the withdrawers' sharing echoes the other's deprivation and attachment needs, which then makes it easier for the other to respond positively. The usually blaming spouse, for example, may say to her engaging partner in Step 6, "I can really relate to your aloneness. I am sad as I hear you right now. I don't want to play a part in you feeling alone. I often feel alone, too. I did not know the depth of this inside you. I am sad, and yet on the other hand, I am so glad that you are sharing this with me."

The process of Step 7 takes the emotional experience of Step 5 and further crystallizes emerging meanings into expanded views of self and other. These new meanings emerge from experientially processing attachment-related affect, now used to restructure the relationship. The new emotional experience of a partner in Step 5 becomes a new interactional event in Step 7—one that redefines the control and affiliation in the relationship.

EXPLORING THE PROCESS OF WITHDRAWER RE-ENGAGEMENT

Withdrawer re-engagement occurs when the more withdrawn partner shifts the focus of their coping strategy from one of emotional elusiveness to one of emotional engagement. As the initial change event in Stage 2, withdrawer re-engagement is an essential first step toward restructuring the couple's attachment bond. The process of withdrawer engagement is outlined by following eight themes that organize the therapist focus through this change event (see Lee, Spengler, Mitchell, Spengler, & Spiker, 2017; Rheem, 2011). These themes illustrate this process sequentially; however, the therapist may return to different themes in a recursive or iterative manner.

WRE Theme 1: Withdrawer's Possible Disclosure

As a result of the exploration and elaboration of Step 5, the therapist wonders how it would be for the withdrawer to experientially imagine disclosing his attachment fears in a vulnerable manner.

> *Example: "Can you imagine, Burt, sharing this pain in your heart with your wife? You just did a great job letting me help you explore your inner world. You let me focus you in the all the places that you have avoided for decades, as you said earlier. All the places of pain and dis-connection from years of feeling alone. How would it be to share some of this pain with Michelle?"*

WRE Theme 2: Distilling Primary Affect (Tango Move 2)

After imagining disclosing vulnerably to their partner, the therapist works with and deepens the emotional blocks that arise in the withdrawer.

> *Example: "When you think about sharing with your wife, what fears come alive, Burt? What do you say to yourself? What's a worst-case scenario that would push*

you back toward avoidance and self-sufficiency? What blocks you from opening up with Michelle?"

WRE Theme 3: Enactment (Tango Move 3)

The therapist requests the withdrawer to share his fears and other primary or core emotion that was distilled through distilling primary affect.

> *Example: "Could you turn to her, Burt, and say to her what you just said to me? You said, 'I'm so tired of feeling small and unsuccessful in this relationship.' Could you turn and share this with your wife?"*

WRE Theme 4: Increasing Experiencing and Additional Enactments

Withdrawing partners often need a series of enactments to deepen their emotional experience to a level that engages a more profound review of their view of self and other. In process research studies of withdrawer engagement, researchers found that often three or more enactments are needed to intensify the emotional experience of a more withdrawn partner (Lee, 2017; Rheem, 2011) such that the "the emotional drip" of one enactment develops the "drip" of the next enactment.

> *Example: "Right, as you said, Burt, you are so tired of feeling small and unsuccessful. The tension that comes from feeling small and unsuccessful is just too much. You're tired of it, and that makes sense. Can you feel that tension now? On this inside of you, what's the sensation of this tension that you've lived with for too long now? Can you share with your wife how this sensation feels and how it has left you feeling?"*

WRE Theme 5: Promoting Acceptance (Move 4, Step 6 of EFT)

After the hard work of the withdrawer, at this point, the therapist turns to the listening partner and often leads with an evocative question aimed at promoting acceptance of the risk the withdrawer just took.

> *Example: "Michelle, what's this like to hear about Burt's feelings . . . small, unsuccessful, and the tension that comes? What's happening on this inside for you as you take in his experience? Help us know how you're feeling . . . "*

WRE Theme 6: Partner Enacts Support and Validates

The therapist facilitates the listening partner to enact their acceptance of the withdrawing partner's disclosure. This reach back by the listening partner is characterized by validation, reassurance, and support.

> *Example: "Michelle, you just said that you would like to know when Burt is struggling. That you haven't known and that it matters a lot to you. Can you imagine turning to him? Could you share, 'I haven't known how small and unsuccessful you have been feeling. I haven't really realized how critical I've been and how sharp my tone has become. I do care and I want you to feel better. I want us to feel better. I'm glad you told me.'"*

WRE Theme 7: Expressing Need (Step 7 of EFT)

The therapist goes back to the withdrawer to elicit a final enactment focused on the withdrawer's attachment needs. More withdrawing partners often need validation and affirmation regarding a sense of their adequacy and personal worth (Lee et al., 2017)

> *Example: "As we linger in this lovely openness between the two of you, your attachment-related needs, Burt, I'm wondering what your need is . . . we've processed you feeling small and unsuccessful. There is tension there for you that grips your body. We also processed your fears of not getting it right, in Michelle's eyes, and how hard that is for you. That fear, that despite your best efforts, she might still be disappointed in you. What is your need that emerges from that fear of disappointing her?*
>
> *"With this lovely vulnerability in your voice, can you share this need with her? You said, 'I need to know that I'm enough . . . my efforts are enough. I will never be perfect, but I care . . . a lot . . . and I need to know that my caring, my love for you . . . that I'm enough for you.' Can you see her eyes and share that with her?"*

WRE Theme 8: Partner Responds to Needs

The resolution to this change event occurs when the listening partner responds to a withdrawer's reach for their attachment related needs with empathy and support. The therapist continues to help the listening partner enact their support and validation of the withdrawer's need for connection and closeness.

> *Example: "I can see this is touching you, Michelle. What's coming alive emotionally as you heard Burt's needs that his caring, his love, he in fact is enough for you? Can you share with Burt directly what you're describing is happening in your heart: 'there's a melting . . . an opening. I had no idea that you (Burt) were so afraid that you aren't enough for me.' Can you share with him right from your melty, opening heart, please?"*

Withdrawer Re-engagement Example

Follow how these themes unfold as the therapist focuses on Moves 3 and 4 of the EFT Tango, inviting the withdrawing partner to take new steps of vulnerability and connection.

Rosalita and Jon have been married for three years, each having children from previous marriages. They presented for couple therapy because of "intense fighting" and lack of communication. In previous sessions, it became clear that Rosalita was the more pursuing partner and Jon the more withdrawing. "I get so mad at him," Rosalita explained. "I hate it, but I do. He's so competent at work, you know, such a leader. But at home with me, he just goes quiet, runs away, acts at times like he's a baby or something." The therapist learned that Jon got nervous when the couple began to argue, and when it escalated, Jon soon learned that he was no match for Rosalita. "I can't stand and fight it out with her anymore. Her tongue is sharp, and her mind is so quick. I don't know, maybe it was because she grew up with a lot of brothers and sisters and learned early to argue well, but I am no match." The therapist, focusing on the present process, finds Jon beginning to touch his core emotions, sharing that he "gets all sweaty in no time," when things are not going well, and a fight ensues. He said, "It's like I almost see white. I get so tense, so afraid, I guess. Being afraid sounds weird, but my heart pounds, and I have to get out of there." He went on to talk about feeling "like I am not much of a husband" and "wondering if she really still respects and loves me."

In Stage 2, the therapist turns her focus on an emerging attachment-related emotion, which follows the EFT Tango, as the therapist highlight's Jon's experience of his fear and sense that he is "not much of a husband." Here is an example of the therapist assembling emotion in Stage 2 with a more withdrawing partner. The therapist focused on Jon's experience when he said "like not much of a husband." The therapist knows that she needs to help Jon feel more deeply to find traction with Jon's inner-world (Step 5 of EFT). Notice how her attention goes to evoking his inner-world through assembling emotion.

Therapist: (using RISSSC manner, especially a soft voice tone) How is it, Jon, on the inside when you hear yourself say "not much of a husband?" What comes alive emotionally?

Jon: (withdrawer, looking down at his hands) Well, it kind of stinks, you know. Like not what I planned on. I'm used to being successful. She's right—at work I do a lot better.

Therapist: (taking his word, "stinks," and conjecturing emotions that might be there, too) Right, "stinks." I get it. Kind of hurts . . . makes you uncomfortable? Any of those words fit?

Jon: Well, yeah, it is uncomfortable. . . . Actually, it's really uncomfortable.

Therapist: (same soft voice tone) Right. Makes sense. Uncomfortable. Maybe so uncomfortable that it may even hurt sometimes?

Jon: Yeah, I guess it does. (looking up a bit) Not like I pay attention to it, but now that we're talking about it, I guess it does hurt.

Therapist: (reflecting the present moment as a way to amplify it) Right, now that we are focusing in this way, you can feel that it hurts. This is the stuff that you try not to pay attention to, right? Like you said, "I don't usually pay attention to my own inner-world." How is it, right now, that I'm focusing you in this way? I'm kind of keeping you focused in a place that you normally would avoid. How are you doing with my focus?

Notice here how the therapist validates Jon's secondary response to felt distress and then promotes safety and goal alliance by checking in with Jon on the process of focusing on an experience Jon typically moves away from. In Step 5, the therapist seeks to distill attachment-related emotion, which requires experiencing these emotions in the present.

Jon: I'm OK. I mean—not great but OK. You've already told me that this is what I need to do to help my marriage, and I want to help my marriage.

Therapist: (validating his efforts, which are framed as strengths either about his relationship or about himself) I appreciate that. So different for you to focus on your own emotion. Not easy. You must really love Rosalita. . . . Well, I know you do, but this is another big sign of your love for her! (refocusing on his inner-world) . . . It does hurt, doesn't it? When you think you're not much of a husband in her eyes, it does hurt. Can you feel that hurt on the inside?

Jon: Right here (touching his hand to his sternum). There's a knot, and it grows.

Therapist: (using repetition to deepen his experience) Oh wow, right. A knot that grows. Grows bigger when there's more hurt?

Jon: I don't know . . . probably . . . yeah, I think so.

Therapist: (his inner-world is distilled enough to make it relational) Does Rosalita know about this knot that grows? Do you think she knows you hurt sometimes when you two are disconnected?

Jon: I don't know if she knows. (looking at her) I guess she doesn't.

Therapist: (WRE Theme 1) How would it be to tell her about this knot of hurt that lives right in the center of your chest?

Jon: (he seems uncomfortable; he's looking down at his hands again) Ummm . . . I don't know how it would be to tell her. I wouldn't want to add more to her load, I guess. I wouldn't want to increase her burden.

This response from a withdrawer is expected and makes perfect sense. WRE is the start of a paradigm shift: from avoidance and self-sufficiency to taking the risk to share with a loved one, a start toward interdependence. This paradigm shift does feel risky to the withdrawer. It is so foreign to their nervous systems. The therapist knows how hard this will be and is gently persistent.

Exercise 6.1. WRE Theme 1

In WRE, before getting to WRE Theme 1 (wondering if the withdrawer can disclose his experience to his partner), a lot of intrapsychic exploration is needed to get the withdrawer in touch with and then describing his affective experience. Please check all the interventions that help the withdrawer go closer to and then make contact with his inner-world.

a. "When we slow the moment down and you say, 'I don't know what I feel,' how it is for you that I'd like to focus there? How would it be for us to linger here?" _____
b. "When you say, 'I don't feel anything,' and I reflect my observation of you looking down and away as you say that you don't feel anything, how it is for you that I'm wondering if we can explore the nooks and crannies of 'I don't feel anything.'?" _____
c. "What comes alive emotionally when I reflect your partner's words, 'I need more!'?" _____
d. "The sensations in your body? When she said, 'I need more,' you felt yourself get stiff? You felt a gripping?" _____
e. "As you shut down, go numb, start avoiding, you notice you're feeling what emotionally? Some kind of pain or fear is compelling you to shut down, do numb, start avoiding?" _____

Exercise 6.2. Engaging and Deepening Core Affect

1. Please write one evocative response to use to assemble and deepen a withdrawer's inner experience.

   ____

   ____

   ____

2. Please write one conjecture you can hear yourself using to encourage continued exploration of the Jon's inner-world.

   ____

   ____

   ____

3. Please write one validating reflection to normalize Jon's experience.

   ____

   ____

   ____

As the session continues, the therapist shifts to distilling Jon's core emotion. The therapist focuses on evocative responses, heightening and empathic conjecture to hold Jon in deepening his experience

Therapist: (WRE Theme 2) Somehow, Jon, you think you should be able to handle it all on your own? You would be less than the man you are if you shared your hurt with her? What comes alive when you think about sharing this knot of hurt with her? (Therapist makes space for his fears as Jon experientially imagines what would come alive for him if he were to take the risk and share his knot with Rosalita.)

Jon: Less of a man, not so self-sufficient after all (with a bit of sarcasm), I guess. Her worst fear coming to life. Maybe my worst fear coming to life! I can't be soft. I can't be seen as soft. Soft is weak. I'm not a weak man.

Therapist: Like a fear of being seen as weak?

At this point in the process, the therapist often conjectures "fear." Adding in "fear" keeps the process focused experientially on affect (afraid of being seen as weak) versus cognitive/perception (I'm not a weak man). Working experientially with fears is our primary objective in both change events.

Jon: Yeah, for sure, fear of being weak. . . .

Therapist: You can feel that fear on the inside, Jon? How does this fear come alive inside of you in these moments?

Jon: (tentatively focusing inwardly) I can feel it. It's a tension that's all over. (his hand going from his chest to his stomach)

Therapist: (soft voice, slow pace) Yes, makes sense. So, the knot in your sternum grows . . . a tension comes alive all over your chest and stomach when this fear comes alive. Fear that Rosalita will see you as weak if you shared more of your heart with her.

As his fear gets named and processed a bit experientially (Move 2), it is time to consider making his fear relational with an engaged encounter (Move 3). With half an eye on the listening partner, Therapist is assessing the partner's readiness to hear from withdrawer. If the listening partner is "with" you and the process, asking for the enactment is a good next step. If therapist isn't sure if listening partner is "with" you and the process (because she is looking out the window and/or getting impatient or reactive in anyway), the therapist processes a possible enactment with each partner first to avoid putting the withdrawer at more risk (doing an enactment with a partner who is spacing out or reacting) by asking the Rosalita: "What's happening for you as Jon is opening up and sharing so vulnerably with us?" Or "How would it be, Rosalita, if I encourage Jon to share his fear and the tension that comes with his fear directly with you? How would this be for you?"

Exercise 6.3. WRE Theme 2, Distilling Core Emotions

In Theme 2, the therapist distills the underlying emotion that would block the withdrawer from sharing with his partner. Check all the possible moves a clinician might make in order to bring the withdrawer closer to his primary emotion.

a. Reflect her observation of water in his eyes. _____
b. Upon hearing emotion in his voice, conjecture that it sounds like there's some sadness or some other emotion there. _____
c. After his partner said, "I care and I'd like to know what he goes through in these tough moments" and you wonder what's coming alive on the inside for him as he heard his partner say, "I care, and I'd like to know what he goes through in these tough moments." _____
d. Normalize how scary it is to start paying attention to pain and fear. Temporarily, this attention will make pain and fear feel worse before feeling better. _____
e. Validate how different and risky it is to open up, so therefore we don't need the withdrawer to take the risk to open up. _____

Exercise 6.4. Distilling Core Emotion

In deepening the withdrawer's affect, common interventions used to encourage continued exploration of his inner-world are

a. Reflect, evoke, reflect. _____
b. Reflect, conjecture, validate. _____
c. Evoke, conjecture, evoke. _____
d. Reflect the cycle. _____
e. RISSSC. _____

As Jon experiences a more clear and coherent sense of his fear, the therapist shifts toward engaging this experience. In Move 3, the therapist engages Jon in supporting and challenging Jon to move into his fear and share it.

Therapist: (WRE Theme 3) How would it be, Jon, to share this fear with her? She's right here. She's open.

Jon: (tentatively looks toward Rosalita) Well . . . I guess I do . . . I do get this tension. . . . I guess I do fear being seen as weak. You seeing me as weak.

Therapist: So brave, Jon. Such a new kind of strength to turn and share your fear with her.

Jon: I don't feel very strong. In fact, quite the opposite. What kind of man needs to share his fears like this?

His wondering or possible distrust of sharing his fear with his wife is normal. On the one hand, showing his weakness is a risk. On the other hand, he's trusting the clinician and the process that sharing his weakness will help them rebuild their connection. This is the classic bind of withdrawers—a personal pact "to never let 'em see me sweat" bumps up against the realities of love, which requires interdependence. This is, in part, why the risk the withdrawer takes is framed as such a strength. It takes all kinds of strength to do something so different emotionally.

Therapist: (reframing his vulnerability as strength) Well, the kind of man who is brave enough to learn a new language to help his relationship feel better. A man who is strong enough to be vulnerable. Just in here, for the time being. A man who is strong enough to let his wife see his humanity.

Jon: (nodding tentatively) If you say so. . . .

Therapist: (more soft voice and slow pace to process the engaged encounter) Right here, on the inside of you, what are you feeling? What are you noticing? You just did something really big, and I wonder how it feels on the inside.

Jon: Humm, I mean, well, it was hard.

Since depth of emotional experiencing is so important to get a revision of Jon's view of self and other, this repetition is vital. The therapist processes the enactment (Tango Move 4) to help the withdrawer to continue to feel what's coming alive after taking such a big risk (in sharing his vulnerabilities in Tango Move 3). This is a good example of the iterative nature of withdrawer re-engagement, including where a withdrawer drips, drips, drips emotion a little bit more with each enactment.

Exercise 6.5. Preparing an Engaged Encounter

The therapist asks the withdrawer to take one of the hardest steps—engaging their emotions and needs. What does the therapist need to be aware of as he or she sets up an engaged encounter? (Check all that apply.)

a. That the listening partner isn't zoned out, reactive, or impatient. The listening partner needs to be neutral, at a minimum, and more ideally, open and receptive. _____

b. That the withdrawer has some experiential contact with his emotion. It is important that these enactments not be cognitive. To create a bonding moment, the withdrawer has to be in contact with some of his vulnerability. _____
c. That the withdrawer's affect has been distilled and the actual enactment is a simple, clear statement. _____
d. That the listening partner has already softened and shared her vulnerabilities. _____
e. That there is time to process the engaged encounter with both partners. How does it feel to share? How does it feel to hear? _____

Personal Reflection

Therapists may worry when setting up an enactment or actually asking for one. Therapists worry about the enactment falling flat (not enough emotion to *move* either partner), the enactment will have too much emotion, and the partners will get reactive, or the message will be too cognitive or too complicated. Take a moment to feel into your worries about setting up and asking for engaged encounters.

Write your worries here:

____

____

____

As the therapist shifts focus to increasing the withdrawers presence and experiencing of these new emotions, the therapist returns repeatedly to the emerging fears and needs as they slowly unfold in session. This repetition deepens the withdrawer's experience and focuses the partner's felt awareness on emerging views of self and other. This is the heart of the fourth theme in withdrawer re-engagement.

Therapist: (WRE Theme 4) Right, right. It was hard, wasn't it? So outside your norm. Could you turn to her again and tell her that it was hard to open up to her about the knot of hurt in your chest? Could you?

Jon: (tentatively turning to wife) This stuff is really hard. I'm not used to opening up . . . to anyone. It is hard, but I want us to feel better together.

Therapist: (re-focusing him on his actual affective experience to make sure this gets shared, too) It is hard to tell her about the knot of hurt in your chest? Right, Jon?

Jon: (looking back at Rosalita) Yes, it is hard to tell you about this knot of hurt in my chest. (sighs) I just never knew that it would help anything if I told you. (shifts in his chair) But it's true . . . my chest tightens so much that sometimes I feel like I can't breathe. That scares me even more. It is a knot that is almost always there. It's a place I don't want to pay attention to but then, in here, it's what we do here. (half smiles at the therapist)

Therapist: (staying in touch with his affective experience to continue to prioritize it, knowing we will probably need yet another enactment) So good, Jon. So well done. (softly and evocatively) How is your chest now? How is the knot?

Jon: Not so bad, I guess . . . it's there but not as a tight, I think.

Therapist: (WRE Theme 4, third time) Right, right. It's there but not as tight. I hear you. There're times when this knot of hurt grows, and I've just never told you that I have a knot of hurt (as if I'm Jon). Can you turn and tell her, "I've got this knot of hurt when we get disconnected?"

The therapist keeps the focus on his pain and fear. With each iteration, the engaged encounter is more specific and with more depth. We want him to be "associating" with and "self-descriptive" about his inner-world, according to the Short Form of the Experiencing Scale (ES; Klein, Mathieu, Keisler, & Gendlin, 1969).

Jon: (to Rosalita, with a flushed face) It's true. I have this knot of hurt when we get disconnected. It's right here (touching same place again), and it doesn't feel good. I don't like it.

Therapist: So strong, Jon. So strong.

Exercise 6.6. Repeating Engaged Encounters

In WRE, there is a need for repetitive, iterative, deepening enactments to increase depth of emotional experiencing for the withdrawer. In both studies of WRE, repetitive enactments were shown to increase depth of experiencing, which is important to ensure there is enough depth to get revision of view of self and view of other. The clinician's repetitive focus is based on which important factors? (Check all that apply.)

a. Enactments can be evocative, and more emotion comes alive for the withdrawing partner, often with engaged encounters. _____
b. As more emotion comes alive, the clinician can distill and deepen it with the client. _____
c. With iterative enactments, the withdrawing partner can move from "associating" (ES Level 4) to "exploratory" (ES Level 5) to "affirmative" (ES Level 6) with emotional distilling and deepening done between enactments. _____
d. To push the withdrawing partner into deeper emotions before he's ready to go there. _____
e. Repetitive enactments stretch the withdrawing partner's window of tolerance bit by bit, which helps the withdrawer not recoil from increased experiencing. _____

Exercise 6.7. Focusing on Engaged Encounters in Withdrawer Re-engagement

The content of these repetitive engaged encounters are (Check all that apply.)

a. The client's affect. _____
b. The client's body response/sensations. _____
c. The client's old avoidance behaviors. _____
d. The client's fears. _____

e. The client's view of self/other (VOS/VOO). _____
f. The client's experience in the present moment. _____
g. The client's thoughts. _____

Personal Reflection

Of all the possible answers in Exercise 6.7, which content areas are hardest for you to work with? And how do you make meaning about why these are the hardest ones?

____

____

____

At this point, the therapist turns to Rosalita to process experientially how Jon's experience is impacting her. This is an important shift in the process as the therapist moves to Step 6 of promoting acceptance. We need to hear how she's experienced his sharing (Tango Move 4) and to facilitate her acceptance of his sharing (if/when possible), which is the focus of Theme 5.

Therapist: (with curiosity) How was it, Rosalita, to hear about Jon's knot of hurt? He was so strong to turn to you and share his knot of hurt so openly. How does this touch your heart?

Rosalita: Um . . . um . . . I didn't know he had that. I didn't know, which is strange not to know. But, like you said a minute ago, I'm open. I want to know about him. I want to know what he is going through. I'm open to it . . . especially the softer stuff. That is what's so different in here. At home, we aren't really soft with each other. I do think it will help me . . . to know. I do think it will help us know each other better again.

Exercise 6.8. Interventions and Promoting Acceptance in Withdrawer Re-engagement

Name the main interventions the therapist uses to explore Rosalita's emotional response to Jon's sharing. (Check all that apply.)

a. Evocative responses _____
b. Conjectures _____
c. Track and reflect the cycle _____
d. RISSSC _____
e. Reflect primary emotion _____
f. Reflect to validate _____
g. Reflect to slow process and place emphasis _____
h. Reflect secondary emotion to contain _____
i. Catch the bullet _____

Exercise 6.9. Reasons to Process and Promote Acceptance

Check all the reasons it is important for the clinician to process with Rosalita.

a. For Jon's sake, it is important for him to know how his partner is experiencing the risk he took in sharing his inner-world with her. _____

b. If her acceptance isn't there or her response is below neutral, these are very important data for the therapist, who will need to process the blocks to acceptance. _____
c. She may feel very confused hearing such new data from her husband. The therapist expects to help her makes sense of her confusion, dissonance, and blocks. _____
d. It creates more safety for the withdrawer if he's not the only one processing emotion. It is ideal to have both partners deepening their emotional experience somewhat simultaneously. This lowers the risk for each partner of feeling too vulnerable and too exposed without the other partner risking at all. _____
e. The therapist needs to process with the partner to give the withdrawer time to integrate. _____

Now, after using Move 4 of the Tango to process Rosalita's response to Jon's enactment (Move 3 of the Tango), the therapist wants to help Rosalita enact her acceptance of Jon's sharing. Enactments make important emotional moments relational. This provides clarity for Jon (a noticeably clear signal of acceptance and support from Rosalita), which starts to meet his longings to be successful with her. Equally important, without her enacting her acceptance back to Jon (WRE Theme 6), they would be missing out on a potential bonding moment. Throughout the change events, we always look for moments of vulnerable accessibility with one partner to be enacted to create as many bonding moments for the couple as possible. It takes repetitive, iterative enactments of vulnerability between partners to restructure their bond, the goal of Stage 2.

Therapist: (WRE Theme 6) Could you tell him, Rosalita? Could you tell him that you're open? Could you tell him that you want to know about him, what he goes through?

Rosalita: (to Jon, softly) I do want to know about you . . . even the knot of hurt. It matters to me. You matter to me. We're not the same, and I want to know you again. Especially when something fills your chest with tension and it scares you, I want to know.

Therapist: (validating her reach) So good, Rosalita. So brave. He matters so much to you.

Therapist: (to Jon) How is this, Jon? To hear your wife's openness to you, that your hurt matters to her, how she wants to know you better again? (The therapist uses this as another opportunity to deepen him into his affective experience. More evocative responses to keep his focus on his inner-world, which continues to stretch his window of tolerance.)

Jon: (pensively) It's good. It's good. I guess we got really far apart. Maybe more than I realized.

Exercise 6.10. Enacting Acceptance in Withdrawer Re-engagement

What are some of the important reasons for Rosalita to enact her acceptance of Jon's experience? (Check all that apply.)

a. If she is able to offer reassurance, this becomes a new signal from her to him and is the start of restructuring their bond. _____

b. It is important to give Jon a really clear signal of acceptance and support. He took a big risk in sharing his vulnerabilities, and we want him to get all the comfort and reassurance available to him. _____
c. Enactments between partners are more potent because each partner is hearing from the other partner directly. It creates another possible bonding moment to have Rosalita enact back rather than the therapist speaking to Jon for her. _____
d. It's good to finally give the listening partner a chance to talk. WRE takes a long time, and the listening partner is often waiting. _____

Exercise 6.11. Enacting Partner Acceptance

Write what you would like Rosalita to respond back to Jon. What would she say as she enacts her acceptance?

____

____

____

The therapist is aware that Jon has yet to enact his need which is the culmination of withdrawer re-engagement (Step 7 of EFT). In this enactment, we want his need to emerge from the intrapsychic processing that has just occurred, which has made clear his attachment-related *needs*.

Therapist: And in this place of more openness, Jon, this knot of hurt that has lived in your chest—what is the need that emerges as we focused on your fears of being seen as weak and this tension, this knot tightens your chest and scares you even more . . . your need. . . .

Jon: My need . . . my need is to know that my wife doesn't see me as weak . . . that she still loves me and that I'm enough. . . . (turning toward her) I need to know I am enough for you.

Therapist: (WRE Theme 7) Can you say that to her again, Jon. "I need to know. I need to know that I'm enough for you."

Jon (to his wife) I do need to know that I'm enough for you. That you don't see me as weak and soft . . . that you still love me.

Therapist: Of course, Jon, right. You so need to know that you're enough for her and that she still loves you. So brave in sharing your needs that are at the heart of your fear, yes?

Exercise 6.12. Enacting a Withdrawer's Attachment-Related Needs

In this most important engaged encounter of Jon's needs, what are important characteristics of this enactment? (Check all that apply.)

a. It be made from an emotionally accessible place inside of Jon. _____
b. There be some eye contact with his partner. _____

c. That the client actually shares his need rather than the therapist doing it for him. _____
d. That Jon would tell Rosalita what he has been thinking about lately. _____
e. That the therapist validate Jon for this additional risk he continues to take. _____

Exercise 6.13. Refocusing an Engaged Encounter

If this enactment focused on his need ends up with the withdrawer distancing from emotion and the enactment sounds like a cognitive request, what is the therapist's best next step?

a. Tell Jon that his cognitive request sounds too much like a demand, and he needs to do better. _____
b. Ask Jon why he has the need that he has. _____
c. Go back to the most recent emotion that was alive for Jon and bring that emotion alive again. From the place of having the emotion alive again, invite the need to emerge and be shared from this emotionally accessible place. _____
d. Ask Rosalita if she thinks his need is valid. _____

After asking the withdrawer to take the biggest risk of all—share his needs vulnerably with his spouse, it's vital that the therapist support the spouse in responding to the withdrawer's reach with as much soft openness as possible. It is so different, foreign, and risky for the withdrawer to share his need vulnerably. It is a "reach" from the withdrawer's heart, which the therapist validates as they work with the partner to respond from her heart. The therapist directs Rosalita's attention to her heart as a way to evoke softer emotions. It is important that Rosalita not provide a cognitive response to Jon's emotional reach.

Therapist: (to Rosalita, who's looking right at Jon) And, Rosalita, your heart? How are your husband's needs landing in your heart? You're feeling what right now?

Rosa: (WRE Theme 8, to her husband, who is looking at her cautiously) You are enough (she said with certainty). And I do love you. Always have. We did get really dis-connected, but I never stopped loving you. And the more you share your heart with me, the more you are enough for me. I don't see you as weak, at all, but in your old silence, I didn't know how to see you. The more I know about your heart, the more you are enough for me.

Therapist: (to Rosalita) So true, Rosalita: the more he shares his heart, the better you see him and know him, right. When he shares his heart, he is so enough for you. So true. I get that. I hear you. He takes the risk to share his heart, and it helps your heart not feel so alone. He is with you when he shares his heart, and that changes everything. And, Jon, how is your heart, after hearing from your wife that you are enough for her?

Jon: It feels good to hear.

Therapist: That you're enough for her. Especially when you share your heart?

Jon: Yes, that part! It does feel good to hear that it helps her. She doesn't think I'm weak or soft. That she actually needs to know my experience. I'm surprised, but it's a good surprise. I just never knew or thought that sharing would be helpful to her or me. It is really good to know. . . . I've just always wanted to know how to be successful with her. Feels good.

Exercise 6.14. Processing the Partner's Response to a Withdrawer's Reach

After any engaged encounter, it is important to process what was shared with both partners. Check all the reasons processing with each partner is so important.

a. Enactments are evocative, and it's important to allow time and space to learn what emotions came alive as a result of the engaged encounter. _____
b. It's important to track the minutes spent processing with each partner to make sure it is always equal. _____
c. Since engaged encounters are risky for the one sharing, processing with the listening partner is important to send, if possible, a message of validation and reassurance back to the partner who risked. _____
d. If a message of validation and reassurance isn't possible, the listening partner will benefit from the Therapist's support to process confusion, dissonance, and reactions. _____
e. The therapist's ability to catch the bullet, as needed, helps both partners at an intense, emotional time. _____

Therapist: Right, Jon, such a surprise that sharing your heart actually helps her feel better, and then you feel better. So different than that old worry that you would be burdening her. You've done so well, Jon, staying with your inner-experience, that knot of hurt that grows and how the tension of fear grows in your chest and stomach. You were so strong to share that with Rosalita. When you share, that what gives her your heart, which helps you both so much. And, Rosalita, you were able to take in his hurt and fear and reassure him that he's enough for you. This is the start of your new pattern with each other. All of us who love another need to take the risk to share our hearts, especially when we are in pain or scared for any reason.

This example of the start of Jon's withdrawer re-engagement highlights the classic way an EFT therapist supports the withdrawing partner in finding his emotion and then sharing some of it with his spouse. Throughout Stage 2 of EFT, this process is repeated several times so each spouse builds the capacity to find and share their softer feelings in a vulnerable way with each other. This is the essence of how the couple's bond is re-structured, the goal of Stage 2.

SUMMARY

In conclusion, the withdrawer re-engagement change event process weaves many key elements of EFT together. While the EFT therapist is constantly moving between Tango Moves 2 (assemble and deepen affect), 3 (choreograph engaged encounters/enactments), and 4 (process encounter/enactment), the client's emotional experience is deepening session by session (from Steps 5, focusing on and lingering with primary emotions, to Step 7, the sharing of fears with spouse). As a vulnerability emerges and is distilled in Tango Move 2 for the withdrawer, the sharing of it (Move 3 of Tango) with the spouse often increases the depth of emotional experiencing. This increased depth of emotional experiencing becomes the heart of the engaged encounters, which often amplifies his primary emotion as the withdrawer risks sharing opening and seeing his spouse's eyes and face. Sharing vulnerably with the spouse not only reprocesses old pain and facilitates corrective emotional experiences but also creates bonding moments for the couple as they take in and process each other's experiences (Move 4 of the Tango). As the withdrawer feels his spouse's acceptance (Step 6 of the client process of change), there is revision of the withdrawers' internal working models (VOS/VOO), goals embedded in the withdrawer re-engagement change event.

Shifting paradigms from self-sufficiency to interdependence, as withdrawers do in EFT, is a powerful unfolding of the withdrawer's humanity. Often, it is the first time that the withdrawer has been open and vulnerable. It can be the first time the withdrawer has shared his pain, hurt, and grief. In these sessions, it may be the first time that the spouse of the withdrawer sees their partner's humanity in this emotionally focused way. Where once the spouse feared the withdrawer's indifference, the spouse is now hearing and taking in new, emerging emotion. This is a monumental shift for both spouses and their relationship's pattern of interaction. The slow and deliberate pacing, the narrow focus on his inner-world, and the gentle repetition provided by the EFT therapist are paramount in this unfolding we call withdrawer re-engagement.

ANSWERS AND SUGGESTED RESPONSES

Exercise 6.1. WRE Theme 1

Answer: All responses (interventions **A–E**)

Exercise 6.2. Engaging and Deepening Core Affect

1. Possible Evocative Responses: Her statement, "I need more!" triggered you? What happened on the inside for you, when you heard her say, "I need more!"? Or when you heard her say, "I need more!" you said what yourself? Or when you heard her say that, what did you feel? Something came alive for you on the inside? That was hard for you? Your body stiffened?
2. Possible Conjectures: "That was hard for you, Jon? Is 'hard' a good word? Something came alive, and you're not sure yet what it was? It was hard for you? Uncomfortable? Painful? Do any of these words fit for you? Or "You felt mad, Jon, at her reaction? You're a good man, and you're working hard to be there for her. You felt mad—does that fit?"
3. This is so hard on your heart, Jon. You're a good man, and you are working hard to be there for Rosalita. It makes sense that you aren't sure what you feel when she responds. Emotions come alive so quickly; for lots of us, it's hard to know what we feel."

Exercise 6.3. WRE Theme 2 Distilling Core Emotions

Answer: All responses (**A–D**)

Exercise 6.4. Distilling Core Emotion

Answer: A, B, C, E. These are interventions that encourage exploration of the client's intra-psychic experience, which is necessary to deepen and distill the withdrawer's emotion. Reflecting the cycle, option d, is more cognitive and would bring the client's attention and the process out of experiencing and exploring the client's inner-world.

Exercise 6.5. Preparing an Engaged Encounter

Answer: A, B, C, E. These serve as a checklist for the therapist as you prepare the withdrawer to take the risk of enacting. Option d isn't viable because we work on the withdrawer re-engagement change event before we start the softening change event. Therefore, we don't expect the listening partner to be "already softened," as option d suggests.

Personal Reflection Possible Response: I will do it wrong and make them worse. I won't know what to ask for with the enactment. How do I know that the partner is ready to share? How do I know what to suggest they share? If it goes wrong, I'll feel responsible for them. They're paying me; I'm supposed to be the expert. If they end up escalated again, I'll be to blame. As hard as I will work to set it up well, you never know what they will actually say to each other. It's risky. Why take the risk? I don't like taking the risk. The partner will react, and I will freeze. Then they are worse after the enactment than they were before. How will I calm down their reactivity again if it all goes sideways?

Exercise 6.6. Repeating Engaged Encounters

Answer: A, B, C, E. These responses highlight the need for the therapist to "come alongside" the withdrawer to make the exploring of emotions and needs safer. The therapist's attunement to pacing and the client's felt sense of the process is important. Pushing the client, as option d proposes, doesn't work. The client may get "pushed" into deeper emotion but won't be able to stay there or integrate. The recoiling likely after being pushed into deeper emotion work against the larger process of withdrawer re-engagement.

Exercise 6.7. Focusing on Engaged Encounters in Withdrawer Re-engagement

Answer: A, B, D, E, F. All responses except c and g emphasize the focus areas of potential enactments. Enactments are meant to be emotionally alive, a little bit risky, and emotionally vulnerable in order to reprocess old emotion and to provide bonding moments. There will be no glue or adhesive (necessary for a bonding moment) if the enactment isn't emotionally alive, which makes it experiential. Focusing on the client's old behavior (option c) or the client's thoughts (option g) will decrease emotional aliveness, and the enactment won't lead to a new emotional experience or a bonding moment.

PERSONAL REFLECTION POSSIBILITIES

It's hardest for me to bring my clients closer to their pain and sadness. My head knows that this is the most efficient way to work, but my heart aches at the thought of asking them to go closer to their suffering. What if going closer to their pain doesn't help? It is a bit easier to ask clients about their body/sensations, but then I don't usually know exactly what to do with their answers. VOS/VOO confuses me still. At times, it is really hard to make the distinction between them, but I'm growing in my comfort to explore. It is getting easier to explore these areas with my clients even when I don't know what to do next or how best to use their answers. I'm learning that the process of exploring is the more important piece, and gains do get made even if I'm not clear moment by moment.

Exercise 6.8. Interventions and promoting Acceptance in Withdrawer Re-engagement

Answer: A, B, D, E, F, G. All responses except c highlight the primary interventions the therapist uses to work intra-psychically with a client. Working intra-psychically is required to process emotions experientially. The function of these interventions is to explore the client's inner-world, which is needed to promote the partner's emotional acceptance of the withdrawer's enactments. Response c will provide an exit from any emotion that is alive or starting to come alive, which works against our attempts to promote the listening partner's emotional acceptance of the withdrawer's enactment. Responses h and i are needed when the withdrawer's enactment triggers the listening partner. The interventions of reflecting secondary emotion and catching the bullet function to contain reactive emotion. As reactive emotion is contained, the therapist can work to find the softer, more primary emotions embedded in the reactivity.

Exercise 6.9. Reasons to Process and Promote Acceptance

Answer: All responses

Exercise 6.10. Enacting Acceptance in Withdrawer Re-engagement

Answer: All responses

Exercise 6.11. Enacting Partner Acceptance

Suggested Response: I would ask Rosalita to enact back to Jon: "You do matter to me. You matter a lot. We did get really far apart, and I have missed you. I have missed us. It helps me so much to know more of your inner-world. It calms me." Or "I know I haven't been easy to come close to lately but you do matter to me . . . a lot. I have been feeling really alone, and I didn't realize you felt all this tension. I do care about you and want us to be "us" again." Or "This is surprising and a bit strange to hear—that you're in this much pain. I didn't know. I thought you were fine, and I was the only one in pain. I'm hearing new stuff. It's different and strange but in a good way, I guess. I'm glad we're talking together again."

Exercise 6.12. Enacting a Withdrawer's Attachment-Related Needs

Answer: A, B, C, E. All responses except d are important characteristics of this enactment focused on the withdrawer's needs. It's so important that this enactment be emotionally alive rather than cognitive. Ideally, the enactment of the withdrawer's needs emerges from the processing of his emotion and the expression of needs results from the flow of processing his pain, fears, sadness, and other emotions.

Exercise 6.13. Refocusing an Engaged Encounter

Answer: C. Losing focus and distancing from the emotion are natural and understandable parts of the process. The therapist expects these possibilities! When it happens, simply go back to the last emotion that was alive in the process (as response c suggests). Utilize the interventions that bring emotion alive, distill that emotion, and then request the enactment again! You got this!

Exercise 6.14. Processing the Partner's Response to a Withdrawer's Reach

Answer: A, C, D, E. All responses except b provide rationale for why we process with each partner after enactments. When processing emotion with one or both partners, tracking the minutes spent processing, as response b proposes, isn't necessary or important. While it is always important to keep "half an eye" on the partner you aren't processing with (to track any reactivity or emotional expression), spending equal minutes with each partner isn't necessary in Stage 2. Expect that processing emotion takes time, good pacing, and an unhurried approach, and the time needed could be different for each partner.

7

STAGE 2: SOFTENING

Softening or blamer softening is the second change event required to restructure attachment in a couple relationship. This occurs when the more pursuing or critical partner is now able to ask for contact and comfort from a position of personal vulnerability. As this partner "softens," both partners are now able to more fully engage one another with emotional accessibility and responsiveness, which are the key elements in building and maintaining secure bonds. Powerful bonding events can now occur as partners *own these new positions* and walk through new positive interactional cycles in which they are emotionally accessible and responsive to each other.

EFT Snapshot: Softening

Inez and Fernando announced that they had been caught in the negative cycle that morning, but they let it go in the car on the way to the session. The therapist invited the couple to revisit their distress after recognizing they found ways to exit this predictable pattern. Fernando shared how he had been scanning his email as Inez was preparing to leave for the session. Fernando read a work email that spiraled him into the negative mix of feelings. As he was getting off the computer, Inez spotted an email from their daughter, and she sat down to enjoy the holiday photos that were attached, but Fernando interrupted her to insist they leave or risk being late for their therapy appointment. He snapped at Inez, who, true to her usual form in the cycle, puffed up and shouted at him.

Fernando: Well, I got flipped into that place again. I got an email from someone at—at work. You know, it put me back there. To all the dreadful times I had at work—disrespected, dismissed, struggling so hard to show I'm not a failure.

Therapist: (RISSSC manner) Right. So, you're back in the old place—the disrespecting, the dismissing, the struggle. It's hard to feel that you're enough.

Inez: Well, why can't you talk about that then, instead of going for me?

Fernando: I just tried to get past it. I called you in to see Angela's holiday photos.

Inez: Yes, but, just like you said, you were in that place again.

Therapist: It's hard for you to let her in when you are "flipped into that place"?

DOI: 10.4324/9781003039457-9

Fernando: I never wanted her to see me there.

Therapist: Never wanted her to see that inside you were struggling, that it was so hard for you. Such a tough place. What would happen, Fernando, if she saw that? (empathic reflection, relationship question)

Fernando: I wouldn't be manly, you know? She wouldn't respect me.

Therapist: She wouldn't respect you?

Fernando: Look, the real truth of the matter is that if she saw me, saw how pathetic I really am—she'd probably find someone else. (laughs bitterly) That's why I always came on so strong—never let them catch you with your armor off!

Therapist: (softly) It's hard to trust that if she saw the real Fernando, it's like a part of you says, "If she saw the real me, there's no way she'd stay around. She'd probably head out the door." Is that close? (empathic conjecture)

Fernando: (head down) That's it. That's exactly it.

Therapist: Can you turn and share this directly with her now, Fernando? Would you please turn and tell her how a part of you says, "She'll leave if you admit this. Don't you show her the real you!"' Can you share that directly with her now in your own words please? (restructuring interactions, Move 3)

Fernando: (smiles weakly) Well, yes but no. Yes, I did it again today. I did it again. I know I've done things to hurt her, and I know I can't change the past. But I want to change the future. I . . . I want to make things different.

Therapist: (repeats her request) Can you let her know, Fernando, just how hard it is for you, for you to let her see the guy on the inside, the inside Fernando? (heightening)

Fernando: (turns to Inez) Inside, inside I feel . . . (Fernando pauses) It's hard.

Therapist: It's hard to say?

Fernando: (small voice) Yes.

Therapist: So hard. So hard to look at her and say. . . . (heightening using RISSSC)

Fernando: I . . . I . . . (Fernando pauses again)

Therapist: It sounds like this is really scary—a real risk for you, yes? It's really scary to begin to tell her how low you sometimes feel, how afraid you get that if she really sees you, she may not like what it looks like, and she may head out the door? (empathic conjecture, heightening)

Fernando: Yes, a risk. But Inez, you've taken risks with me. (Inez reaches out to take Fernando's hand.) Sorry, kid . . . (his voice is thick and husky) Thank you. I feel you there.

You know I feel so puny sometimes; it's so damned hard to be me sometimes. Armor. That's what I do—and yes, I see how it pushes you away.

Therapist: So, what do you need, Fernando, when you feel so small and puny? (evocative question)

Fernando: I have it right here in my hand. (He looks tenderly at his wife.) I need for you to hold me. Comfort me like you are now.

Inez: (with tears in her eyes) I am here, Fernando. I am here for you.

Therapist: I see there are tears, Inez, and you look emotional. I am wondering what this is like for you? (evocative question, Move 4, processing encounter)

Inez: I only saw him cry once in his life. When his father died.

Fernando: Did you despise me for it?

Inez: No! You placed your trust in me. I am honored by it. You trusted me. It means so much. I've never felt closer to you than I do right now.

Therapist: When you see his softer, tender side like you do right now, this pulls you toward him? You say, "I've never before felt this close to you." (empathic conjecture)

Inez: Yes, never like I do right now.

Therapist: This tender side of Fernando pulls you in, and you are really here to comfort him. (heightening positive response)

Inez: Right now I feel like I do count.

Therapist: Right. When he lets you in and is vulnerable and shares his needs for you, then you feel like you matter to him. (validation)

Inez: Yes, I feel important to him. And I am not alone.

Therapist: Can you tell him that, Inez, right now? (restructuring)

Softening Event

Research demonstrates that the blamer softening event is crucial to success in emotionally focused therapy (EFT) (Johnson & Greenberg, 1988). Softening events fuel creation of secure relationships in which both partners are accessible responsive and emotionally engaged (A.R.E.). In secure relationships, partners ask for attachment fears to be soothed and attachment needs to be met. In turn, softening events powerfully initiate the bonding process, wherein secure attachment bonds are engaged and the subsequent bonding events that follow result from this change effectively creating more securely attached relationships. The softening event follows the same EFT steps as withdrawer re-engagement, and these steps highlight how the deepening of emotion moves partner's to more poignant awareness of their view of self and other and one's core attachment needs.

EFT STEPS: Stage 2, Restructuring Bonds—Blamer Softening

5. Access implicit needs, fears, and models of self.
6. Promote acceptance by other—expand the dance.
7. Structure reach and respond, express attachment needs, and create bonding interactions.

Once the more withdrawing partner is "engaged" relationally, the therapist focuses primarily on the more blaming partner through deepening an awareness of disowned aspects of self and promoting partner acceptance (Steps 5 and 6). In Step 7, this culminates into the blamer softening event in which the now softened partner, immersed in attachment-related affect, directly shares attachment fears with their partner and directly asks for her or his attachment needs and wants to be met.

The softening process often begins with the softening partner sharing attachment-related fears. These fears have often shut partners down through the years, blocking the healthy integration of emotion-generated meaning, much less the actual sharing of these fears. The primary object is not to gain insight into these fears and blocks but rather to experientially expand the attachment-related emotions that organize and orient partners to what is important. When attended to and integrated, these expanded emotions propel partners to reach to their partner for comfort, acceptance, and love—through fears and all. Living in fear is exhausting and debilitating. It keeps partners alone and unseen. Attachment-related fears are often embedded in internal working models that inform one's view of self and other. Consider these typical Step 7 statements from softening partners:

- Will you be there for me if I show you this weak and fragile person that I hide from everyone?
- Why would you be there for me if I opened up this much with you?
- How can I trust you? No one has ever really been there for me. (view of self and other).
- I know you are there. You are always there. It's just. . . . It's just how could someone really love me? I mean, just look at me. (view of self).

The EFT therapist must discern whether a softening partner is speaking from a view of other (e.g., fear of rejection), a view of self (e.g., fear of abandonment), or both.

EFT researchers identified six thematic shifts found in successful softening events. Bradley and Furrow (2004) followed the therapist focus and interventions when the therapist guided a pursuer through a softening change event. This process is one of preparing for, shaping, and setting up *enactments* in which partners express attachment needs and connect emotionally. The six themes are sequential rather than linear, meaning the therapist is free to circle back through them based on the processing needs of each particular couple (Figure 7.1). The following exercises will lead you through each of these themes as we follow the therapist focus on changing interactional patterns through blamer softening.

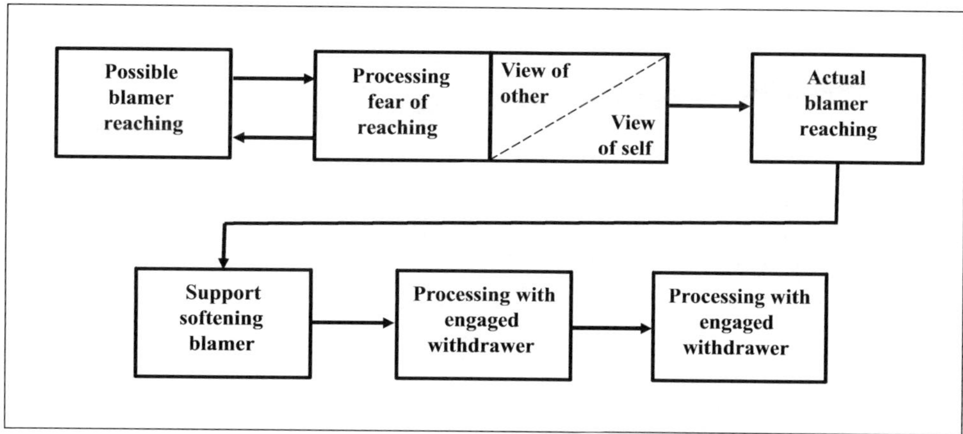

Figure 7.1 Softening mini-theory (Bradley & Furrow, 2004).

Blamer Softening Walk-Through

Marcus and Fresca have been married for 30 years, with three children now grown and out of the house. They are in their mid-50s with middle class socioeconomic status. Marcus has a European cultural background, while Fresca is Hispanic. For Fresca, religion and spirituality were very important, and while Marcus acknowledges that Fresca's Catholic background has impacted him positively, he wasn't particularly religious. They are both second-generation Americans, and both are employed full time. They entered couple therapy reporting ongoing marital conflict for "as long as we can remember." Fresca reported battling with an eating disorder for years, for which she had attended therapy and her struggle with depression, along with a sense of "almost just giving up on us." Marcus described having severe anxiety, to the point at times that he could barely get up and go to work. He also reported being hospitalized for his anxiety several years ago. Each partner acknowledged their struggle to count on the other for emotional reassurance or trust.

As they progressed through Stage 1, both partners were able to clearly describe their cycle. A typical example began with Marcus getting frustrated at Fresca and raising his voice. Fresca responded by trying harder to abate the growing intensity by offering answers she felt were more clear or effective in addressing his concern. Fresca shared: "Even then though, right at the beginning of these times, I feel myself starting to tense up. It's like, 'Oh no, he's building anger here. I've got to defuse it, or he'll explode into me." Her efforts to stop the ensuing "volcano" rarely worked, and Marcus reported that he just wanted her to pay attention to his efforts and support. "Half the time she barely notices that I am asking her for help or that I can't find something." Marcus quickly escalated into anger, criticizing and attacking Fresca. Fresca used to fight back at some point, but for the past ten or so years, she has been just given up and stayed silent. "He rages on for some time, but eventually, he stops. I just let him go. There is no stopping him." At an underlying level, Fresca was very lonely and a felt a sense of being deficient, often saying to herself: "I can't please him. I can't do it right. I come away feeling like an idiot over and over. That just hurts too much, so I've learned to put up the wall and shut him out."

Moving into Stage 2, Fresca began to engage Marcus with her needs. Fresca touched a deep sense of wanting more in the relationship. She realized that she was not perfect but that she was not deficient either. She was tired of walking on eggshells over his anger, and she wanted him to stop attacking her. Marcus was able to solemnly hear her and stated that he wanted that, too, but that he was scared. "I don't know if I know how to stop myself in my negative ways, but I want to. I can see how much this means to you, how much we mean to you." In withdrawer re-engagement, Fresca turned to Marcus and stated, "I am tired of being lonely in our marriage. It doesn't have to be this way. I don't want to hurt like this anymore. I want you to work with me rather than pushing me away with your anger. I need a husband that will love me. One that will hold me when I feel alone or scared. I want you and no one else. We can do this."

In turn, the therapist began to focus more on Marcus and his nagging pain and fear of getting older. He wasn't happy with how much he had done with his life, how much he had saved for his family financially—and he wasn't getting any younger. He reported hearing the "Tick! Tick! Tick!" of the "clock of life." "It's screaming at me, 'You've failed to make enough to support your wife and family! What good are you after all of these years?'" So, when he saw bills to pay or something broken needing replacement, he would quickly go to Fresca to ask how they could possibly owe so much or how something else could yet again be broken. He was quickly overwhelmed often responding with intense anger.

At a core emotional level, Marcus felt like he had failed as a provider to his family and that there was no time left to amend that. Marcus had always been taught by his father that the most important thing in life was being a financial provider. When this sense of failure hit him, he felt panicked in the pit of his stomach. On top of this, the couple's cycle had become so negative and rigidly set over the years that Marcus doubted whether Fresca really loved him. The therapist supported Marcus in sharing these fears with his wife: "I can't say I would blame you if you didn't love me. I haven't been very supportive, either emotionally or financially. Why would you love such a loser and wimp? I get all mad at you, when underneath I feel like such a loser."

Fresca had no idea these emotions were behind Marcus' angry attacks. "I never see this side of you," she responded. Later she reflected on her Hispanic background as being helpful to her in this specific situation: "You know that my Latino heritage really puts family first, and I want to understand this better, to be there for you, and support you." The therapist helped reinforce how important this was to her, how her cultural background well prepared and spurred her on to have a secure connection with Marcus, and that she desperately wanted him to feel safe in sharing with her. "In fact," she said, "these are the same kinds of fears and emotions I have. This lets me know that we are more similar than I ever knew. And that I am not alone in my pain in this relationship." Fresca's support set the stage for the therapist to move toward blamer softening. The therapist wondered if Marcus was ever able to share his attachment fears with Fresca, to really reach for her as his ally.

Theme 1: Possible Blamer Reaching

The therapist often "choreographs" entrance into the softening event by asking the couple to imagine engaging with one another from a new level of vulnerability. The stage is set when the couple has re-entered a recent episode when the more blaming partner has gotten angry, sullen, or sad, the effect of which usually shuts down hopes of mutual accessibility and responsiveness. Often, the result of this interactional sequence breaks the emotional connection between partners. "I told him I could handle it," a typical engaged partner says, "but he just kept getting angry. I wasn't withdrawing, but I wasn't going to allow him to just run over me either. I asked him what was going on, could we talk about it. He just got more angry and eventually went silent. Like we've talked about in here, at these times he won't really let me in. So, I said, 'forget it.' We haven't really been 'connected' since then, and it has been three days."

At this point in the therapy process, the negative interactional cycle is nothing new to the couple or therapist. In Step 7, the therapist briefly re-enters a recent salient episode by reflecting reactive behaviors and underlying emotions but then quickly follows this with an evocative inquiry that explores a new kind of relational possibility—one indirectly aimed toward the more blaming partner. "When you get like this, when you are so overwhelmed, so panicked, could you ever turn to her and say, 'I am so panicked right now. This fear is really welling up inside of me'? Would that be too hard for you? What would that be like, to let her in, to reach to her for then?"

The therapist usually uses a "first-person" stance or "proxy voice" that allows the more-blaming partner to experientially take on this possible position and being to imagine leaning into this experience. This has the effect of experientially preparing the couple for what is next without creating an interpretive or skills-building context.

Earlier in the week, Marcus had learned that their house had termites and needed extensive treatment. The costs of this had sent him through the roof. On top of this, his car's engine was skipping, and the mechanic suggested it was time to look for a new car. Marcus had again gone a rampage, attacking Fresca for not staying on top of when the house needed insect treatment. She had remained engaged, however, stating that she was sorry that she missed it, but that he missed it, too. "I see that you're angry," Fresca had replied. "And that's okay. I am angry, too. What I don't want is you going on and on at me. I want you to stop. This gets us nowhere, and we both know that. Let's tackle this together. First, though, what is going on for you besides the anger?" At that point, Marcus "shut down" and refused to talk. Marcus is well aware of his affect, but he is unable to take an interpersonal step and enlist his wife as an alley against the fear and loathing of himself.

Therapist: Marcus, you know, you guys have come a long way. You are not fighting nearly as often, nor as intensely. Fresca, you really stood your ground when Marcus got upset this time. I think it's great how you were able to, in effect, see through his anger and not withdraw. Marcus, you were able to stop attacking when she did this. But there still seems to be one aspect missing.

Exercise 7.1. Possible Blamer Reaching

Check the responses an EFT therapist might make to help Marcus begin to imagine reaching to Fresca in times of severe distress. The therapist wants to know if he has considered sharing with her during these times and what that prospect is like for him. Look for responses that assess and yet invite him to experientially imagine this new way of interacting with his wife. (Check all that apply.)

a. "Could you ever turn to Fresca and share with her about how overwhelmed you feel in these times?" ____
b. "Marcus, Fresca wants to be let in when these worries and fears invade you. This week she stood beside you and said, 'What's going on besides the anger?' On another level, she is saying, 'Let me in.' Right, Fresca? (she nods). She's saying, 'I want to be there and help you.' What would it be like for you to try to let her in during these times?" ____
c. "Marcus, if you used 'I' statements and Fresca assured you that she would only listen and reflect back to you, would you try communicating like that with her next time?" ____

d. "You can't let her in because she will only make fun of you, call you a loser, remind you of how you've failed. This is what you heard all through childhood, and you're convinced that's what you would get from her." ____
e. "Fresca didn't withdraw. My sense is she wants to be there for you when you are overwhelmed, vulnerable, afraid, and all. What would it be like to risk sharing your fears with her then? What would it be like to begin letting her in?" ____
f. "What thoughts came into mind when Fresca asked you what was going on besides the anger?" ____
g. "Marcus, have there been times when you were able to let her in? Let's look at what was different about those times." ____

Exercise 7.2. Exploring a Possible Blamer Reach

Continuing in this scenario, the therapist asks the more blaming partner to imagine making a bid for his attachment needs to be met. Choose the EFT response that best accomplishes this.

a. "What happens inside as you consider opening up to her during these situations?" ____
b. "Do you ever turn to Fresca and share what's going on inside for you?" ____
c. "The cycle between you has changed, guys. Fresca, it's great how you stood your ground. It seems that you didn't let Marcus' anger push you to withdraw. Rather, you asked him to stop the anger and include you in what was perhaps underneath and bothering him. You want him to let you in, yeah? Do you hear her right now Marcus?" ____
d. "Marcus, during these intense situations, do you ever think of turning to Fresca and saying, 'You know what, hon, I'm struggling with all of this anxiety about this termite situation and the costs. And I am really dejected about the car. I'm still caught in all of that, you know, all those feelings that come up for me about money and my worth to you and the family. I am having such a hard time with it right now.' That would have been really hard for you, yeah?" ____

Exercise 7.3. Forming a Possible Blamer Reach

When a more blaming partner reports, "I let him have it. I did. I hate that I did. I just get so upset with him. I just feel like he should be able to do this right! I know I am driving him away, but at the time, my anger just overruns my fear so fast." "It's easier for you to run to your anger," the therapist responds, "than it is to risk letting him in on the fear and pain that is going on inside of you. And so you guys get stuck here yet again, right?" (brief summary of blamer's cycle and underlying emotion)

Write your own processing possible blamer reaching responses to this vignette. First, create your own brief reflection of the blamer's cycle and underlying emotions.

Create a brief cycle summary with underlying emotion.

____

____

Now write a brief "first-person" dialog using proxy voice that experientially walks the more blaming partner through inviting the other to come close and comfort during overwhelming times. When finished, compare your responses with sample responses given at the end of this chapter.

Create a first-person dialog (proxy voice) inviting the other in.

____

____

Theme 2: Processing Fears of Reaching

Most partners respond that they do not invite the other in mainly because it's too risky and they are afraid. They sometimes report having done this in the past or that it is something they could try. Regardless, the EFT therapist takes them at their word and responds in a manner that moves them forward to risking this in session. Degree of fear varies among couples, which is largely related to the level and duration of distress, but there is usually some form and level of fear blocking possible attachment bids. This does not apply to any situation in which distress occurs but rather in interactions when attachment insecurities get primed and are up and running between mates. This may or may not happen in a discussion about taking out the garbage, for example. Fighting and disagreements are normal, perhaps even healthy at times.

It's the habitual negative cycle that spins out of control when attachment-related fears and insecurities are triggered. Empathic conjecture/interpretation and heightening are both used at this point. If fear has been previously recognized by the more-blaming partner as blocking in these specific situations, then heightening the attachment-related fear is in order. If fear has yet to be uncovered, the EFT therapist often uses empathic conjecture/interpretation to help the client deepen and assembler their experience (Move 2). Insight is not the goal here. In fact, an insight-oriented interpretation at this point can shut down experiential processing, yielding more-cognitive responses such as, "Oh, I'd never connected that with my past before" or "Yes, you are right on." Instead the EFT therapist focuses on deepening emotional experience and assembling the pursuing partner's attachment-related fears. Empathic conjecture/interpretation of fear is followed with heightening to make it more vivid and alive in the session. New meaning crystallizes from the slow processing of attachment-related affect that has previously been pushed out of awareness.

In session, Marcus states that he never really considers sharing or letting Fresca in when times get intense. "It's not safe enough for me to let her in during those situations," he reports, shaking his head demonstratively. He then talks about how she has hurt him in the past and that he wouldn't risk showing his vulnerability by asking for anything when he's really feeling that low. "When I am that overwhelmed and low, she could really hurt me if I let her in on how I am actually feeling" he says. "I can't see doing that. The stakes are just too high." This signals the therapist to move into processing fears of reaching—fears that serve to block and shut down attachment longings for support, comfort, and reassurance (Move 2).

Exercise 7.4. Processing Fears of Reaching

In these exercises, you will be asked to identify typical EFT responses when beginning to process fears of reaching for support. You will then practice writing your own similar responses.

Based in Marcus' responses in the previous scenario, choose the EFT responses from the list. (more than one correct answer)

a. "I don't know, help me out here, but it sounds like you are dealing with this all alone." (Marcus nods yes) ____
b. "Have there been times when you have been able to let her in? What was different about those times?" ____
c. (slower) "It's like one part of you says, 'Well that would be pretty scary to do because suppose I did it wrong or suppose I got aggressive like I have in the past or suppose I just lost it and looked like a real 'loser.' Right? That goes through you?" (he nods, slowly and softly) "This would just be too risky . . . too scary." ____
d. "Okay, I don't think you should let her in. Neither of you can handle it. It's just too much. I want each of you to promise me that you will not talk about what is really happening for either of you when these kinds of situations arise." ____
e. "You guys have made real progress here. But it looks like there needs to be this one more step. Fresca, you are there, standing with Marcus, asking to be let in. But Marcus, you get scared, right?" (he nods; softer) "Help me understand this fear, what happens inside when you are really overwhelmed and Fresca says, 'Hey Marcus, here I am. Please let me in. Can you hear me?' What happens?" ____

Exercise 7.5. Processing Fears of Reaching and Empathic Conjectures

A more-blaming partner may respond to the EFT therapist's imaginative inquiry (e.g., "Have you ever turned to him and . . . ") with "I can't let him in, not then. I would never reach for him then. I just can't," shaking her head vehemently. While this partner has globally talked about her fears before, she has never shared that fear blocks her from reaching during these specific and intense situations. Based on attachment theory, the EFT therapist hypothesizes that unprocessed fear is indeed often shutting her down. Now, select two empathic conjecture/interpretations from the selections that best seek to help the client take one step further into her experience.

a. (softly) "It seems to me that you get to this point, when he is there wanting to understand, and you either show anger or go silent. I don't know, help me here if I am wrong, but I am wondering if there is a part of you that really gets scared during these moments. A part that that says, 'You had better not risk this.' Is that close?" ____
b. (softly to engaged withdrawer) "It must be terribly difficult for you to want so badly for your wife to let you in when she is struggling so, only to have her get angry or shut you out. How do you cope with this?" ____
c. (softly) "I am going out on a limb here a bit, so please help me out. I wonder if a part of you really gets scared when he is there and you are faced with all of these things that overwhelm you. I mean at a level that perhaps you rarely allow yourself to touch. I wonder if this fear tells you that you had better not open up to him. Can you help me here?" ____

d. (softly) "It seems to me that you say you want him to be close, but then when there is a chance, you sabotage it. You are withholding yourself from him. I think you are being dishonest with your husband. Let's not waste our time here. It's time to come clean like adults." ____

When the more blaming partner responds "Nooooo. I haven't let her in when I am getting that angry. I go from overwhelming shame and feelings of worthlessness to anger so fast. To show her that vulnerable side, that weak part of me—that's not what she wants and needs from me. Who would want that?"

Write your own brief summary reflection, including an empathic conjecture to help this client begin to take one step further into his experience of fear that is blocking possible connection with his wife. When finished, compare your responses with the sample EFT response provided in the answers section.

____

____

____

____

Exercise 7.6. Processing Blamer Reaching With Heightening

Now imagine a more blaming partner is well aware of attachment-related fears that shut her down, and the therapist moves directly to heighten these fears. Key secure attachment descriptors are often woven into the processing to further prompt the surfacing of healthy attachment wants and needs (see "trust" and "rely"). The therapist continues to stress what is possible—the risk of reaching for comfort and security.

> *"No way," a more blaming partner says, "I don't reach for him. That is just too scary." "I see," the therapist responds. (slower and softer) "It's just way too scary to risk beginning to trust and rely on him. It's just not safe. A part of you says, 'Don't you dare!'"*

Write one of your own heightening responses to this scenario. Remember, the client is aware of fear, which signals the therapist to heighten rather than empathically conjecture/interpret.

____

____

____

____

Following your response, suppose the more pursing partner looks to exit processing their fear and says, "Yeah. It's too risky. But it wouldn't help anyway." "It wouldn't help anyway?" the therapist responds. "Help me understand." "What good would it do?" the more-blaming partner responds. "I mean, he'd either belittle me, or ignore me, something like that."

Exercise 7.7: Processing Blamer Reaching With Heightening Empathic Conjecture

Choose the EFT response that deepens the more blaming partner's fear of reaching using an empathic conjecture followed by heightening.

a. "It's just too scary. You just can't bring yourself to risk." ____
b. "Help me out here, but it's like this part of you stands up and says, 'Don't you dare share how afraid or scared you are! If you show him your "underbelly" he'll belittle you or ignore you.' Right? This part piles on and says, 'What good would it do anyway? Don't you dare do it. He won't be there. He won't care. Don't you hope for that.' It's just too scary for you let him in. The stakes are just too high, too painful." ____
c. "You're so disgusted at him that you aren't convinced turning and sharing this with him would do any good, right? You've tried this before, and he only dismisses you. Time and time again, you've risked with him, and he just doesn't get it. He'll never get it." ____
d. "This is the point in the cycle where you guys never seem to be able to 'break through' and risk sharing your underlying emotion with each other. You usually choose to attack him, which covers up your fears. All he sees is your anger, though, which compels him to protect and withdraw. This keeps both of you 'locked out,' so to speak. Suppose I had a magic wand, and I waved this magic wand, and a miracle occurred. The miracle resulted in this dilemma being solved. Suppose now that happened. What would now be different? How would you know that this dilemma between you was solved?" ____

Staying on track is also part of the processing fears of reaching theme. Sometimes when a more blaming partner is asked if he ever considers reaching for support at home, he will report that he has reached for his partner and that this is nothing new. This can be a way of trying to sidestep having to risk, even risking imaginatively in session. Such responses attest to the power of the softening event. Usually, the kind of reach that the therapist is talking about is not the kind the client reports. In these cases, however, the EFT therapist briefly assesses this by tracking what was said, how it was said, and how it ended. These interactions can indeed be attempts for attachment, but they often lack the kind of attachment-related processing that is the key to change in softening events. In session, the therapist recreates the interaction and then intensifies it in the same manner as is being described in this chapter.

Processing Views of Self and Other

When attachment-related fears are heightened in Step 7, they emanate from the more-blaming partner's negative views of other and/or views of self (see Figure 7.1). It is important for the therapist to recognize and attend to these distinctions. Responses resulting from negative views of the other usually have to do with the fear of the other partner showing contempt, criticizing, pouring shame on them, or abandoning them. Responses resulting from negative views of self are more likely rooted in an inherent sense of deficiency, worthlessness, feeling unlovable, and self-shame. As one client, speaking from a positive view of other but a clear negative view of self, sobbed, "I know he will be there. He always is. My fear is, who would really want me? Just look at me!"

The EFT therapist starts processing fears emerging from a negative view of other, and for many couples, this seems to be enough. But for some couples, a negative view of self must be heightened and processed through as well. Note in the following exercise how the EFT therapist often uses "parts" language to separate out healthy attachment longings from the fears that block moving to get them met. At times partners will tie in attachment fears to how a parent was so condescending to them, so distant or neglectful. The therapist naturally honors such insights and memories to help shed light on and heighten the difficulty and fear of reaching to the other in the present relationship.

Exercise 7.8. Processing Fear of Reaching

Choose which of the following heightening responses address negative views of other and which address negative views of self. Enter "self" or "other" for each response.

1. "It's so hard for you to risk turning to her. The stakes are so high. She could really hurt you. She means more to you than anyone else, and you desperately want to reach to her, for it to be safe. But the part of you that is afraid keeps saying, 'Don't! Don't! Don't!'" ________
2. "You see him standing there, arms open. He's saying, 'Risk it honey. I'll be here for you. You can count on me.' But a part of you is saying, 'No, I can't risk it. He won't be there. No one has ever truly been there. It's too scary, too risky, it could hurt too much.' Is that close?" ________
3. "You're saying, 'I know she is there. I believe her. It's not that, it's that no one has really ever been there and cared for me.' A part of you says, 'Maybe there's something wrong with me. Maybe I am too strange, kind of unlovable.' Is that some of what goes on?" ________
4. "You're saying, 'I see you there, and I hear that you want me to risk letting you in. But I am so afraid. My parents let me down and hurt me so badly. I risked with my father, and he left me all alone, crushed. I vowed that I would never let anyone hurt me that badly again. And here you are, asking me to risk with you? It scares me to death.' Am I getting it?" ________
5. "Of course, this is very hard for you. Of course, it's very scary. How could it not be? Bill has not been there in the past. For years you've had to go at this all alone. When you were sad, he was not there. When you were in pain, he was not there. You learned to cope without him. You gave up on your dreams for the two of you. Now, suddenly, he says that he is there and that he wants you to let him in, after all these years. A part of you says, 'He will hurt me again. I can't count on him. Play it tight to the chest, play it safe.' Right?" ________
6. "Bill is here asking you to reach for him, to count on him, to let him in. But no one has really ever cared that much for you. No one has ever really cherished you just because you are who you are. Your mom died at an early age, and you two weren't close. Your dad drank and abused you. That's what men have done to you for most of your life, right? And so now as Bill stands here wanting you to

share your heart with him, to risk sharing your fears and longings with him, you find it very hard to believe that he really wants you, that he really loves you. It's so scary for you to let yourself even begin to believe that anyone could possibly love you wholeheartedly. Am I hearing you?" ________

Marcus stated that he never turns to Fresca and shows his "soft side." "No," he reported, "I only get aggressive with her." The therapist heightened based on a possible negative view of other: "So, what you're saying to Fresca is (slowly), 'Fresca, when these fears come up for me, when I start to feel caught in all of this stuff about that I don't feel somehow in control of my life or that I haven't been able to do some things in my life that I wanted, I still feel somehow out of control around money, it still scares me—when I am struggling with all of these feelings, it's still really hard for me to reach for you. I am just not sure if you'll reject me or get angry at me or call me weak.' Yeah?"

Now imagine Marcus responds: "Yes, I am scared that she will see me as wimpy . . . small. Who wants that? My mother always told me that I'd never be able to make any woman truly happy." (he cries) "I sometimes think I am just so sick, so weird, somehow wired differently than others. Fresca tries, she really does, but I don't know why she really cares at all."

Exercise 7.9. Processing Blamer Reaching With Heightening

Using the previous transcript, use "parts language" (i.e., "One part of you says . . . but another part says. . . .") to (a) briefly reflect Marcus' fears/negative view of other and (b) heighten his fears/negative view of self. Try to incorporate "first-person dialog" as part of this heightening. Seek to bring the attachment fears and longings to a "boiling point." (c) Finish with an evocative response (i.e., "Is this close?"). When completed, compare your responses with one provided in the answer section.

- Briefly reflect fears/negative view of other (use parts language).

  ____

  ____

- Heighten fears/negative view of self (use parts language).

  ____

  ____

- Provide a brief evocative response.

  ____

  ____

The more-blaming partner needs to deeply experience attachment-related fears in the session—in other words, they need to become real and alive. This process has to reach a "boiling point," so to speak, before moving forward. The duration of this, of course, varies among couples. If sufficient heightening is not accomplished, the softening may take on a more cognitive emphasis, which pulls them out of immediate emotional experiencing. As demonstrated in the next list, the words used and the tone taken vary among couples. For some couples, perhaps less distressed ones, it is not as scary to share and open themselves up during softening events. For others, the process proves very difficult and requires more heightening and more processing.

To this point, the softening partner has only spoken directly to the therapist, which is not sufficient in EFT. In fact, this only clarifies what needs to be shared and asked for from the other, now-engaged partner. In preparation inviting an engaged encounter (Move 3), the therapist briefly summarizes work just completed in the processing fears of reaching to set up a possible softening enactment. The therapist summarizes Marcus' experience "So, to even consider turning to Fresca and saying, 'Honey, I am just so scared right now. I am overwhelmed, I need a hug, a little reassurance. I am really doubting myself.' That is really scary for you. This fear sort of paralyzes you; it keeps you alone in your doubts and fears, yeah?"

Exercise 7.10. Summarizing the Processing of the Pursuer's Fear of Reaching

Which of the following are typical therapist responses best summarize a pursuer's fears of reaching before initiating a softening enactment?

a. "If we're going to be truthful here, you have to be honest with her. The fact is you don't trust her. You're not convinced that she has changed. You are being just selfish enough to not give her the chance to hurt you again, is that it?" ____

b. "You never show him this part of you, this part that says, 'Don't you dare open up to him again. You'll get stabbed in the heart. It just hurts too much to risk.' You never let him in when this part raises its head. You never say, 'I am really scared right now that you can't be trusted. Could you please reassure me now?' You never say that, right? Because that is just too scary, too . . . precise . . . too . . . on the money?" ____

c "She has asked for your forgiveness many, many times. She has done as much as she can to prove to you that she is trustworthy. And yet, you stay here, unflinching. Unforgiving. What will it take from her for you to honestly forgive her? I can't make you do it, and neither can she. You have to take the risk." ____

d. "So, this is very dangerous territory for you, yeah? You see that she is here, right now, wanting you to come out and be with her. A part of you sees that and for the most part believes that. But there is this other part that really protects you, and it is screaming, 'No one has ever loved you. No one ever will. The only safe game in town is to hide, whether in anger or silence.' Right? So this indeed is dangerous territory." ____

e. "Bill, I'd like for you to play her father for a minute. Elisa, look at him now. He is not the way he was before; he is your father, there to accept you and hold you. Do you see that in your father's eyes now? Bill, what did you feel as Elisa was doing this?" ____

f. "This week, Lucinda, you noticed at one point when the cycle was starting to happen that you felt afraid that Juan may leave again. But this time you didn't attack him or go silent. This time you said, 'Honey, I am getting scared that you might leave me. The rational side of me knows that we are just arguing, but there is another part of me, a bigger part, that is scared. Could we stop arguing for now and could you reassure me?' How was that for you, to risk reaching from within your fear?" ____

In the space provided, try out your own summarization of the work just completed in this therapist theme as illustrated above (i.e., "So to even consider turning to Fresca and saying . . . is just so scary . . . ").

____

____

____

____

____

____

Theme 3: Actual Blamer Reaching

The process of a softening partner turning toward their partner and reaching for accessibility and assurance amid their attachment fears and longings is in many ways the capstone of EFT. In this engaged encounter (Move 3), the therapist gently directs the now softening blamer to listen to and *enact* attachment needs and longings and to reach directly to her partner for comfort and assurance. This is one of the simplest directives the EFT therapist makes, but it is also one of the most intense, both for the couple and therapist. Having heightened the attachment-related affect, the therapist gently asks the softening partner to turn and share this with his partner using a restructuring and reshaping interactions intervention.

The softening encounter often starts with having the pursuing partner share directly with the other how scary it is to envision openly turning to the other. Typical wording of the intervention could include: "Marcus, would you please turn now and share this with Fresca, in your own words," or "Marcus, could you begin now to tell Fresca how scary it is to even think of turning to her during these times? Would you please share this with her now?" This intervention is short, direct, and to the point. The groundwork has been laid, and the time to risk and reach is now. Often, the softening partner then needs time to integrate newly emerging meaning brought into awareness from the processing of attachment-related affect before beginning to directly address their partner. Initial research shows an average of 8 to 16 seconds of silence is common, authenticating the intensity of the moment (Bradley & Furrow, 2004). The therapist respectfully stays out of the way unless this partner gets stuck and asks for aid.

The "softening reach" is actually worded within each couple's own language and rhythms. It doesn't, for example, come off as dry as our academic description of "asking for attachment needs and wants to be met." It must be affectively charged for the message to come across experientially. In real-world language, the softening reach often begins with the seemingly small yet transforming step of directly facing one's partner and revealing, "It's so scary to think of turning to you and letting you in," or "I am really afraid to share this with you. I don't ever show this part of me." The therapist often aids the softening partner to articulate attachment needs and wants with their partners, which usually follows the immersion into and sharing of one's attachment-related affect. In the case of less distressed couples, the softening reach may move directly into the articulation of attachment needs and wants more fluidly, such as "I need you to be there and help me with these fears, with these doubts. I've carried these with me my whole life, and it's terribly hard to share them with you. But I want to let you in . . . and for us to face this together." If the softening reach is not affectively charged and, for example, seems very cognitive in nature, the EFT therapist often returns to further heighten views of other and/or self.

Exercise 7.11. Softening Reach Enactments

From the list, choose the EFT responses typically used in the actual blamer reaching theme (more than one correct answer).

a. "Could you please turn to him and share with him how scary it is to reach out to him in these situations—in your own words?" ____
b. "Could you tell her, please?" ____
c. "If you were to reach out to him, what do you think he would think and say?" ____
d. "You've shared with me how afraid and paralyzed you get by this fear. But it's one thing to tell me, and quite another to tell her. Would you please, just now, turn and share this with her?" ____
e. (to engaged partner) "What do you think is going through her mind as she considers reaching out to you?" ____
f. "Could you turn to her now and tell her how much you desperately need and want her to be there for you now, in your own words, please?" ____
g. "I'd like for you to turn to him now and risk letting him in. Will you please now, in your own words, share with him what it's like for you to even consider turning to him when you are so afraid and how he can help you in this." ____

Exercise 7.12. Practicing a Softening Reach

Using the following example, practice forming a blamer softening reach.

"So, to even consider turning to Fresca and saying, 'Honey, I am just so scared right now. I am overwhelmed. I am struggling with these frightful doubts about whether you really love me. I need a hug, a little reassurance. I am really doubting myself.' That is really scary for you. This fear sort of paralyzes you . . . it keeps you alone in your doubts and fears, yeah?" "Oh yeah," Marcus replies, looking down. "That would be huge." Now write a softening enactment reach.

____

____

____

____

Theme 4: Supporting the Softening Pursuer

The fourth theme in the process of blamer softening focuses on Move 4 of the EFT Tango. The therapist stands behind and supports the blamer as they risk, as the following example shows. Marcus gathered himself, turned directly to Fresca and slowly shared, "This is really hard for me. I really doubt myself, and I doubt that you will even want me if I show this weak and scared part of me to you. If there's any way. . . . I'd just love for you to grab my hand or hug me sometimes when I am afraid or acting stupid because of all of this junk. I'd love your reassurance. But it's so scary to ask you for it; to even do this right now is all new territory for me. And I am scared right now that you'll laugh at me, or think, 'Who is this weak man I married?'" Fresca warmly replied, "I love it when you show this part of you to me, Marcus. If you ask, I will do all I can to comfort you."

The therapist first moves to "shore up" the softening blamer's new interactional stance just taken in the relationship with support, which emphasizes the importance of the relational step just risked. The therapist briefly reflects with an attachment-related affect and present focus. (therapist, softly) "I think that was great, Marcus. You really risked. You opened up and shared with Fresca what you need and how scary that is. Borrowing your own words, that was 'huge.'"

The therapist then aids the softening partner in processing their own internal responses to the softening reach with an evocative response intervention. "What was it like for you, Marcus, to turn and say that to Fresca? What's happening inside now?" This helps the softening partner organize arising new meaning stemming from the attachment focused interaction. (Again, this demonstrates the inextricable interactional systemic, and intrapsychic experiential focus of EFT.)

Exercise 7.13. Supporting Softened Pursuer

Select the EFT supporting softening blamer responses that best support Marcus following his reach to Fresca.

a. "That was really something there, Marcus. You really did it. You jumped out there and risked. What was that like for you?" ____
b. "I want to recognize what Marcus just did. Marcus, I think you really risked here, you really risked with Fresca. You asked her in. How was that inside for you?" ____
c. "Marcus, what you just did really was different from the way you learned to interact growing up. You would never have said that to your members of your family. You're really starting to stand on your own two feet." ____
d. "What could Fresca do to help you do this more? What would you like from her to help set the stage for you?" ____
e. "You just opened up to her, Marcus. You let her in on your fears. You asked her to come stand with you. How was that for you? What's happening inside now?" ____
f. "Fresca, what was it like to hear this from Marcus?" ____

Now write your own supportive response while also considering how you might validate Marcus' response to your support.

- What would you say to support Marcus after his reach?

____

____

- What would you say to validate Marcus' experience if he shared that he felt "uneasy" making this request?

____

____

The therapist then briefly reflects the softening partner's response, anticipating moving to getting clear support from the other. "It was scary, but . . . it felt really good," Marcus replied. "It felt good to finally come clean with her about my insecurities and fears." "It feels good to open up to her like that," the therapist reflects and then turns toward the other.

Theme 5: Processing With the Engaged Withdrawer

The softening event continues as the therapist turns to process the softening reach with the other partner. The specific focus is the immediate affective response of the engaged partner to the softening partner's reach from within attachment fears and needs. Again, the softening reach pulls for comforting responses. The objective here is to help the engaged partner clarify and organize immediate emotional processing into a direct response of accessibility, responsiveness, safety, and comfort to the softening partner. The therapist carefully creates the context by slowly reflecting the salient attachment themes of the softening reach, followed by an evocative response intervention. "Fresca," the therapist slowly says, "Marcus just shared how afraid he gets, scared that you will see him as weak or somehow lacking. And how he desperately longs for you to accept and comfort him . . . to be there for him regardless. He really risked sharing this with you just now. What happened inside as he let you in like this?" (Therapist taps hand just above her own heart as she says this.)

Exercise 7.14. Exploring the Engaged Withdrawer's Response

From the list, choose the EFT responses explore the engaged withdrawer's experience of the engaged softening encounter. Hint: Look for evocative responses and questions:

a. "Fresca, has he opened up like this with you before?" ____
b. "Marcus, what did Fresca do that helped you risk and share like this?" ____
c. "What was it like for you, Fresca, as Marcus shared with you how afraid he gets, how this fear grips him and tells him that you'll look down on him as somehow weak? What happened inside as he showed this part to you just now?" ____
d. "What happened inside, Fresca, as Marcus just risked sharing with you how much he desperately craves your acceptance and reassurance? It's like you have this balm of healing that he longs for, but a part of him is so afraid to ask for it. What was it like inside hearing this?" ____

e. "Fresca, can you now accept what Marcus just said? Remember, this is about accepting the differences between you. You accept that his needs are different than yours. You don't have to agree with what he said, but it's important that you each accept your individual differences in needs and perspectives. Can you state back to him his needs now from a stance of acceptance rather than blame or defensiveness?" ____

Now write your own supportive response while also considering how you might validate Marcus' response to your support.

- What would you say to explore Fresca's response to Marcus' softened reach?

  ____

  ____

- What would you say to reflect and heighten Fresca's response if she tearfully shares that she felt a "deeper love and appreciation" for Marcus through his vulnerable reach?

  ____

  ____

"It was great," Fresca replies. "I don't see him as weak. In fact, when he shows me his heart like this, I want to be with him. I want to comfort him." The therapist then reflects Fresca's response, often with a sense of intrigue, framed such as "Let me see if I get this. When he opens up and shows you these parts of him that are afraid and uncertain, when he says, 'I need your acceptance and comfort,' this actually pulls you toward him?" This reflective/questioning response is important because it keeps the process flow going naturally toward asking this partner to now reach directly back to their partner with support.

Exercise 7.15. Processing and Assembling the Engaged Withdrawer's Response

From the list, choose the EFT empathic reflections/questioning responses that help in processing with engaged withdrawer.

a. "What have you done in the past that has worked when he says these things?" ____

b. "When you hear him open up, it actually pulls you toward comforting him." ____

c. "Am I hearing this right? When in fact he shows you his fears, you want to then come and comfort him?" ____

d. "Can you tell him that you will accept that he feels insecure sometimes?" ____

e. "Wow. I find this incredibly interesting. When he dares to show you his fear and his vital need for your reassurance and comfort, things that he fears will send you packing, it actually moves you toward comforting him?" ____

Now write your own empathic reflection or evocative response to invite Fresca to further explore her experience building on her response to Marcus described above.

- What would you say to further explore Fresca's response to Marcus' softened reach?

____

____

- What would you say to heighten Fresca's response if she tearfully shares that she felt "more important to Marcus" because he shared this vulnerable need?

____

____

- What other response might you offer Fresca to further assemble her core emotional response to Marcus if she wanted to reach out and hug him but wasn't sure if this is what he wanted?

____

____

Theme 6: Engaged Withdrawer Reaching Back With Support

The final step in the softening event involves unfolding the processing momentum built thus far. The softening reach has now been briefly processed intrapsychically with the engaged partner, and the therapist moves to the interpersonal, reaching back to help the engaged partner support the softening partner. "Yes!" Fresca says adamantly. "It makes me feel close to him. Like I can come be with him. I have something special to offer him." The therapist responds with a restructuring interactions intervention such as, "Would you please tell him this in your own words right now? How when he risks like this and lets you in, that this makes you want to be with him even more? Would you please turn and directly share that with him now in your own words?" The therapist creates an engaged encounter (Move 3) focused on the engaged withdrawer's processing of the softening event as a whole and the pursuer's more vulnerable reach for support.

Exercise 7.16. Enacting the Engaged Withdrawer's Response

- What would you say to reflect or heighten Fresca's response if she tearfully shares how much it meant for him to turn to her and share this vulnerable need? How would you focus and highlight her emerging awareness and openness?

____

____

The therapist deepens Fresca's experience highlights an emerging confidence in Marcus (e.g., "He is truly relying on me.") and shifts her experience toward her hopes that he truly values her. She in turn responds: "I wish he would turn to me like this more often, I would be there for him."

- What would say to create an engaged encounter focusing Fresca's openness and engagement?

____

____

BLAMER SOFTENING MISSTEPS

Blamer softening is the more challenging of the three EFT change events with couples. Bradley and Furrow (2007) highlighted common missteps they found in reviewing unsuccessful softening attempts. These missteps provide the EFT therapist reviewing softening attempts that go awry or fail to promote the impact consistent with this "watershed event" (Johnson & Greenberg, 1988).

Missing Attachment Focus

Attachment theory provides a critical lens for the EFT therapist in making sense of the emotions underlying the blocks that organize relationship distress. As the therapist comes alongside a couple's core pain and fear, we need to be working though these blocks using an attachment frame. Rather than focusing only on the emotion (e.g., sadness), the EFT therapist locates that sadness in a relational frame often including a focus on the attachment significance of that experience. For example, Marcus' expresses fear of his inadequacies and how they leave him feeling unworthy. More than focusing solely on his fear of being abandoned places that fear in relationship to Fresca. "Marcus, in these moments, the fear takes hold, a fear of not only being alone but also of losing Fresca and all she means to you, yes?" This empathic conjecture primes the attachment significance of his fear. The EFT therapist embraces the attachment context as a foundation and frame to reflect, reframe, and heighten the primary emotion that becomes the main message of our engaged encounters throughout Stage 2.

Self-Assessment: When processing emotional experience, do I frame the present experience of my client in relational terms or an attachment context, priming a client's experience with key attachment themes and words?

Attachment-Related Affect—Distance

Throughout EFT Stage 2 change events, therapists have to hold the client's primary emotion like a sculptor holds clay. If the therapist is emotionally distant from a partner's affect, so also will that partner. As clinicians, we take up the client's pain first, picking it up (metaphorically speaking), and passing it back and forth between our hands, shaping experience. We hold it, we let ourselves feel the lure of it, we imagine it were our own for a moment. We hold it in ways that help it come alive by holding in an attachment context for the client.

In softening events and throughout the whole of EFT, we go into the emotion and use it to choreograph new experiences for each partner and their relationship. When we find ourselves talking about the emotion or educating our clients about emotion, we need to shift levels and go into the emotion, experientially. The therapist works not only from a perspective of emotion as "allowable" (Bradley & Furrow, 2007, p. 36) but also shifting to actually prioritizing and privileging emotion experientially. In EFT Tango, this is the crucial work of assembling and deepening emotion, which harness the power of relationally engaging underlying models of self and other in a transformative way.

The only way to get limbic revision is by making sure we are working experientially. Essentially, that the limbic system is open and active and therefore able to be revised as a result of new experiences, or as Bradley and Furrow (2007) suggest, the emotion-focused path is working, ". . . from the inside out—letting the emotional unfolding lead the way" (p. 37).

Self-Assessment: When focusing on a partner's underlying view of self or other, do I deepen the present experience of my client and foster a deeper engagement of their vulnerability through intensifying attachment-related affect?

Attachment-Related Fear Allergies

Overlooking fear or acknowledging but not accessing fear can be a type of "fear allergy" for some clinicians. Talking over fear, teaching or explaining fear, or patting down fear are all strategies we use to combat fear in our lives. Today, the science is clear: We need to go close to our clients' fears, hold them, take them in experientially ourselves, and let them come alive in order for the client to make and then deepen their experiential contact with their fears. As we, together—clinician and client—make experiential contact with the client's fear, the fear become less potent, less overwhelming, more friendly. As the fear becomes less overwhelming, the client and their partner grow confidence and competence in working with this fear together. In exploring and engaging this fear, the client's need emerge, and this explicit need re-orients the client and their relationship to what's most important. Helping our clients find their fear (experientially!) and take the risk to go close to it again and again changes it! Our fears feel smaller and get less scary and continually orient us to our needs.

If you notice that it's hard for you to go closer to your own or your client's fears, practice evoking, reflecting, and heightening fear in the context of its attachment significance: a current or historical relationship. As we know from Bowlby (1988), unprocessed fear blocks our expressions of vulnerability and reaches for connection. In Stage 2 sessions, you will want to cultivate your courage to go close to your client's fears as they come alive in the current relationship and work with the fears experientially. Let the fears grow, come alive, and be shared—this is the ultimate reach in the Stage 2 change events!

Self-Assessment: When are you likely to mis-attune, disengage, or dismiss a partner's fear in session? What is happening inside in you in one of the moments? Reflect on this experience and the triggers and your actions in responding to a partner's fear. What it be like to go the other way in this moment and to lean into processing or deepening your client's fear?

Unacknowledged View of Self/View of Other

In Stage 2, the EFT therapist is focused on eliciting problematic views of self or others. These underlying perceptions organize the social and emotion responses partners share in more vulnerable experience of their relationships. Pursuers' core emotions are commonly informed by a negative view of self and are ironically maintain a preoccupied focus on their partner's insecurities and shortcomings. In Stage 2, it is crucial for the therapist to evoke and heighten a partner's fears in response to a negative view of self or other, as the processing of these experiences promotes an internal awareness of one's attachment-related needs and wants. The therapist's ability to help clients fine tune their experience with a level of specificity or granularity that promotes their ability to more effectively use these experiences relationally.

One of the most effective ways of working with a negative view of self and view of other is "parts" work. Working with "parts" helps to tease out competing or "opposing" parts (Greenberg, Rice, & Elliot, 1993) and normalizing the reality of "parts," particularly when taking risk to do something new and different or when feeling vulnerable. Working with "parts" of the client's experience assists the therapist to enter in and move with a client's more defensive responses. As we get traction going into a client's defenses, we tease out and learn more about each salient part that clarifies and distinguishes important elements of the client's experience. The therapist is listening for, evoking, and conjecturing the client's fears related to both view of self and view of other to get these fears distilled and deepened for the engaged encounters of Softening events. These fears connected to differing views of self, often deeply held, often outside of awareness, and when unprocessed, keep us in our protected states. Processing them is pivotal to assist the client in stepping out of a protected state and into taking the risk of reaching vulnerably with engaged encounters throughout the Softening event.

Self-Assessment: Reflect on a partner who has shared a negative view of self and a negative view of other. What are the differences in the you notice between the two? Which of these fears do you find most compelling, most informing to the clients' struggle to connect? If you were to help your client differentiate this fear more clearly, what would you say or where would you focus your work in session?

No Softening Reach

Many clinicians haven't known how necessary it is to have the blamer actually make the reach of their vulnerable attachment needs to their partner! In the flow of the session, the clinician might actually share the pursuer's need with their partner or turn to process the pursuer's need with the partner before actually asking that partner to make the reach him- or herself. Couples may simply assume because the pursuing partner shared their need that their partner has heard and acknowledged their need, but as Johnson (2020) has recently highlighted, there is no substitute to the blamer actually reaching in the softening process! As intimate partners, this vulnerable reach is pinnacle in intimacy: open hearted, vulnerable, leading with fears. There is no substitute or better way to get a bonding event, which is required to restructure the couple's bond!

In promoting an effective softening encounter, the therapist uses "proxy voice" or a first-person stance to heighten and empathically conjecture about the pursuer's attachment-related emotions and needs. This enables the EFT therapist to work from a deeply attuned, empathic place, where the therapist is "with" and close to the pursuer's vulnerability. Blamer softening involves the therapist choreographing a change event and then following through by directing the pursuer to vulnerably reach to their partner with their need. At the heart of the transformational power of a softening change event are the actual reach and response of attachment needs, and the therapist leadership makes this possible by leading the partners through their fear to find each other.

Self-Assessment: What markers do you look for in a session focused on pursuer softening that help you know to direct the pursuing partner to share their attachment needs? What's it like for you to direct a reluctant partner to share their vulnerability in a moment like this?

Personal Reflection: After reviewing these missteps, which two are you most likely to be challenged by in your work in Stage 2? Reflect on your own attachment strategies and how they might influence your work with more pursuing partners, especially when the focus around sharing vulnerability may prove to be a profound and intensely challenging. Share your insights with an EFT colleague or supervisor.

SUMMARY

As you have learned from this chapter, the therapist's presence is of import throughout the Stage 2 change events. Not only is the therapist an active choreographer of the change events, but the emotional stance of the therapist facilitates the clients getting to and lingering with their deeper emotional experience. Sufficient depth of emotional experience is required for limbic revision (for each partner) as well as the restructuring of their bond (for their relationship). The emotional presence of the therapist needs to be congruent with the context and process of each of the change event sessions. Specifically, while processing client's vulnerabilities throughout the change events, the emotional presence of the therapist as described by softened voice quality was associated with the depth of the client's experience moment-to-moment and successful softening change events (Furrow, Edwards, Choi, & Bradley, 2012). The therapist using softened voice qualities, conveying warmth, support, and safety, more frequently facilitates the deepening of the client's emotional experiencing. The therapist's softened voice is the clearest signal of safety (Porges, 2016), which allows for the client to follow the therapist into deeper emotional waters. The safety created by the vocal quality of the therapist helps both the withdrawer and the blamer take the risk to reach toward the partner from a deeper, more vulnerable place, the essence of the Stage 2 change events.

ANSWERS AND SUGGESTED RESPONSES

Exercise 7.1. Possible Blamer Reaching

Answer: A, B, D. Incorrect and why: c (too skills based); d (too interpretive); f (focus on thoughts to the exclusion of emotion); g (finding an exception)

Exercise 7.2. Exploring a Possible Blamer Reach

Answer: D. The therapist uses words as if she were the client. By taking this "first-person stance," the therapist is imaginatively walking each partner through what a secure interaction can look and feel like for them. The first-person stance more deeply involves the client. This anticipates the therapist asking the more-blaming spouse to indeed reach later in the session. They experientially "try it on" before they actually are asked to risk reaching in reality. Note: c does not anticipate Marcus reaching to his spouse. It could, however, be followed by a response akin to d, which then puts it squarely into the initiation of Step 7.

Exercise 7.3. Forming a Possible Blamer Reach

"I was wondering—when you start to feel really upset over this Tom, when you start getting scared that Rebecca really doesn't believe in you or fear that she really doesn't want to see this relationship work."

Do you ever turn to her and say, 'Rebecca, I am starting to get really scared right now. I am having all of these doubts about whether you really care about me and whether you really want this to work. Could you just give me a little hug right now, just let me know that I am not alone here?' What would this be like for you to try this, Tom?"

Exercise 7.4. Processing Fears of Reaching

Answer: A, C, E

Exercise 7.5. Processing Fears of Reaching and Empathetic Conjectures

Answer: A, C

Exercise 7.6. Processing Blamer Reaching With Heightening

Suggested Response: So, when you feel this shame about yourself, like you are just not cutting it, feeling worthless, rather than reaching for her and showing that you are hurting, you show her anger. It's like it's just too scary to show her that side of you—the side that hurts so much. Part of you says, 'She will see me as weak—a big baby'? So, you hide it from her. It's safer that way. You stay alone in your pain?

Exercise 7.7. Processing Blamer Reaching With Heightening Empathic Conjecture

Answer: B

Exercise 7.8. Processing Fear of Reaching

Answers: 1, 2, 4, and 5: negative view of other; **3** and **6**, negative view of self

Exercise 7.9. Processing Blamer Reaching With Heightening

Suggested Response: "So, there is a part of you that fears Fresca's possible responses if you reach out to her. She could reject you; she could shame you. But then there's this other part that wonders if you are somehow wired differently, if it's possible that someone like Fresca could really accept and love you, right? This part is about you. It says something akin to 'Your mom was right. You are not someone who a woman will love, you can't make a woman happy. If you show Fresca all of you she will be disgusted, appalled . . . ' Am I hearing you right?"

Exercise 7.10. Summarizing the Processing of Pursuer's Fear of Reaching

Answers: A, B, D, F. Note: Answer **F** is an example of a couple that begins to soften at home before an occurrence in-session. When this happens, the therapist "reenters" the episode with the couple, slows it down, and heightens the attachment-related affect. A more heightened and processed softening event is the goal.

Exercise 7.11. Blamer Softening Reach

Answers: A, B, D, F, G. All but c and e, which are both questions and not direct requests.

Exercise 7.12. Blamer Softening Reach

Suggested Response: Marcus, could you turn to Fresca and share that when this fear of whether Fresca really loves you takes hold, you get paralyzed by your fears, and what you need most in that moment is her reassurance and a hug> Could you tell her now about your fear and what you need in this moment?

Exercise 7.13. Supporting Softened Pursuer

Answer: A, B, E. The other responses are not as effective: c (too insight driven); d (fails to process softening reach); f (moves to other partner too quickly).

Exercise 7.14. Exploring the Engaged Withdrawer's Response

Answer: B, C, D. Answer a focuses on Fresca's behaviors rather than her experience. Response **E** focuses on her intentions and not on processing her experience. The response also may be heard as an expectation and directive to share an unprocessed experience.

Exercise 7.15. Processing and Assembling the Engaged Withdrawer's Response

Suggested Response. "Fresca, when Marcus turned to you asking for reassurance, this deeply touched you. It's like he really opened his heart to you, and you felt like he really needed you in a way that you felt special, important, like you truly mattered in his world. What's happening as I say this to you?"

Exercise 7.16. Enacting the Engaged Withdrawer's Response

Suggested Response: "And so you say, 'I wish he would turn to me more often. " What would it be like to turn to him now and share this, to say to him 'I want us to be able to share this way, I feel closer to you, and you are not weaker; we actually become stronger!' So in your own words, could you share this with Marcus?"

8

STAGE 3: CONSOLIDATION AND COMMON EFT IMPASSES

Following the key change events of Stage 2, the couple moves to the final emotionally focused therapy (EFT) stage before terminating treatment. In Stage 3, the therapist supports the couple's finding new solutions to past problems and consolidating their new, more responsive positions through creating new relational narratives that integrate the couple's revised views of self and their relationship.

EFT SNAPSHOT: CONSOLIDATION

As the weeks progressed, Inez and Fernando grew in confidence as they were able to readily identify and interrupt their negative cycle. When they caught themselves beginning a cycle, they would stop and sort out their deeper emotions rather than getting caught in the cycle and their defensive surface emotions. Jane joined the couple in reprocessing difficult incidents, linking them to their cycle and then helping them to access, share, and respond to their attachment-related emotions and needs. She also highlighted and validated the couple's progress. The couple started coming every second or third week, and after session 18, they decided to wait four weeks before returning to their next session. At session 19, they shared that the past four weeks were the closest month of their relationship; things were going extremely well between them. Moreover, Inez had joined a fitness center and was feeling much healthier and trimmer, and Fernando, who had been trying to lose weight for some time, had now lost 15 pounds.

Fernando: But ironically we got into a fight an hour before we came here.

Inez: I just thought, "Let's wait and talk about it with Jane." He told me I need to lose weight." (She begins to tear.) That hurt because I have been trying, and personally, I can see the difference!

Fernando: I didn't just say it like that! I asked you not to buy peanuts. I can't resist them. I told you, I'd like your support in losing weight, and you could use to lose a few pounds, too.

Inez: Well, last time I lost 10 pounds you told me I was fat. I thought, "Why bother?" and gave up. You'd never find me attractive anyway.

Therapist: You worry he won't find you attractive?

DOI: 10.4324/9781003039457-10

Inez: I know I am not attractive to him. After all, once he told me, "Never gain weight. I won't find you attractive; this is simply a fact." And if that's not enough, we haven't had sex for years. (Fernando flushes, looks down at his hands.)

Therapist: So, Fer . . . " (Inez interrupts)

Inez: No!! Wait! I have to say something. It's not all his fault! I pushed him away for years when I was in menopause. I didn't want to deal with it all.

Therapist: Aha. So, Inez, you want to help Fernando here?

Inez: Yes! I know how that would upset him, if he thought I was blaming him for us never having sex. That's not fair. (turns to Fernando) I wanted to be sure you understood. I know I was at fault, too.

Therapist: But what's on your mind today is about feeling closer and yet fearing that you guys have maybe lost the physical part?

Inez: (looks tearful again) I never forgot what he told me.

Fernando: What can I ever say that will counteract that? You say some stupid things when you're in your 20s. For me today, attraction is about whether I get whacked over the head, not listened to or ordered around; then sure, that's not attractive to me.

Inez: Well, that's not happening these days, is it?

Fernando: No. And I want you to know how much it meant to me, just now, when you said it wasn't all my fault that our sex life went down the tubes.

Therapist: That was a tricky moment back there?

Fernando: It would have been. Could have felt like a whack—that's when I would get into my wobbly place.

Therapist: So, what I'm getting today is that you are understanding each other's vulnerable places and helping each other out more, is that right? (Fernando and Inez both nod their heads.)

Therapist: And it sounds that, although you can still get into a fight, somehow it's at a different level than it was before?

Fernando: I'm trusting Inez more now, too, trusting she does value me. (turns to his wife) And you know, kid, that can be a real turn-on for me.

Inez: (reaches out and touches Fernando's knee)

Therapist: That feels good to hear, Inez?

Inez: (nods, tearing again) I'd like for us to be close again.

The session continued with the therapist facilitating a discussion of their sexual relationship in which Inez acknowledged the distance that had come between them sexually. The therapist highlighted Inez's engagement as she owned her part in this, which opened an opportunity for the couple to discuss their fears and desires for greater closeness and physical connection. The couple also identified that differences in household responsibilities and expectations had become a problem following Fernando's retirement and Inez's depression. They recounted how they found a solution to the stalemate that had left the couple frozen in avoidance.

Following 18 sessions, Inez and Fernando were now able to discuss the difficult issue of the loss of their sexual relationship without splintering into the rigid positions that defined their insecure pattern. The couple avoids the pull of this cycle as tender issues of physical appearance and intimacy are discussed, finding instead openness around their fears and needs. The couple is effective in discussing these issues as the increasing security in their relationship creates greater confidence to face past concerns and both discover that in facing these challenges together, they find more room for trust and closeness in their relationship.

In their final session, they proudly announced that they had cleared years of junk from the basement without a single episode of conflict. Time was spent describing the journey that the couple had made together in therapy. The therapist validated the courage and strength each possessed, often enduring times that seemed almost unbearable. The couple booked a session for three months ahead, but they cancelled this session two weeks before it was scheduled. Soon thereafter the therapist received a card from Inez and Fernando, thanking her for her help and telling her that things in their relationship were going very well. As this final EFT stage concludes, the couple leaves therapy with a new story of their relationship, one that is founded on a sense of safety and awareness of their relationship that is secure, safe, and sound.

KEY MOVES IN THE PROCESS

The goals of Stage 3 include helping couples find new solutions to long-standing issues in their relationship and helping partners consolidate the gains they achieved in therapy. In Step 8, the therapist supports the couple as they discuss issues of concern in an atmosphere of safety given the changes the couple has made in their relationship. In Step 9, the therapist's goals include identifying and supporting the healthy patterns of interaction and helping the couple articulate a shared narrative that characterizes the progress the couple has made in gaining a more secure relationship. The therapist reinforces and supports the success of the couple in enacting secure patterns characterized by increased accessibility and responsiveness. The couple's story provides a reference point for their reflection on the ways they have found to leave the "problematic cycle" and take risks to connect in new ways around issues that pulled them apart in the past.

EFT STEPS: STAGE III, CONSOLIDATION

8. Facilitate new solutions to old problems.
9. Consolidate new positions, positive cycles, and stories of secure attachment.

In Steps 8 and 9, the therapist typically observes several key shifts that occur in the couple's relationship. The EFT therapist builds on positive interactions and newfound security, fostering greater confidence in the couple's renewed bond. At this stage, partners often sense more freedom to revisit their concerns and raise long-standing issues that may be difficult to resolve. The therapist promotes exploration and discussion of these issues and encourages the couple to create their own solution. As security builds in their relationship, there are greater resources for exploration and creative efforts at problem solving even in the midst of working through difficult issues.

For example, a previously withdrawn partner now may feel safe enough to discuss an issue that he previously avoided. The therapist meets the partner's effort with support for the risk that asserting his concern represents. Similarly, there is support for the other partner in helping receive this concern in a way that promotes availability rather defensiveness. The couple is generally better able to address the issues in their relationship with less reactivity and therapist helps the couple's solidify of a more accessible and responsive positive pattern. The therapist guides the couple through these interactions, focusing on the present moment, assembling emotions, and often heightening more positive experiences as the couple share together and make sense of a strong emotional bond. As couples grow confident in their relationship changes, they will describe ways in which they are engaging new patterns in their relationship, both inside and outside therapy. The therapist helps the couple stay on track and promotes a more secure bond through highlighting the couple's healthy patterns and encouraging them to continue taking steps toward greater security in the relationship. As termination approaches, couples indicate that they no longer need therapy. They are clear about the changes they need to make in their relationship and what they have accomplished. The therapist responds to the couple's initiative by validating the couple's strengths and encouraging them to continue their commitment to emotional engagement and maintaining a secure bond.

Step 8. Facilitate New Solutions

In Step 8, the focus of sessions is often more pragmatic. Consider the following session in which Bob and Sharon return to a discussion of financial concerns, which were a common source of conflict. Initially, Bob and Sharon's arguments about bills and savings would trigger their cycle in which Bob would criticize and blame Sharon for mismanaging their finances and Sharon would either withdraw in self-blame or fight back by being critical of Bob's neglect of the family. Through working through their previous pattern of insecurity, both found a more positive cycle of support, especially though understanding the underlying threats that triggered their defensive pattern. Sharon began to talk about her fears of being rejected by Bob because of the shame she felt. Similarly, Bob softened, identifying his need to control Sharon resulted from his fear that she would reject him and leave. Together they found greater security through being more responsive and accessible to the other's underlying emotions as well as the issues at hand. Here is an example of Sharon returning to the financial issue in Stage 3.

Sharon: One of our bills was past due last month. It was on the counter when Bob came in. We didn't talk about it. He just opened it and left it on the table.

Bob: Yeah, I didn't know what to say. It just seemed best to keep quiet.

Sharon: So, I figure that it really bothered him, but he didn't want to risk a fight, so he kept it to himself. Still, I felt the tension and left it alone because I knew we would be talking to you. (Bob stares at the floor.) I wish he had said something to me.

Therapist: What's it like for you, Bob, to hear Sharon say she wished you had said something even it if you were feeling upset?

Bob: I don't know. I mean, I believe her, but it's hard for me to believe she wants my anger. Things have been good, and it's just a late notice. Why spoil what we have worked so hard to accomplish with a picky comment? I should be bigger than that—you know, let it go because we have something better now.

Therapist: Sure, it makes sense that you would want to protect your relationship from the return of the cycle that could easily take over and you have that part of you that says you should be able to manage your anger and be a bigger man. But being bigger means you have to hide this part of you.

Bob: I suppose that's it. It's hard 'cause I don't want to hurt Sharon, but we need to do better handling the money.

Therapist: Right, of course; you don't want to hurt Sharon, and it's not you pretending it doesn't matter. This is your way of protecting her, protecting what you have now. Does she know this?

Bob: (looking at Sharon) I don't want to hurt you, and I don't want to go back to the way things were. I just don't know what to say.

Therapist: When Bob says he doesn't want to hurt you? That he doesn't want things to go back to the way they were? What's this like to hear?

Sharon: Yes, I don't want it to go that way either. I am scared, too. When I saw the bill, I felt this pit in my stomach. I could hear his anger—my fear—I started to cry. It's been so sweet lately, and I just couldn't handle thinking that we were going to lose it.

Therapist: Lose it?

Sharon: The softness, the closeness, the sense that we are in this together.

Therapist: (softly) Can you tell him—can you tell Bob about that fearful part that worries that you might lose the closeness, the softness, the togetherness you have? Can you tell him?

Sharon: (in tears) I am sorry about the bill. It's my fault. I am afraid. I don't want to go back to the way things were. I want what we have now. I don't want to lose what we have.

Bob: (reaching out to touch her as she cries) I know. I feel that, too. I found the bill, and I was frustrated, but not like before. I just did not know if I started to talk about it if you would feel attacked and then disappear. The cycle. I was afraid that we'd go right back, you know. I don't want that. I want you to know that I am here for you. We can figure out the money situation. We just need to talk about it, together.

Therapist: (silence, then softly) So when you both turn toward each other and let the other know that you care, things will be okay. A past due notice doesn't mean that the cycle takes over. When you show your fears about going backward, you actually move forward. You both show that you are concerned—new possibilities emerge. Like you, Bob, inviting Sharon to talk with you about the late notice. Does that seem different to you?

Bob: Yes, I am more concerned about her than the late notice. I mean, it still matters, but I am thinking about her first.

Therapist: How about you, Sharon? Can you tell him what feels different?

Sharon: I feel responsible for the bill but not like before. When we first started, the late notice meant that I was a bad person in his eyes, and now it's regrettable and a problem, but it doesn't have to come between us. That's the way I feel now, more secure. I can make a mistake, and maybe it's okay. (laughing) For Bob at least; maybe not for me!

Step 9. Consolidate New Positions, Cycles, and Stories of Secure Attachment

The final step of the EFT process focuses on the integration of more secure patterns into the everyday interaction of the couple. As Bob and Sharon work through a past issue, the couple is moving into greater confidence in their newfound availability. The therapist's primary goal is to identify and promote healthy patterns of interaction, most commonly those that are characterized by partner accessibility, responsiveness, and emotional engagement. This is typically summarized in story or narrative form, in which the couple is able to put in context the changes that they have made and the new understanding of their relationship. There are three important elements in this narrative. These include

- Differences between how they previously reacted toward one another and how they respond now
- Shared understanding of the deeper emotions underlying each partner's actions in the cycle
- Ways the couple has found to exit their cycle and connect to one another

The couple's goal is the development of a coherent narrative that brings together each partner's past and current experiences of the relationship. Achieving a shared story about their relationship further enables the couple to appreciate what they have experienced and most important the strength of their commitment. The coherence of a couple's narrative is a common indicator of attachment security in attachment research (Hesse, 1999). This process enables the experience to be more fully integrated into the lives of the individual and the couple (Greenberg & Angus, 2004). The couple's story provides a way for each partner to make sense of his or her experience by tying together the emotional themes of their journey toward a more secure connection. As Dickstein (2004) noted, the attachment story of more secure couples is most likely to include each of the following:

- Awareness and understanding of the couple's ability to handle negative affect
- A clear expression of the value they both place in their relationship and attachment-related experiences
- Limited defensiveness when discussing relationship problems or negative issues

- Ability to reflect on how they each contributed to the changes in the relationship
- Ability to reflect on the personal growth as a result of relationship change

Together, these markers provide the therapist with the means to assess the security of the couple's relationship in narrative terms.

Personal Reflection

Think of a couple you believe have a secure bond. Which of the following attributes stand out to you about their relationship and how they talk about their relationship?

Rank the following from 1 to 5 with 5 being most obvious to 1 being least obvious.

_____ The couple's acceptance and understanding of negative emotions
_____ The ways they talk about their relationship, including examples of accessibility, responsiveness, and emotional engagement
_____ Their willingness to take on difficult discussions and limit defensive reactions
_____ Each partner's awareness of how they can influence their relationship positively
_____ Each partner's awareness of personal growth as a result of their relationship

The EFT therapist may reflect on a couple's strengths and invite focus on their new attachment-related story. The therapist will

1. Help couple review changes in their relationship—what has changed?

   "So, when you look back at how you faced this big decision together, what seems different? What changes have you both made that made this possible?"
2. Encourage them to contrast emotional experiences associated with past behaviors and more recent responses.

   "Before, you felt like you had to hide because the fear of being exposed as unworthy was too much, but now you hang in there because she is there for you, and you know that now."
3. Focus on ways that they have found to exit the cycle.

   "And you see the cycle and how going on the attack will take you farther away. You step back then ask her a question rather than fire an accusation. That's amazing that you can do that even when the heat is on."
4. Emphasize the couple's courage to take risks.

   "It is sometimes hard for couples to take those risky steps. To share and to reach out to the other, especially when there has been a history of disappointments. You both show a lot of courage in being there for each other even when things get difficult."
5. Highlight the potential that these changes have brought to providing support for one another in the future.

   "You have both found a way to make sure the other knows that you are in this together. That's a powerful thing, especially because of times when this bond of yours is tested, like last week's situation. But you have this history, this bond you have shared, and that says there is another way, another option, another opportunity to be there for each other rather than against each other."

Termination

Upon reaching Step 9, the couple moves toward termination. The EFT therapist commonly addresses a number of common issues at the close of treatment. For some couples, the end of therapy prompts concern about what may happen to their relationship once they discontinue regular therapy appointments. Using evocative responding, the EFT therapist helps each partner explore and share these fears. It is helpful for the therapist to direct the couple to addressing these concerns on an ongoing basis.

Some couples fear a relapse into their old cycle. Using validation, a therapist can normalize their concern and remind the couple of the ways they have exited the cycle in the past. The therapist should focus the couple on the ways that they can respond to one another to head off the escalation leading to the start of the cycle.

Attachment Rituals

At termination, the therapist can promote the couple's effort to be proactive in maintaining their emotional connection. The therapist can help the couple identify and develop rituals that symbolize their connection and promote security in their relationship. These prescribed actions are called "attachment rituals" because they provide regular reminders of the secure connection the two partners share. William Doherty (2001) describes a marriage ritual as a joint activity that a couple repeats on a regular basis that is meaningful to both partners. These activities may be simple or elaborate and may vary from once a year to every day. Rituals are an important resource for couples in maintaining their connection to one another (Crespo, Davide, Costa, & Fletcher, 2008).

Attachment rituals help couples focus on specific actions that symbolize partners' attachment to each other. The most common rituals mark times of greeting and times of leaving. How a couple says good-bye at the start of a day or how they greet each other when they return embodies the meaning and value of the relationship to each partner. These gestures are "meaningful" exchanges that provide an unspoken language for the attachment of the couple.

Examples of Attachment Rituals

- Kissing and hugging partner good-bye and hello
- Letter writing and leaving notes for each other
- Participating in religious rituals: praying together, attending religious events, or sharing sacred readings together
- Reading a book together
- Saying hello and asking about the other's day
- Calling during the day to check in
- Spending part of a morning together in bed talking and holding each other
- Making a conversation ritual—a daily time to talk about the day and catch up with one another
- Maintaining a regular date night
- Developing a hobby that both share
- Taking a class together or learning a new skill together
- Finding someone in need and working together to serve or help
- Having a ceremony to renew vows

Constructing an Attachment Ritual

The therapist can begin constructing these rituals by asking the couple how they plan to maintain the connection that they have worked so hard to create. The couple can be asked to create a list of ways they can remind themselves and their partner of the importance and closeness of their relationship. The therapist may ask a couple to consider how they can express their recognition and support for their partner when she returns from work or he leaves in the morning. The therapist helps the couple identify particular patterns of behavior or symbols that communicate to both a sense of the couple's ongoing emotional connection. It is only a ritual if both partners know what the action or symbol means. Attachment rituals may include specific romantic activities like an anniversary or a weekly date, but often the power of attachment is communicated in daily routines or connection rituals that communicate each partner's significance to the other. The most powerful rituals are based on the symbols and practices that are unique to a particular couple.

Questions a therapist may use to identify an attachment ritual include

- What does your partner do on a regular basis to show she or he is there for you?
- When do you make time to remind yourselves of the connection you share?
- If you could not use words to tell her/him that you really cared for him/her, how would you show it? Be creative!
- How would your partner know you were on his/her mind when you were away?

As a couple near termination, therapists may also want to find closure on issues outside of the relationship that have arisen in the process of therapy. Partners may confront individual issues in the process of therapy that require further attention. The therapist may work with the client to address the issue with the other partner or extend a series of individual sessions for the partner. For example, Sean and Linda had bitter conflicts over their competing work schedules and responsibilities. As they reconnected, they were better able to differentiate their intimacy fears and needs from their work habits. Sean reorganized his priorities and his time to better accommodate the needs of their relationship. At the same time, Sean felt increasingly conflicted by his tendency to define his worth by his work. He recognized some of the insecurity that he carried into his marriage was also defining his work behavior. He asked the therapist for some additional time to explore the "cycle" in which he found himself at the office. Additionally, some therapists may refer Sean to individual therapy to maintain clarity in the focus and treatment contract.

COMMON INTERVENTIONS USED IN STEPS 8 AND 9

As the therapist facilitates further consolidation of the couple's newly engaged patterns, the therapist will work to keep the couple on track and highlight the gains the couple has made. Four interventions are commonly found in Steps 8 and 9. In the next examples, note the differences in how each intervention is used in the latter stages of EFT.

Reflection and Validation

These interventions highlight the ways the couple enacts new patterns and engages new responses. The therapist uses these interventions to keep the couple available and responsive as they encounter responses from one another that may prompt more defensive responses. Consider the following example in which the therapist validates a client's experience and reflect on a husband's ability to remain engaged.

Therapist: Jose thinks many husbands would have found that difficult to hear, but you hung in there. When Sofia said she sometimes found it hard to trust your word, you didn't go on the attack but asked her to tell you more. You really showed her you cared about her concern.

Evocative Responding

This intervention helps the therapist slow down the process and keep partners focused on their experience. If the therapist notices that the client is flirting with taking an old position in the problematic cycle, then she can intervene and process the partner's experience using an evocative response.

Therapist: Can we come back to that? I want to make sure we don't miss you, Sofia. It's like you were right here and then you disappeared. Jose started talking about your family, and it was like we lost you. Can you help me? What happened for you when Jose started in about your mom and sister?

Reframing

In the consolidation stage, the therapist will often actively reframe the new and positive actions of each partner as a change from the problematic ways of the past. Emphasis is placed on the "way we are now" as opposed to the "way things were before."

Therapist: So, when Sofia talked about the time she needed for work and she reminded you that her first priority was to see how this impacted you, Jose, you could hear that. You didn't attack like in the old arguments. Right? You heard her concern, and you were both able to talk this through. This didn't get the best of you as a couple.

Restructuring Interactions: Narratives and Engaging Encounters

Building on these moments, the therapist may also summarize the changes in the couple's patterns in greater detail and then invite the couple to create their own version of a "before-and-after" account of their relationship changes. This intervention helps the couple label these changes and furthers consolidation of the new patterns they have embraced.

Therapist: And that would have triggered a big fight weeks ago, but things are different now, that's not what happened?

Sofia: It's almost like I was waiting for him to criticize, but I put down my guard. I thought, "We can talk about this." I know he cares.

Therapist: So, you saw the familiar pattern from the past but chose to trust what's new for both of you. Can you tell me what made the difference?

Sofia: I guess I know what happens when we fight, we never get anywhere. And I thought about Jose saying he cares about me and us and sometimes doesn't know how to show it. I just thought, "Give him a chance. Look at this as coming from his caring side rather than the critical side."

Therapist: And you trusting him this way says a lot about where you are now compared with where you have been. Can you tell him, "I know you care, and I see the risk you are taking in telling me these things"?

Exercise 8.1. Reviewing EFT Micro-Interventions and Consolidation

Match the therapist statement with the intervention listed.

1. "That was nice, Brandt. You were able to see your tendency to react to Sally's silence by pursuing her, but you were able to go to your feelings of concern and give her the space to respond. Can you tell Sally what has changed for you in the relationship that makes it safe for you to share your feelings more? How have things changed? What's different?"
2. "It is quite amazing to watch you two handle a hot issue. It's like I am waiting for the old cycle to kick in, but you both went a different direction. You stay connected, and that must take a lot of courage and trust to stay with each other even though the stakes are higher."
3. "And that is the way things used to go. You guys would get scared and overwhelmed, and the music of that old dance would take over, but now you feel safer and trust your connection more. Now you can see that old dance and feel powerful enough to risk and put on this new music, the music that leads to getting close and reaching for each other. You expect a more secure relationship, a safe relationship for your future."
4. "Tom, it seems like we lost you there, when Sarah started talking about your work pressures and missing you. It is like you started backing away. What happens for you when you hear her share this? What's it like to hear her missing you?"

Reframing ____

Evocative responding ____

Reflection and validation ____

Restructuring interactions ____

Exercise 8.2. Practicing EFT Interventions and Consolidation

Read each of the following situations and then form a therapist statement for each of the following Step 8 and 9 scenarios.

Mario and Luisa are discussing their plans for changing their son to a parochial school, when Mario increases the intensity in his voice and states definitively: "We must do what is right for our son, and I think there is only one option!" The therapist senses Luisa backing away from the discussion as she disengages, staring out the window while Mario continues his justification.

1. Form an evocative response that would encourage Luisa to process her experience and to keep engaged with her present experience.

____

____

Luisa shares that she found Mario's tone threatening, as if he just wanted her to agree with him because he thought he was right. She felt her opinion did not count. Mario responds, "Oh, I didn't mean it like that. I just feel strongly about this, and I don't see any other way, but you are his mama, and you see his world differently than I do. I want to know what you think, no matter how strongly I feel."

2. As the therapist, form a statement that includes a reflection and validation to highlight the new position that Mario takes in response to hearing Luisa's experience.

____

____

Luisa responds to Mario: "I guess sometimes it is hard for me when you come on strong, and I hide. It helps to know that you want to hear my thoughts and concerns. I like your strong voice, and sometimes I just don't know how to respond. This is an important issue, and I also have strong feelings about this as well."

3. As the therapist, you want to punctuate the real change in the couple's typical pattern of attack/withdraw. Now form a reframe statement to help the couple reflect on the new way that they are relating to each other and the ways in which they are building a more secure relationship.

____

____

4. At the end of the discussion, the therapist wants to further consolidate the new positions that Luisa and Mario have taken. How would you encourage the couple to create a statement that characterizes how their relationship is different after the work they have done?

____

____

Notice how you could then use this statement to help them choreograph an encounter based on their new shared experience.

Consolidation With Fernando and Inez

Briefly review the case of Inez and Fernando at the beginning of this chapter. Respond to the following questions that will lead you through the creation of a narrative summary of the couple's new relationship pattern. First, recall that at the beginning of therapy, Inez was in a more withdrawn position. The underlying emotions that colored her distance and avoidant stance include feels of sadness and shame and an underlying fear of abandonment. Ferdinand's reactive position in the couple's negative cycle was more often as the pursuer. He feared losing Inez, which was compounded by his own fears of rejection and felt inadequacy as her husband. He also felt shame in response to his own failures in the relationship.

Exercise 8.3. Consolidation With Inez and Fernando

How would you describe the couple's understanding of their relationship as a result of treatment? Answer the following questions about the changes that have occurred in the couple's cycle.

1. Thinking back on Inez and Fernando's rigid positions that defined their relationship, identify the positions and each partner's underlying emotion.

   Inez (position) ______________ (underlying /core emotions) __________________

   Fernando (position) ____________ (underlying/core emotions) ________________
2. When Fernando sees Inez's withdrawal, he now knows she may be experiencing? ____.
3. When Inez withdraws feeling criticized, what does Fernando know she may need? ____
4 When Inez senses Fernando responding with a defensive attack, she now knows he may be experiencing ________________________________.
5. How have Inez and Fernando found ways to exit their cycle? Name one way the couple has found to exit their cycle. How would you describe this to the couple?

   ____

   ____

   ____

6. Now imagine you are their therapist, and it is now the 20th session. The couple just recounted their daughter's surprise at the cleaned-out basement. Now construct a brief summary of their relationship that validates the daughter's surprise but also expands to include their success in strengthening the bond and avoiding the problematic cycle. Try to include as many of the following elements in your narrative summary.

   - Changes in the relationship
   - Emotional experience with their old cycle and new relationship patterns
   - Ways couple has come up with to exit their cycle
   - Ways these changes will help them in the future

   ____

   ____

   ____

   ____

   ____

   ____

Exercise 8.4. Attachment Ritual

Describe an attachment ritual you might suggest for this couple as a way that they can remind each other of the closeness they have achieved through all their hard work.

____

____

____

Exercise 8.5. Reinforcing New Pattern

If in the closing session, Inez raised concerns that the old cycle would return, how might you respond to this concern? What would you say to the couple?

____

____

____

Exercise 8.6. Termination and Transcript Review

Review the transcript of Fernando and Inez at the beginning of this chapter. Check all of the following indicators of termination that apply to this case. Which of these does the therapist see?

a. Reduction in negative affect ____
b. Increase in positive cycles of interaction ____
c. Expression of emotions and responses to partner's emotions ____
d. Increase in accessibility and responsiveness between partners ____
e. Partners ask for what they need in a way that encourages partner's response ____
f. Partners make more positive attributions about responses of partner ____

Common Impasses in EFT Practice

Impasses in the EFT process can erode hope yet also be one of the most powerful forces to fuel change. Consequently, it is important to move beyond impasses as quickly as possible. Impasses can occur at any phase of therapy. They appear most often during Stage 1, assessment and stabilization, and in the restructuring processes of Stage 2. A less common type of impasse occurs when clients fail to generalize changes from inside the therapy room to outside the therapy room. We briefly review common warning signs, causes, and impacts of impasses on clients and therapists

Impasse Indicators or Warning Signs

The following are five areas where a therapist may question whether an EFT impasse is at work. We have also included questions that may signal a possible impasse.

- Alliance Block: Is my alliance with imbalanced? Have I overidentified with one partner, family member, or aspect of my client's experience?
- Disengagement: Has my client become more experientially avoidant in our session? Do they seem disengaged and less invested in treatment?
- Lack of Change: Has the treatment process stalled? Do my sessions appear unproductive and treatment progress and process lack clear direction? No change is evident.
- Lack of Hope: Am I questioning my clients' ability to change? Do I question the viability of a couple's relationship or the competence and caring of parents or other family members?
- Therapist Lack of Confidence: Do I feel lost in the EFT process or less confident in my ability to provide a clear focus to the in-session process?

Common Causes of Impasses

EFT impasses occur for different and sometimes overlapping reasons. These treatment blocks may result from a therapist's lack of awareness, understanding, and skill in applying EFT. Other impasses are rooted in lack of client goal alignment. Listed next are some common cause reasons clients and therapist find themselves in a stalled EFT process.

- Absence of Experiential Focus: The client(s) or therapist lacks an in-depth, experiential sense of the problem cycle(s). A client's experience is not clearly ordered. Similarly, the therapist EFT Tango process lacks emotional, depth almost becoming only a communication or cognitively focused exercise. The therapist may focus on problem solving for the client or become distracted by content. This is particularly easy to do in EFT with individuals.
- Unprocessed Emotional Experience: The emotions that drive negative patterns have not been fully accessed, assembled or deepened, or shared. This may include unprocessed trauma or attachment injuries that block access to a client's vulnerability.
- Lack of Safety: The therapist does not intervene in escalating conflict soon enough, and sessions lack felt safety.
- Client Shame: Shame blocks client from seeing how important they are in helping their partner or child heal.
- Attachment History: Client(s) lack experience in being in a secure relationship and consequently do not have a personal map for what a secure relationship looks like. In a similar way, a therapist's attachment history may contribute to a difficulty in promoting felt security.
- Modality Differences: The therapist has limited understanding of the EFT model and how it applies across different modalities (e.g., emotionally focused individual therapy [EFIT], emotionally focused couple therapy, emotionally focused family therapy [EFFT]).
- Confidence in EFT Skills: Lacks skill and confidence EFT interventions, including heightening, accurate empathy, empathic conjecture, validation, and RISSSC. The therapist may also not regularly follow the EFT Tango or have difficulty tolerating intense emotion or working with a lack of emotion.

- Outcome Focused: The therapist gets caught in doubt about her or his own ability to effectively bring about change. The therapist lacks confidence in the potential for healing and change and loses a process focus.
- Problem Focus: The client and therapist get caught in the restricted views of problems and potential for healing that can come from diagnostic labels. In a similar way, a therapist may be caught in a negative cycle, including blaming or pathologizing one person or becomes caught in hopelessness.

Resolving Impasses

There are a number of ways a therapist may address an impasse in the EFT process. When confronting an impasse, the therapist may shift their focus, making the impasse explicit or seek additional resources through an individual session or supervision. A number of strategies are listed next for addressing an impasse in the EFT process.

Make the Impasse Explicit

Here the therapist reflects, validates, and heightens the emotions and interactional elements of the impasse. The therapist comments on the process of how the client(s) are not moving to a different position and puts the impasse in the context of attachment needs and relational cycles. The reflection emphasizes each person's emotional experiences (or the parts of a person's emotional experiences) and how their responses tie into the cycle. This is Move 1 of the EFT Tango—focusing on present process. Promoting acceptance, the EFT therapists does not blame clients for an impasse, as clients have often been caught in various elements of the cycle for many years without really understanding or knowing how to change. The EFT therapist assumes there is always an inherent logic informing the impasse and by patiently searching, a way through the impasse will appear in session.

In mirroring the present process, the therapist holds the impasse up to the light and presents it multiple times, at multiple levels, from multiple angles. The idea is that the client(s) not only identify the action tendencies, the perceptions, and the vulnerable soft core and secondary reactive emotions in their stuck cycle, but they also experience each of these as a relational process through their own experiencing and that of others. As the impasse and the dilemma it presents are repeatedly processed, different elements come forth that lead to breaking up the impasse. Change results from experiencing fully the responses that threaten a coherent sense of the self and one's relationships with others. These responses are experienced as compelling and legitimate in the moment.

Ramona and Mike were stuck at the stabilization stage with their therapist. In deepening the elements of the cycle and elaborating their stuck positions, the therapist talked about how they both "launched missiles at each other" when they were hurting. This then led each partner feeling hurt, violated, and more alone. Through de-escalation, Ramona, who was the pursuer, said to the therapist, "When you talked about how, when we are hurt, we launched missiles at each other, I saw what we were doing and how I launched missiles. Mike also saw this and how it just led to more hurt. After that whenever I felt he was being mean and I wanted to get back at him, I had an image of me launching a missile at him and him sending missiles back, and I stopped."

The EFT therapist may use transparency to make the impasse more explicit. The therapist and couple may talk about the fact that "*we* are stuck," not just that "*they* are stuck." It is important to avoid overdoing this response such that clients lose confidence in treatment. The power of the therapist's confidence is essential, especially in communicating to clients that there is a way forward.

When facing a severe impasse, the therapist may heighten a client's fear and desperation as a last-ditch effort to create a shift. Sometimes acknowledging and highlighting fear and desperation helps clients take the risks needed to move forward. For example, Maria and Toni and their therapist faced an impasse in softening a pursuers angry attack. The therapist would help Toni, a withdrawer, come out and engage, but Maria would in turn attack him for being untrustworthy and further her criticism by stating she could never trust him because of his emotional absence and overworking.

After several months of processing and working to get past this point, the therapist knew she must do something different. She spoke to Maria and Toni openly about how they were stuck (Tango Move 1). The therapist also shared that she felt stuck. "I have thought a lot about how we are stuck, and I think perhaps part of the problem is I have failed to understand how dangerous this is for you, Maria, to again risk getting close to Toni, even though a part of you longs to be close." The therapist focused on validating the part of Maria that said "this is dangerous—don't trust him—he will disappear again, and the pain will be unbearable" (Tango Move 2). Maria expressed her "terror" of getting hurt again and what that would mean and how it would feel. When Maria said, "I think you are getting me," the therapist had her share the pain and the terror directly with Toni (Tango Move 3). Toni responded with deep regret over how his overwork had left her alone and abandoned and in massive amounts of pain. He also said he wanted to be with her and would wait as long as needed so she could see he really was there for her (Tango Move 4). The therapist summarized (Tango Move 5) what had just happened without pushing Maria to open up more to Toni.

In the next session, the therapist shared she had thought all week about Maria's "terror" of opening up and her good reasons for this fear. The therapist conjectured about Maria's confusion in seeing her husband come out to meet her like she had always wanted but not trusting it was safe enough to believe he would really stay (Tango Move 1). The therapist further validated the part of Maria that wanted to reach out and connect, "and yet there is a part of you that longs to be close and be comforted like you used to be." Maria agreed. The therapist said she wanted to honor both parts and that perhaps it was her hope to get Maria to risk connecting with Toni, but she should not push. It was okay for Maria to hold in this place of mistrust and then conjectured about how for now that was safer than connecting.

Maria then talked about how she wanted to be close to Toni and how she could feel it this longing but also felt the terror. Again, the therapist validated and deepened this (Tango Move 2). The therapist had her share this with Toni (Tango Move 3). In tears, Toni shared he wanted to be that safe place for her, reassuring her that he would wait as long as needed, even though he longed for the closeness they once had (Tango Move 4). The therapist again heightened Maria's fear and honored that it was okay for her not risk taking this step (Tango Move 2). Maria also cried expressing her conflicted experience, saying: "but I do want to be close to him." The therapist had her share this with Toni (Tango Move 3), and Maria turned and said, "I do want to be close—I need you—please hold me" and then reached for Toni. He embraced her and held her as they both sobbed. Following this the therapist processed their experience and explored the emerging warmth and peace both found in this moment (Tango Move 4). The therapist summarized how Maria had faced her terror and had reached and trusted and Toni was there and felt wonderful and how amazing it was to see her do this (Tango Move 5). The therapist also suggested that the hurt part of her would be scared again and that this was normal and OK.

"Slicing It Thinner"

Slicing it thinner involves the therapist's asking the client to take very small risks—slicing risks small enough that the client can take them. Similar to a present process focus that makes an impasse explicit, the therapist works to focus on slicing a client's experience thinner while doing the Tango. The therapist invites a new experience through helping the individual, couple, or family fully experience what is happening around the impasse for each of them and how that translates into actions and patterns (Tango Move 1). The therapist focuses on blocks to risk taking. Acceptance of the reasons behind why a client does not want to take risks and validating these reasons is key to really accessing the core blocking emotions. The therapist then assembles the core softer emotions, perceptions, interactional strategies or action tendencies, and other aspects of the cycle that are related to the impasse (Tango Move 2) in preparation to get the client to risk sharing them (Tango Move 3). Once there is emotion in the room that has been assembled and organized, the therapist invites an enactment of this experience (Tango Move 3).

For example, after processing and deepening fears of losing the other partner, the therapist could say "Can you tell him how scared you are of losing him?" If the client refuses, the therapist then explores the block with questions like "help me understand . . . this hard . . . what is getting in the way of telling him you are afraid of losing him." The therapist then slices it thinner by saying, "Can you tell him 'I have to protect myself—it is too scary to tell you how much I need you'?" (Tango Move 3). The therapist can then process how it was to share the fear of sharing softer feelings and elicit a response from the partner (Tango Move 4). If the partner's response is positive, the therapist then heightens it and gets the partner to share directly (back to Tango Move 2 and 3). For example, if the partner says, "I love it when you share your softer feelings. I think it takes a lot of courage and I need to know that you need me," the therapist can reflect and heighten it by saying, "Can you hear that he sees this type of sharing as courageous, and he needs to know how much you need him?" (Tango Move 4). If the client has a hard time accepting it, the therapist can slice it even thinner by saying something like, "Can a part of you take in that he needs to know you need him and he wants you to share your soften feelings?" The therapist can then work with the part that does accept it and the part than does not. When the block(s) has been worked through, the therapist goes back to having the client directly share by saying, "I think your partner needs to hear it directly from you. Can you tell him you are scared of losing him and you really do need him?" (Tango Move 3), process this (Tango Move 4), and summarize what was just done (Tango Move 5).

Disquisitions

Disquisitions are dramatic narratives that capture distressed clients' dilemmas and hurts. As a disquisition involves a story that reflects a client's attachment dilemma, it can be used to help the client see this dilemma more clearly and so move past the impasse. One of the advantages of disquisitions is that clients can see their situation in a different and less threatening light. The key to using disquisitions when at an impasse is making sure that the disquisition really captures the reason for the impasse, which means the therapist must have a good idea of what is happening with the client(s).

Consider the example in a case in which a husband refused to acknowledge his wife's pain and loneliness, and the therapist formed the following disquisition to engage the impasses. "For some reason, you remind me of a couple I once worked with. The wife kept talking about how unhappy and lonely she was and kept asking for change. The husband had a hard time believing that she was really that upset and that they had serious problems. Funny thing about that case, the wife finally gave up on him and filed for divorce. The divorce was very painful and involved a lot of conflict and legal battling. I saw him months later, and he said, 'She really was upset. I should have taken her more seriously. Now I have lost my marriage and family and everything.' For some reason, you guys really remind me of that couple. I am not exactly sure why." In this case, the husband said, "I know why—that is what I am doing." Disquisitions should be used sparingly, but when used at the right time, they can help clients see an impasse differently and move forward as a result.

Attachment History

Bowlby believed that defensive or non-feeling responses were always "perfectly reasonable" if one understood a person's attachment history (Bowlby, 1988). Doing a brief attachment history is part of the assessment process. However, an in-depth attachment history can often provide important clues that can help in breaking through impasses. See Chapter 4 and Appendix A for a list of possible attachment history questions. Blocks often occur because of past relational trauma, including attachment injuries, major attachment violations such as child abuse, and the lack of a consistent or safe attachment relationship growing up. Doing an attachment history can emotionally unblock people and help partners and families understand behavior in attachment contexts, which can depersonalize painful interactions.

For example, during EFFT, a therapist was having a hard time getting a father to see his children's need for his emotionally engagement. In a family session, the therapist did an in-depth attachment history focusing on the father's relationship with his parents. The father talked about how his father was drunk, angry, working, or watching American football. The father talked about getting his first football jersey and pads when he was about 8 years old. It was a big deal for him, and he was sure his dad would be proud. With great excitement, he ran up to his father to show him, and the father shoved him away and said, "Get away from me, boy—you think you are tough, but you don't know what tough is." As the father talked about this memory in session, he started to tear up and he talked about how he learned he should not rely on others and that part of "being tough as a man means not talking about feelings." The therapist was able to process this, and the father said, "I can see that what my father did to me was wrong, and now I am doing it my children, and it is hurting them like it hurt me. I want to change." The mother cried, and the kids cried and talked about they wanted to be closer.

Attachment histories can also help clients find safe attachment relationships from their past that they can use as a resource for building the current relationship. For example, one woman in identified her relationship with her grandmother as being secure and safe. After talking about her relationship with her grandmother for a bit, the therapist asked the woman what her grandmother would say about the couple's present dilemma and what she could do to change it. With much emotion, the woman replied, "She'd say, 'Trust him. Try it. He's soft—he won't hurt you or take advantage'" (Johnson, 2004, p. 315). This facilitated her softening.

If clients do not have an image of a secure attachment, the therapist may have to "seed" the attachment. Understanding a person's past allows the therapist to see the risks involved and to see implicit needs and so say, for example, "You would never turn to him and say, 'I need you; come and be with me.'" In seeding the attachment, the therapist acknowledges difficulties and paints a picture of what a secure attachment would look like in current relationship(s). Attachment histories can be particularly helpful in EFIT because they can help the client and therapist see patterns that would normally show up in the therapeutic alliance.

Repairing the Alliance

A positive therapeutic alliance is essential to the change process in EFT, and alliance problems can easily create impasses and can flow from impasses. In either case, it is critical that alliance problems are repaired. It is important for the EFT therapist to be particularly sensitive to this issue because alliance problems cannot always easily be detected. More subtle breaches in the alliance can be identified through examining the therapist's feelings about each client, viewing a recording of therapy, asking for feedback from all clients involved in the therapy, or presenting the case to a supervisor or colleagues and asking them for feedback.

For example, Juan was working with a heterosexual couple in which the wife felt deeply violated because of the husband's pornography usage while she was pregnant. She experienced it as a major violation of their marriage. In response to her pain, she frequently blamed and shamed her husband. For months Juan validated and assembled her pain and sought to stop her from verbally attacking her husband in session. He tried everything he knew to help her see how damaging her name calling, yelling, and threats were. In the process, the wife felt Juan was not understanding her experience, and she started telling Juan he was not a good therapist. Juan became frustrated and did not look forward to their sessions.

Repairing the alliance can be done in multiple ways. As with other aspects of impasses, the solution often lies in going back to the basic processes of therapy. It is especially helpful to walk around in the client's emotional experience through empathic reflection, empathic conjecture, and validation. Working to really understand the client's world helps the therapist gain greater empathy and promotes a client's sense that the therapist cares and stands with them. Sometimes a breach in the alliance can best be repaired through a direct therapist apology. The therapist could say something like "I am sorry. I don't think I have really understood" or "I am sorry. I think I have pushed too hard—that is not what I want to do."

In the case of Juan and his clients, he talked openly about how he was afraid that in trying to stop the blaming and shaming, he had hurt her, and he may not fully understand her experience. He sincerely apologized. They then discussed what she felt he was not getting and how he could validate her pain while also helping her change what she was doing with it. She suggested that in the future, if Juan saw her shaming her husband, that the best way to respond would be to say "I think your pain is very strong, and you need to be seen right now. I want to see you and help you know you are not alone." Juan did this, and it made a big difference in the therapy.

Individual Sessions

The use of an individual session or two when doing couple or family EFT can be a helpful tool in resolving impasses. In couple therapy when an individual session is conducted with one partner, it is also offered to the other to create balance and avoid aligning or being perceived as aligning with one partner. Individual sessions can be used to repair alliances, uncover and help people approach disclosing secrets, and process specific emotional responses that block emotional engagement. Although repairing the alliance in a conjoint session can demonstrate the power of an effective repair for all involved in the therapy, at times the time and safety of an individual session can be more effective. It provides time to help the client feel heard, understood, and cared about.

Secrets that involve major violations of trust typically require disclosure to promote openness, reduce shame, and create safety and trust. If secrets are not disclosed, they tend to lead to blocks, particularly when working to restructure in Stage 2. However, secrets need to come out at a time and in a way that is respectful and healing even though the disclosure is often painful. An individual session can provide the safety to discuss the secret and how and when the client will reveal the secret and how to respond to and help heal the pain of those who have been violated.

Finally, individual session can provide the safety to access and processes emotions, such as shame, that can block engagement in the EFT process. Attachment issues, past and present may be explored, perhaps through imaginary encounters with the attachment figure. For example, a client might be asked how a safe attachment figure, such as a grandmother, might view the client in her present role as a mother. With the help of the therapist, she might be able to construct a more compassionate, positive view of herself in her present circumstances. This type of intervention will only have power if the client becomes emotionally engaged in the process (Johnson, 2019).

Recording, Self-Observation, and Case Analysis

Often when learning EFT, the therapist can stray from the model. It is enormously helpful to video record sessions, observe them, and code them. If video recording is not available, audio recording can be used. When reviewing the video, the therapist can look at how often the EFT Tango and various specific interventions are being done. It then can help to look at an EFT training video and notice how often the therapist is using various specific micro- and macro-interventions and then compare your work with these examples.

Writing up the session for the file can be a valuable learning tool. It is often a time of reflection when the therapist can process the theory and interventions used in the session along with progress that was made and new understandings that were gained. Students of EFT have found the Training Note Form (see Appendix C) helpful in writing up session notes. The sheet is only intended as a guide for training since different therapy contexts and agencies require different types of case notes. The other side of this form can also be used for taking notes in session. The form attaches to a clipboard with the backside up, and the therapist writes down key metaphors, phrases, and emotions used in the session by the client(s). A simple pad of paper with a line drawn down the middle can also be used for in-session notes. The advantage of taking notes in session is that it highlights for the therapist and the client's key metaphors, phrases, and emotions that are used in session. These can then become part of the case file and can be reviewed before the next session. Additional resources for self-supervision of your EFT casework are available on the EFT Workbook eResource page (www.routledge.com/9780367483425).

Supervision

There are now many certified EFT supervisors (see www.iceeft.com) in the world providing EFT supervision in a variety of languages. They are trained to approach supervision using the EFT supervision model (Palmer-Olsen, Gold, & Woolley, 2011; Woolley, Faller, Palmer-Olsen, & Vitoria, 2016). Typically, these supervisors focus on developing a strong alliance with the therapist, working on conceptual development and integration, creating new experiences, and assisting the therapist in working through self of the therapist issues (Woolley et al., 2016; Zeytinoglu-Saydam & Niño, 2019).

When approaching a case, an EFT supervisor may try to understand if the therapist needs help in one of three major areas:

1. Conceptualizing the case. Is the therapist understanding how the problems presented in therapy is understood from an attachment lens and how EFT therapy can bring about change?
2. Accurate assessment. Is the therapist accurately assessing interaction processes and patterns (e.g., pursuing, withdrawing) and the emotional experiences of clients and where they are working in the model?
3. Intervention. Is the therapist effectively using the micro and macro EFT interventions (e.g., empathic conjecture, heightening, and assembling and deepening emotion)?

It can be helpful for the therapist to use this basic framework in approaching a supervisor for help. For example, if the clients are not accessing emotion in session, focusing on a lot of historical information about the case (which helps with conceptualization) may not be helpful. Instead watching a section of video where the supervisor can see failed attempts to access emotion can lead to the supervisor focusing on how to intervene in a way that results in here-and-now emotional experiences in session. To make supervision as effective as possible, it is helpful to write out the case in detail. Therapists should write out the emotional cycle and the emotions that you have been heightening and working with along with the places you feel you may be getting stuck and need help. Peer consultation and can also be very helpful. This involves sharing videos, discussing cases, and reviewing training films. In some EFT communities, peer supervision groups meet on a monthly basis for video review and peer consultation for difficult cases. For a list of EFT centers and communities, please refer to ICEEFT.com.

Exercise 8.7. Exploring a Stage 1 Impasse

The following exercises explore working through an impasse in Stage 1 using the case of Ruben and Natasha, who are stuck in stabilization.

Ruben works a great deal and is rarely home. When he is home, he doesn't talk much unless they are in an argument, at which time they both yell. Natasha works a part-time job and is the primary caretaker for their two daughters. She has become more and more angry with Ruben's absences and his excuses. The therapist has repeatedly identified the cycle and has reflected it back, but the clients continue to argue and fight, often in session. One day they came in and started into their usual pattern:

Natasha: You worked late every night this last week, and I've had it. Don't tell me that you are going to change because you always say that, and you never do. I can't believe anything you say these days. How can we have a marriage when you are never around, and I can't believe anything you say?

Ruben: I am sick and tired of you complaining. All you do is complain. Maybe if you didn't complain so much, I would come home more.

Natasha: Oh, so you are blaming it on me, are you? You say you are going to come home, and you work every night and through the weekend, and you blame it on me? Well, one of these days, you are not going to have me to come home to if you don't change.

1. What are likely to be core, vulnerable emotions for Natasha?

____

____

____

2. What are likely to be core, vulnerable emotions for Ruben?

____

____

____

3. Which of the following interventions are not useful in slowing down the interaction?
   a. Evocative responding ____
   b. Reflecting the cycle ____
   c. Reframing ____
   d. Enactment ____
4 What type of intervention might you use to make the impasse explicit?
   a. Evocative responding ____
   b. Reflecting present process ____
   c. Empathic conjecture ____
   d. Reframing ____
   e. Enactment ____
5. Write a sentence or two that might help make the impasse explicit. Compare your answer with the example given in the answer section.

____

____

____

6. How could the therapist set up an engaged encounter to help make client responses that contribute to the impasse explicit and deepen them?

____

____

____

Exercise 8.8. Exploring a Stage 2 Impasse

The following exercises explore working through an impasse in Stage 2 using the case of Jose and Rosalita who are stuck in withdrawer re-engagement. Jose and Rosalita met, fell in love very quickly, and married six months later. They are in their fifth year of marriage. Jose is an auto mechanic, and Rosalita is a schoolteacher who has been teacher of the year twice in the past seven years. Rosalita is earning about twice as much as Jose. Jose withdraws, and Rosalita has been pursuing him with anger and blame. Much of the past five years have been characterized by angry confrontations followed by Jose leaving for several hours. She does not know where he goes and fears he is seeing another woman. He promises he is not seeing anyone and that he just goes for long walks, drives in the car, or sometimes goes back to work. After eight sessions of EFT, they are starting to see their cycle and are fairly stabilized, but Jose is distant and not re-engaged in the relationship. For ten more sessions, the therapist tries unsuccessfully to get Jose to re-engage and recognizes they are at an impasse.

1. What types of fears might be holding him back?

 ____

 ____

2. If he is afraid of her anger, what are two ways to reflect this fear in order to deepen it?

 ____

 ____

After 16 sessions of EFT, Jose is beginning to come out and be more present and engaged. The difficulty now is in getting Rosalita to soften. She says she is having a hard time believing that his change is really real, that he sincerely wants to be there, and that he is actually afraid of her rather than simply uncaring.

3. What might be an underlying emotion that could be preventing her from softening?

 ____

 ____

 ____

4. In trying to get Rosalita to soften, you do an individual session with both Rosalita and Jose. What types of interventions and topics would you focus on in your individual session with Rosalita?

 ____

 ____

 ____

5. What types of topics and interventions would you focus on in your individual session with Jose?

 ____

6. Write a possible disquisition for the couple designed to help Rosalita soften and reach for Jose.

____

____

____

____

____

____

____

SUMMARY

The exercises in this chapter review EFT steps to consolidation which is the final stage in the EFT process of change. The EFT therapist builds on the corrective emotional experiences that couples have found through the process of withdrawer re-engagement and pursuer softening. New cycles of secure connection promote each partner's accessibility, responsiveness, and emotional engagement, and in turn the couple is better able to revisit perpetual conflict issues that are commonplace in romantic relationships (Gottman & Levenson, 1999). The EFT therapist facilitates new solutions through engaging positive cycles of security the couple has established through Stage 2. Consolidation also includes a focus on investing in the meaning and actions that strengthen the secure bonds between partners. Attachment rituals provide specific practices the rehearse, remind, and renew a couple's common intentions and resources found in the ability to rely on one another as a secure base and safe haven.

It is important to remember that the EFT model provides a map for change, but every individual, couple, and family is different and unique. These differences can lead to impasses in the EFT process. A therapist must learn about the uniqueness of each person and the process of change with each individual, couple, and family, which is always somewhat different. In some ways, every couple also brings out different elements of the therapist's training and experiences. These may provide important clues in understanding client, client therapist, and therapist processes. It is critical for the therapist to pay attention to all of these levels of process and to be open to the uniqueness of every individual and every relationship.

ANSWERS AND SUGGESTED RESPONSES

Exercise 8.1. Reviewing EFT Micro-Interventions and Consolidation

1. Restructuring (focusing and complementing—creating enactment)
2. Reflection and validation (new patterns and responses)

3. Reframing
4. Evocative responding

Exercise 8.2. Practicing EFT Interventions and Consolidation

Suggested Responses

1. "Okay, Mario, can we come back to that? Luisa, it seems like something just happened. It's like you kind of disappeared. I am wondering what changed. What's it like for you now?"
2. "So, you heard her concern, and you let her know her voice is important to you. You invited her back to the discussion, and that is not always easy to do, especially when her experience of your words was so different than you intended."
3. "So, when you hear Mario saying he wants to hear your voice, you feel important and like your ideas matter and you matter. This helps you move toward him and share appreciation for his strong ideas and those of your own. It's like you are working together on this rather than letting the strong ideas divide you. You are making sure the other person knows he or she is important."
4. "So, you have both come a long way to changing your pattern and staying out of the cycle that was ruining the love you share. How would you say you are different? What has changed for you?"

Exercise 8.3. Answers Consolidation With Inez and Fernando

1. Inez: Withdrawer, sadness

   Fernando: Fear of abandonment, shame
2. Pursuer. Note: Fernando was initially in more of a withdrawer position, but then Inez began to withdraw from the relationship after burning out from her initial pursuit of Fernando. Fernando's anxious response to her withdrawal prompted his pursuit. Shame, inadequacy, fear of rejection, and fear of losing Inez
3. Fear, sadness. She needs support, reassurance, and comfort.
4. Shame, fear of rejection
5. Inez refers to Fernando's remark from years ago, and how it hurt her. But she softens her response by acknowledging the ways she has shut him out on her own account. Fernando responds with regret over his remark and is able to own his fears and immaturity. Fernando also shares how he was drawn closer by Inez acknowledging that part of the distance between them was a result of her own choices.
6. **Suggested Response**. "So, it really surprised your daughter that you could both do this. You have come a long way. The cycle kept you at a distance, and there was no way you could work together without facing those patterns. There were times when the distance was so great, and you seemed to be headed for separate lives. The concerns seemed to drive you apart, with Fernando pulling away from you, Inez, as you both tried to connect through the frustration you were feeling

and the fears that you had that you might be unwanted and rejected in this relationship. Yet you have been able to see the soft side of your hurts and fears and to express this to one another. You've been able to see the cycle and slow things down, seeing your partner's needs and fears and moving to support each other. Whether it's the basement or talking about your sexual relations, you are finding a way to stay connected even when dealing with issues that have been around for a while. It's risky, and it's normal to find yourself in the pattern again, but you also have the experience and awareness to see the cycle and make yourself more available to the other. That is quite remarkable."

Exercise 8.4. Attachment Ritual

A number of rituals would be helpful. It may be helpful to suggest a ritual involving physical intimacy that builds on the hard work they have done to reconnect in this area. A meeting/greeting ritual in which the couple kissed or hugged hello/good-bye would serve as a sign that they want this connection and they can stand up to the fears that used to keep them apart.

Exercise 8.5. Reinforcing New Pattern

"Sure, that makes sense after living with this cycle for so many years, it's hard to believe that it wouldn't come back in some way. Yes, there may be times when you see the cycle start to raise its head, but you now know how to recognize it. Like when you want Fernando's attention and it's frustrating that he doesn't appear available, you also know ways to exit the cycle. You can check it out with him, letting him know what you need. You both found ways to stay connected even though you are discussing threatening issues. Now you know the feelings that escalate the cycle. Getting those out and into the open will help keep the cycle from taking over. Just like when we talked about Fernando's comment about weight—that was a tough issue—but you both found a way to stay connected through it. It was scary, but you did it."

Exercise 8.6. Termination Review

All are indicators of termination in EFT.

Exercise 8.7. Exploring a Stage 1 Impasse

1. She may be feeling abandoned, hurt, and afraid of not mattering and of losing him permanently. She may use the words lonely, disrespected, betrayed, or unloved.
2. Fear of failure and inadequacy, hurt, and sadness are probably primary emotions for him. He may be afraid of her anger and attacks, of being unloved, and of not being good enough or capable of meeting her needs.
3. **Answer: D**. The problem with enactment is that unless they are very tightly controlled, enactments at this stage tend to simply allow couples to enact their present cycle and the secondary emotions that are being expressed with it.

4. **Answer: B.** Reflecting present process and possible enactment if they enact the impasse and the therapist keeps the enactment slow enough so that the clients can reflect on the impasse and not escalate.
5. **Possible Response:** Therapist says in a voice that becomes softer and slower through the interventions: Natasha, if I am getting this right, it is very painful for you when he doesn't come home. You end up feeling very lonely and scared, but you don't talk about the loneliness or the pain. You get angry, and somehow then in an attempt to get him to be with you, then you complain and criticize. Ruben, correct me if I am wrong, but when she criticizes or complains, that is not easy for you to hear—very painful in fact—and you tend to withdraw as a way to protect yourself and get away from the problems and avoid another fight. Once you are in the fight, you try to get it over as quickly as possible because you fear that it will get out of hand. The more scared and angry she seems to be, the more desperate and angry you get, and you withdraw. Is that correct? But that just feeds the cycle. Both of you are stuck in this cycle where you get hurt and are afraid and lonely and to deal with that you attack or withdraw or fight, which means that neither of you end up feeling safe or loved. You are stuck in this pattern where neither of you get your needs met, and it is very hard to move forward to rebuild the relationship, something both of you very much want to do. Is that it? Do I have it right?
6. **Possible Response:** Therapist: I get the idea it is very hard for you when she is so angry—it sounds to you like she's telling you that you have failed in this relationship and that you can't measure up and that you are not going to make it with her. So, you clam up and avoid. Is that it?

   Rubin: Yes . . .

   Therapist: Can you tell her "It is hard for me when you get mad"?

   Rubin: No. I don't want to say it.

   Therapist: I get the idea this is very painful, very painful, to tell Natasha that you are learning you have failed with her. Perhaps you even feel sad about it.

   Rubin: (Shakes his head yes and starts to tear)

   Therapist: Sad, yes, you do feel sad. Can you tell her about that sadness, the sadness that comes hearing you have disappointed her? Can you tell her about that sadness?

   Rubin: OK.

Exercise 8.8. Exploring Stage 2 Impasses

1. **Suggested Response:** There could be many fears, including a fear of more fighting, fear of exposing himself and finding out Jose is unlovable or a failure for his wife, fear of being judged, fear of being vulnerable, fear of not knowing how to

engage, fear of being seen as emotionally weak, fear of being misunderstood, fear of being verbally overwhelmed by her ability to talk, or fear of losing her by any of the above happening.

2. **Suggested Responses**
   - You are very concerned about another fight, and these fights are very painful for you—is that right?
   - When you think of coming out and really opening up, you are afraid she will just attack again, it will be overwhelming, and it will just hurt more than it has.
   - The fear of her anger and disapproval is so intense, so very intense, that you could never turn to her and tell her you need her. It is very difficult for you to even touch that fear it is so strong. It is so much easier to run from it by either withdrawing or attacking. To turn to her and tell that you overwhelmed by her disapproval and feel like a failure with her, that would be far too scary. So, you just turn away or you attack, and that seems less scary than showing how you feel. Is that it?
   - Can you tell her about that fear—that fear that drives you to participate in the cycle that you are both caught in—that fear that makes it scary open up to her, even when you want to? Can you tell her about that fear, what it is like for you when you hear her anger and disapproval?
3. **Possible Response:** She may be afraid that if she softens and becomes more vulnerable, he will abandon her again. She may feel deeply hurt and be afraid that if she opens up, she will just be hurt worse. Deep inside she may have feel shame about herself and may be afraid that if he really knew her, he would not love her or respect her.
4. **Suggested Response:** You might focus on and explore her fear of engaging, when it comes up, what it is connected to, and how she deals with her fears. You could have her imagine herself facing the fear, staring it down, and risking and having Jose be there.
5. **Suggested Response:** You might focus on and explore the cycle and her primary emotions, such as fear and hurt, when he is not present. You could focus on her fear that if she engages, he will not be there. In order to help the fear come alive, you could have him remember a time when he was very scared and help him use that fear to construct an understanding of how she feels about risking opening up to him and being vulnerable with him. You frame her as needing his help and support.
6. **Suggested Disquisition:** I once knew a couple that for some reason remind me of you two. They both desperately loved each other, but the husband was terrified of her anger and disapproval and often tried to escape it though working hard and keeping busy. The more he did this, the more the wife became lonely and hurt and afraid he was leaving her. In fact, she really saw it as leaving her, and she became more and more angry. One day the husband decided that something needed to change. They loved each other a great deal, but he could see how they were both being hurt. The wife did, too. Soon the husband was opening up, and he really hoped she would open up and trust him again. However, she was so scared that he wasn't going to really be there or want to be there if she opened up, that she refused to open up. It was so hard to see him as anything other than the man who had betrayed her and left her alone when she needed him. Despite his pleadings

for her to open up and be close, which she had always wanted, she refused. It was too risky. It was too risky that he wouldn't be there, or he would stay there for a short time and then leave again. No matter how hard he tried and how much he pleaded for a chance to be there, she didn't risk it, even though she was desperate to be close to him. Finally, he went away in sorrow that there seemed to be no way for her to give him a chance. When he did, she said, "I knew he wouldn't be there; I am so glad I didn't risk it." I wonder why you two remind me of them.

SECTION III

EFT APPLICATIONS

9

EMOTIONALLY FOCUSED INDIVIDUAL THERAPY (EFIT)

This chapter reviews the application of the emotionally focused therapy (EFT) model, well known as a couple intervention, for individuals dealing with depression, anxiety, and the aftereffects of traumatic experience. As outlined in *Attachment Theory in Practice: Emotionally Focused Therapy with Individuals, Couples and Families* (Johnson, 2019) and in Brubacher (2017, 2018), emotionally focused individual therapy (EFIT) is a model of intervention based on the perspective on health, dysfunction, and growth offered by attachment science and on an integration of experiential (Rogers, 1961) and systemic (Minuchin & Fishman, 1981) interventions. The great strength of attachment theory is that it seamlessly integrates inner experience and relational pattern (Bowlby, 1969, 1988) and shows how each defines the other through the process of affect assembly, regulation, and expression. EFIT is inherently relational, always seeing the individual evolving in the drama of one's intimate connections. Individual therapy as a modality has often taken individual functioning out of this context, which from the EFIT perspective is like taking a fish out of water—its evolutionary context—and expecting to really understand how a fish actually functions.

EFT TASKS AND GOALS WITH INDIVIDUAL CLIENTS

In this section we explore the EFT tasks and goals as they apply to EFIT. As with any modality of EFT, the tasks follow a similar function. The tasks orient the therapist to the core elements necessary in the EFT process of change.

Task 1. Creating and Maintaining a Therapeutic Alliance

The EFT therapist stance is best defined by the acronym ARE. The therapist is accessible, responsive, and engaged, entering into attuned connection in the manner of a good parent who is intent on creating a secure bond with the individual client while at the same time attuning to the client's experiences with key figures that populate their world. Therapist attunement is essential to alliance maintenance and repair, which is necessary in the EFT therapist's effort to sustain an ongoing emotional balance and focused genuine presence. Repairing ruptures and realigning misattunement strengthens the therapist's alliance and promotes client's exploration and felt confidence in this unique therapeutic bond.

DOI: 10.4324/9781003039457-12

Task 2. Accessing, Assembling, Expanding, Distilling and Deepening Emotion

Accessing, assembling, expanding, distilling, and deepening emotion occur particularly in Move 2 of the EFT Tango; however, the therapist is constantly tuned to emotional cues and almost invariably follows the emotional charge in session. The therapist helps an individual to discover how their emotion is constructed, often distilling reactive emotional experiences down to a core threat or perceived danger that underlies the more surface coping responses such as rage, numbing, or despair. In this process, the therapist helps clients experience and process emotions embedded in anxiety and depression in new ways, opening pathways for more effective emotion regulation and expression. The therapist follows the map of the unfolding process of emotion and basic attachment needs and fears, provided by attachment science and the accumulated clinical wisdom of EFT.

Task 3. Restructuring Key Interactions and Key Ways of Engaging

In Task 3, the EFT therapist restructures key interactions and key ways of engaging with emotion, both when intense unwanted emotion is triggered intrapsychically and by significant others. It is as necessary to shape *interpersonal change events* with individuals as it is with couples and families. The shaping of these interpersonal encounters crystallizes stuck places, core vulnerabilities, and automatic ways of coping and responding, and it structures new corrective emotional experiences that change individuals' key inner dramas. It is in reshaping these inner dramas that an individual's sense of competence and worth can be discovered and consolidated.

The Goals of EFIT

EFIT is oriented to helping clients create *emotional fitness*, which is the capacity to recognize and use one's emotions as a reliable guide and to function with flexibility, connectedness, resilience, and efficacy. The EFT therapist always attunes to individuals in their attachment, relational contexts, viewing individuals as essentially co-regulating beings—functioning optimally when they have one or two others on whom they can depend. Depending on others is what Bowlby (1988) called *effective dependency,* an ingredient essential to health and well-being. The state of optimal dependency involves having positive views of some others as trustworthy and dependable and a view of self as lovable and competent. The specific goals of EFIT include:

- To offer corrective emotional experiences that positively impact models of self and other and shape new responses to self and other.
- To offer transformative moments where vulnerable emotions that are frightening, alien, and unacceptable are encountered with balance.
- To facilitate clients to move into the accessibility/openness, responsiveness, and full engagement that characterize secure attachment with others.
- To help clients to shape a coherent sense of a worthy, competent self who can deal with existential dilemmas and become a fully alive human being.

The therapist follows the five moves of the EFT Tango to reach each of these goals. The Tango moves organize a repetitive process with different levels of intensity that guide the entire process of change. Each move includes experiential and systemic interventions guided by a consistent focus on attachment themes and experiences.

Exploring the EFT Tango in EFIT

We now provide a snapshot of how a therapist helps an individual move through the EFT process of change using the five moves of the EFT Tango. In this brief example with Stephen, we observe how the EFT therapist reflects the present process in an early stage of EFIT to begin *stabilizing* stuck patterns, accessing underlying or unexpressed core emotions, and moving slowly toward *restructuring* Stephen's experience. The therapist focuses on using newly discovered and distilled emotional experience and engaging the present process to shape new ways of interacting and regulating emotion, concluding with *consolidating*, integrating, and celebrating change. Reading Stephen's example, you can move through the EFT Tango and complete each exercise to explore the EFIT process.

Stephen: (speaking fast and directing his gaze at the carpet.) I know I am hard to deal with sometimes. I get very hyper. Wired. Have to be the best at what I do—and my sports things, and—well, everything. Have to be on the go. Busy. High energy. My wife says I am too much. Like—I want us to make love every night and then some. But she goes and sleeps on the couch. I get pretty angry, and then we really fight. She even mentioned divorce. She won't talk to me for days. You know she was engaged to my best friend, and he dumped her, and then she agreed to go out with me. He is one of the richest men in the country now. Somehow, I persuaded her to marry me, but . . . My mum used to tell me "You'd better knock yourself out and find some magic or you'll be a nothing like your father." But I am fine. I just want some help with all this not being able to sleep and freaking out when I lose a case in court. Maybe I just need to try harder or get some sleeping pills—half my firm are on them. Some of them are really effective these days. . . . What was I saying? Oh yes (pauses) I get so angry. So, I go work out at the gym. If I stand still . . . well . . . no point, is there? Just emptiness there.

Exercise 9.1. Move 1—Mirror the Present Process

Which of the following therapist responses best illustrates a focus on the present process? *Hint: The best answer will reflect in the present moment how Stephen copes and the emotional impact he is experiencing using this coping pattern.* Choose 1 answer: _________

a. Therapist: You have this strong need to achieve, and it's so hard for you when you lose a case in court—that you go home and put even more pressure on your wife to be affectionate and sexual with you. And I imagine that pressuring your wife to respond is making her frustrated with you. What do you think?
b. The therapist offers a mindfulness exercise to help Stephen calm down and sleep. After practicing the mindfulness exercise with him several times, the therapist assures him this will help him to sleep. Stephen is also given an exercise to use to help him go back to sleep, should he awake during the night.
c. You sound very wound up even now as you talk! So, caught up in this fear of losing—this sense of being a loser running, running at full speed, performing, pushing yourself continually to achieve—to avoid that emptiness of being no more than your dad? You push your wife to show desire for you, and she then moves away, and you end up feeling more unsure than ever that you matter to her, so you push again. The more you push, the more she turns away and the more frantic you become. In spite of your speed and your efforts, anger and emptiness lie in wait for you.

Exercise 9.2. Move 2—Affect Assembly and Deepening

Building on the present process that the therapist reflected, consider which of the following therapist responses best focuses on assembling Stephen's emotional experience. *Hint: The most useful intervention here might include reflecting key elements of his emotion (trigger—bodily arousal—meaning made—action tendency) into a coherent statement that highlights his core attachment panic.* Choose 1 answer: ________

a. "What do you think it means that you cannot slow down and sleep? Did you receive messages, for example, that you have no right to slow down until you achieve more? It must be very difficult to feel continual pressure to push yourself to be bigger and better—fearing failure in your wife's and mother's eyes."
b. The therapist focuses specifically on the trigger for his speed up, "You've said that you get especially wound up when you lose a case—you've said you feel like a loser, in fact. You talk about 'freaking out' when you lose a case." Stephen introjects, "I'm dizzy—perhaps I am just not good enough—sexy enough—clever enough." The therapist responds, "So your natural tendency is to run as fast as you can to avoid the danger of losing, of failing. This emotional music has taken over, and you are wired and angry all the time, dizzy, running from the fear of the 'emptiness'—of not being good enough—that waits for you, yes?"
c. "You have a hyper speedy talking style! You are obviously trying to prove to your mother that you are not the failure she predicted. Your need to prove you are of more worth than your father is repeatedly getting in your way! Can you imagine how much easier life could be if you were to recognize that you have already achieved much more than your father ever did, even if your mother fails to recognize this obvious fact?"

Exercise 9.3. Move 3—Shaping an Encounter

Review the following three encounters that an EFT therapist could shape to help Stephen disclose his newly discovered emotional experience. The therapist could shape an encounter with the therapist, between two parts of Stephen, or with an image of his mother. Read each response and see if you can identify how the use of these encounters could expand Stephen's exploration of his pattern of pressure (e.g., the treadmill of emptiness on which he is stuck). After reading each possible therapist response, jot down a new discovery Stephen might make from each encounter. The discoveries may be about how he constructs his world and how he engages with himself, with others, and with his own emotion. Now imagine what it is like to be Stephen engaging in each of these encounters.

1. Focus on Therapist Encounter: "What happens when I tell you how exhausted I feel listening to you? How hard it must be for you to come in and tell me about these feelings rather than just stay on the treadmill? This strikes me as a lot of courage and insight on your part! What happens to you as I when I say this? Can you hear me when I say this?" (He says, "No. Really only wimps come for therapy.") In this encounter with the therapist, Stephen is likely to discover

   ____

   ____.

2. Focus on Encounter Between Parts of Self: Now can you find an image of your agitated self—demanding you perform—in court? Can you close your eyes and touch your tired, freaked out, almost empty self? Can this tired, empty self tell the on-the-go, run-faster part of himself how tired he feels, how he longs for him a break? In this encounter between his tired self and his run-faster self, Stephen is likely to discover

   ____

   ____.

   Focus on Encounter with an Imagined Other—his mom: "Can you picture your mom—the mom whose message you hear on a daily basis, saying 'If you don't knock yourself out, you will be nothing'?" The therapist wants to explore his emotions in that moment and explore how he might respond to her. In shaping the encounter, the therapist asks Stephen to close his eyes and picture his mother. "What does she look like? What is she wearing? Where is she? What happens inside of you as you look at her like this?"
3. After Stephen has an image of his mother in his mind, he blurts out: "I get dizzy . . . . I start spinning, my heart fills with anger and determination, and I want to say, 'I'll show you! I'll prove to you!' (His shoulders slump. He gasps.)—I feel like collapsing! (He begins to sob.) I just want you to see me—to see that I am someone good!"

   In this encounter with an image of his mother, Stephen is likely to discover

   ____

   ____.

Exercise 9.4. Move 4—Processing an Encounter

From the options, choose the response that will be most helpful to Steven to process his experience of the encounter with *his imagined mother. Hint: The most useful intervention will include an evocative question about his present moment experience and a reflection of what he has just done. Choose 1 answer:* ________

a. "You have hurt for so long about the fact that your mother missed seeing your goodness! Telling her how angry you are about this is a very good thing to be doing. It is helping you understand more about the hurt under the anger. Continuing to express your anger and hurt will be a very good thing."
b. "What happens inside Stephen as you tell this image of your mother how her threat that you will be nothing has driven you to work so hard to prove she was wrong—and then to collapse in tears telling her you just want her to see you are someone, someone filled with goodness?"
c. "Your mother's threat has driven you all these years and still drives you to push yourself relentlessly. And it now drives you to push your wife as well. You want your mother to know she has created a very negative impact on your work and on your marriage!"

Exercise 9.5. Move 5—Integrating and Validating

Here the therapist summarizes what the client has just done by validating and highlighting any new emotional elements and celebrating the process. Review the following therapist responses and choose the one that best summarizes and integrates Stephen's in-session experience based on the encounter processed earlier. Choose 1 answer: ________

a. "Wow—it took a lot of courage Stephen to put words to this anger while looking directly at this image of your mother's face, and in taking that big risk, you discovered this noble, lifelong yearning to be seen as good enough—as a man of goodness! In expressing that longing to her, you were also able to take in her response."
b. "What would it be like to go home and tell your wife about this? Perhaps she sees you in a similar way as your mother does, and this would be good for you to practice confronting this them of others seeing you as a failure."
c. "Do you think you can practice sharing like this more in your life out of my office? It would be good to also practice what you say to yourself in these moments. Practice seeing what is true about you before you react to other's negative opinions and reactions. Then we can see how this goes."
d. "Stephen, you have made good progress identifying your attachment emotions and how they help you see yourself and others in a new way. It is important to remember that these emotions are a valuable part of who you are even if others don't see you that way."

Exercise 9.6. Formulating a Reflective Summary

In this exercise, you are to practice forming a reflective summary that clearly captures the essence of Stephen's experience. Pause and take time to attune to Stephen's experience; then formulate a one sentence reflection for each of the following elements. Try to stay close to his experience using his words and form a statement that captures each of the following:

1. His sense of self (e.g., how he sees himself).

____

____

____

2. His ways of dealing with emotion that trap him in his distress.

____

____

____

3. His strategies for connecting to a primary attachment figure (e.g., informing his key interactional pattern).

____

____

____

4. His core underlying emotions.

____

____

____

EFIT PROCESS OF CHANGE

The EFIT process of change follows the identical EFT Stages also used with couples and families. These include the first stage stabilization (also referred to as de-escalation in EFCT), followed by the second stage of restructuring (new ways of engaging with and seeing self and other) and the third stage of consolidation.

Stage 1: Stabilization

In the first few sessions in Stage 1 of EFIT, stabilization, the therapist does as Rogers suggests (1961, p. 24) and enables the client to "discover the order in their experience," normalizing and validating the client's present ways of experiencing and creating their world. The therapist joins with the client in an accessible, responsive, and engaged manner, shaping a safe haven–secure base alliance as together they uncover patterns in internal and interpersonal experiences that leave the client stuck in apparently unsolvable dilemmas. (Consider the client who says, "I can't stand to be so alone, but I can't and won't let anyone close"). The therapist gives specific focus to reflecting present process as it evolves, including ambivalence and dilemmas, and to making emotions more specific or *granular* and more acceptable to the client.

The goal of Stage 1 is to shape less reactivity and numbing and move toward greater emotional balance. The sessions become a secure base where clients can be more open and explore internal and interpersonal patterns, their distress makes sense to them, and they can begin to accept and own their emotional experience. In Stage 1, as in all stages of EFIT therapy, the EFT therapist uses the macro sequence, the EFT Tango, and the micro-interventions of empathic attunement, empathic reflection, validation, evocative questions focused on present process, interpretations (conjectures), and heightening of emotional experience, as well as reframing and setting up new kinds of interactional dramas with key figures in a client's life or parts of the client's self.

Beginning EFIT Stage 1

In the initial sessions of EFIT, the therapist focuses on building an alliance and assessment. An experiential therapist is always more focused on the client's evolving personhood than on placing people in diagnostic categories. Assessment and treatment are continuous and overlapping. The first concern is to help people feel safe and guide them to clearly formulate their goals for therapy. Fortunately, the de-pathologizing attachment framework of dysfunction and health strengthens the therapist's capacity to help clients feel acceptable and safe, to identify their strengths and vulnerabilities, and to formulate goals that are relevant for therapy.

The EFT therapist, doing EFIT listens to the client's story of who they are, their attachment relationships, and key events in their life. The therapist pays attention to the picture of self and of others that emerges in the client's narrative and in how this person engages with the therapist while sharing their story. Specifically, the therapist pays close attention to how a person deals with vulnerabilities, including patterns of secure, avoidant, or anxious strategies for affect regulation. The therapist also listens for themes in a person's life story, present dilemmas, the key figures who populate the client's world in memory or present-day experience, cognitive openness and level of flexibility, and ways of engaging others that emerge from the client's relationship history.

As an attachment-oriented clinician, the therapist notes the apparent level of secure attachment or anxious or avoidant strategies the client reports. The therapist also notes signs of the dominant models of self and other. The manner in which the client tells their story is key. More securely attached clients tell more coherent organized stories that include specifics rather than offering general, almost impersonal narratives, and they can show emotion as they tell the story. We also especially listen for positive moments or bonds that can serve as a resource as the client moves through therapy. For example, a beloved grandmother who offers the client some level of comfort and connection can be evoked in a difficult session. Achievements, especially when the client felt a sense of competence or personal worth, are also noted. These times evoked the client's sense of resilience and can be used throughout therapy as resources.

Exercise 9.7. Attuning and Exploring in Beginning Sessions

Please read the following scenario once and then read it again and see if you can identify at least one example of each of the following five elements *to attune to in early sessions*, as they emerge in the client's narrative.

Key EFIT Elements to attune to in early sessions:

1. Client's manner of engaging with the therapist and with others.
   Example: Talking rapidly and nonchalantly
   Example: ______________________________
2. Patterns (repetitive internal/interpersonal cycle) of affect regulation.
   Example: ______________________________
3. How client deals with vulnerabilities (getting overwhelmed, minimizing).
   Example: ______________________________
4. Signs of dominant models of self (Am I lovable and competent?) and of other (Are they reliable, trustworthy, and responsive?).
   Example: Model of Self______________________________
   Example: Model of Other______________________________
5. Achievements, moments of competence or personal worth.
   Example: ______________________________

Rose: (talking rapidly and nonchalantly) Most of the time I feel nothing. (Clutching her belly, she continues.) Today would have been my mom's 60th birthday—and I should be happy for her—but I feel nothing. (She chuckles.) I wanted to grow up to be like her—

confident, assured, beautiful, successful—and I'm none of that—I'm alone—depressed—not at all motivated to look for a job. No interest in using my hard-earned MBA. I did well in that program and used to be proud of it. I'm numb mostly—I don't really know—I never felt much—there was never room to feel. She died when I was ten years old, and from that day on, I had to be responsible. Dad said we were strong—we were literally the Strong Family—(sarcastic sneer), and nothing would get us down. Any time I got sad or felt afraid, dad dismissed my fears—"You're ok," he'd say. "We're showing the world we won't let this get us down. We'll stick together. Your little sisters need to see you're strong. Your mom would be so proud to see you show the world we are managing just fine—to see what a great job you are doing with your little sisters!" I think I must have been shattered to lose my mom—but who knows. (another nervous chuckle, continuing to clutch her belly) Well, Uncle Billy noticed—he always called me Little Rosie—I think he got I wasn't a grown up, liking this responsibility. I think he got that I was terrified! Oh, it's silly to be talking about this really—I'd rather we move on—help me get my act together, if you can. I need to find the courage to start job hunting again. There's no room for this silliness.

Now reread the scenario and jot down at least one example of each of the *elements to attend to in early sessions*, listed earlier.

Exercise 9.8. Identifying the Repetitive Cycle

What is the client's repetitive internal, interpersonal, or *within-between* cycle? How would you describe it? (Take note of ways the pattern in her inner experience reflects and is reflected by her relationships with her dad and with the therapist.)

____

____

Exercise 9.9. Finding Emotional Handles

Name some emotional handles—evocative words, phrases, or images—a therapist could repeat to open doors to assemble and deepen the client's emotional experience.

____

____

____

____

Key Elements a Therapist Attunes to and Explores in Beginning Sessions

The previous scenario illustrates the initial focus of the EFT therapist in Stage 1 of EFIT, stabilization. In promoting stabilization, the EFT therapist assesses and explores the following five key areas.

1. *Ways of regulating emotion.* The therapist is tuning into the *process* of affect regulation and looking to identify how the client's habitual ways of dealing with difficult emotions feeds back into chronic mental health and relationship problems. This is <u>the protection/prison cycle</u>. Remembering Ps helps here: The

pattern of emotional *protection* becomes a constraining *prison*, a *problem-perpetuating process.* Melissa outlines that from early childhood when "overwhelmed," she has dismissed and "detached from" her hurts and fears and grasped intellectual control, also focusing on helping others, judging her own pain as just "whining." This "worked" and stopped her from going "crazy." But it now leaves her always vigilant and alone. It has become an ever-turning wheel in which she is always "struggling, on guard, and trapped." This feedback loop maintains her pain and fear, feeding into her lack of emotional balance, destroying any sense of contentment, and preventing new corrective experiences from being taken in and integrated. The client's usual coping mechanism, a once healthy response to vulnerability without solution, has now become chronic and debilitating. This coping is at once validated and also described as part of the present problem.

2. *Within-between cycle.* The therapist also seeks out and outlines the cycle of inner turmoil and distress and the interpersonal problems the client describes, linking these together in a within-between cycle. Melissa says there has never been "anyone to protect/hold me," and so she focused on staying in control and taking care of others. After all, as a small child, she had been ordered by her abusive mother to "take care of your 2-year-old sister." She does not turn to others for support and so carries the load of her trauma and depression by herself, worrying more and feeling more "on edge." Her aloneness and inability to trust and turn to others, such as her husband, feed her sense of being constantly flooded and abandoned. She dismisses her pain as "whining" in much the same way as her mother did.
3. *Emotional handles.* Core evocative words, images, and metaphors that capture a client's vulnerabilities are emotional handles that open the door to what Bowlby called "frightening alien and unacceptable" emotional realities. For Melissa, the handles that emerge in the first two sessions are "exhausted," "trapped," "on the wheel." She tells me that she dreams of a bear in her dreams, and he is always just about to eat her. This bear feels like her fear. These handles are noted and used throughout therapy to assemble emotion and deepen emotional processing.
4. *Key elements of emotional disorders* (Barlow, et al. 2011). The therapist takes particular notice of key elements of particular problems such as depression, anxiety disorders, and post-traumatic stress reactions (Johnson, 2019). Bowlby's description of depressed clients as feeling lonely, unlovable, unwanted, and helpless is pertinent here, as well as the well-known correlates of problems such as depression: Loss, a sense of failure, and self-criticism. The key elements of dysfunctional anxiety are also noted (Barlow et al., 2011) in the unified protocol for emotional disorders, namely, intense unacceptable negative emotion that is lacking in clarity, vigilance for threat that biases perception, intensifying attributions, and fear of fear itself as well as avoidance strategies such as suppression. Post-traumatic stress disorder, even if manifesting below clinical levels, is also characterized by emotion regulation problems such as those mentioned here. The therapist also notes issues such as flashbacks of overwhelming experience and overall numbing. In general, the therapist is looking for triggers that push the client into a sense of danger and helplessness and how ways of coping with this experience block any revision of working models of self and other and block engagement in new corrective experiences, thereby restricting the client's sense of choice and agency.

For example, Melissa is always on guard, trusting no one, keeping everyone at a distance. The therapist listens carefully to evoke from Melissa some specific triggers in her present life that signal danger to her—"*When* do you get a sense you must run from danger?" The therapist also attunes to any moments that Melissa can slow down and describe specific moments that feel unsafe.

5. Specifying goals for therapy. In addition to attuning to the four key areas already discussed, the therapist guides the client into specifying the desired outcome for therapy. Melissa says in session one, "I want these strange flashbacks to my childhood to stop. I am on guard all the time." She also says, "I am exhausted. Always in control—holding everyone up." By the end of session two, with the therapist's help, she can be more exact, using the therapist's summary of her problems. "I want to get off the wheel of worry and vigilance and feel safe in the world. I want to stop dismissing my hurts and listen to what is really important for me." The more the goals for therapy are explicit, concrete, realistic, and stated in a positive frame of what the client wants, rather than what the client does not want, the better.

Exploring the EFT Tango in Stage 1

The EFIT therapist creates and maintains an alliance in which the client feels safe to explore their experience, moving toward the goals specified with the therapist in Step 1. Repeating the moves of the EFT Tango, through Steps 2, 3, and 4 of EFT Stage 1, the therapist and client shape the emotional balance that characterizes the change event of Stage 1, stabilization. The case of May, suffering from depression, provides an opportunity for you to experience and apply the Tango through the stabilization change event.

Practice: Tango Move 1. Mirroring the Present Process

Exercise 9.10. Identify Emotional Handles and Signs of Bodily Arousal

Underline key phrases in the example that focus on emotional handles and key bodily arousal you would attune to as therapist to accurately reflect her present process.

May: Well, I guess I am depressed. Down. No energy. My boyfriend says I am depressed. (She giggles.) I just had a run-in with my boss. She said I was too anxious and not focused enough, and I guess I do worry about things. (Begins to cry.) My boyfriend Tim says he is busy with his job, but . . . I think maybe he is getting ready to move on. Used to call him all the time, but now am just sleeping a lot, watching TV, and eating bad stuff . . . bit pathetic . . . but I am fine really.

Exercise 9.11. Empathic Reflection of Present Process

In the following example of mirroring her present process, underline and number the words and phrases by which the therapist reflects:

1. Her specific triggers (danger cues).
2. Her action tendencies.
3. Her emotional response.

You are tired, depressed, barely any energy for anything, and very worried—your boyfriend is so busy, you're worried he may be about ready to move on, and. Describing those worries brings you to tears—and then you brush it off and say, "I am fine really—it doesn't really matter."

Exercise 9.12. Validate by Linking Trigger and Action Impulse

Create a validation that links triggers (danger cues—related to her job, Tim, and mom) with her present moment action tendencies and emotional distress. You could begin with, "Of course . . . "or "I hear the struggle" or "It makes so much sense." Then add the trigger, her behavioral impulses, and her emotional distress:

____

____

____

____

Exercise 9.13. Finding Interventions

Identify the following micro-interventions in the transcript below.

> Select the following therapist interventions and enter the corresponding number in each blank in the transcript below.
>
> (1) Evocative question with an attachment image.
> (2) Validating experience.
> (3) Reflecting and offering a reframe towards a goal/longing.

Therapist: It's hard to know how to believe you can move forward in your life. ______

May: Oh, well. (smiles and flips her head in the air) I never seem to get it right anyway really—I am just waiting for Tim to tell me we are done, and may-be I don't want that job anyway. . . . My mom says I just need to grow up and stop being a drama queen. We fight a lot. So, I just left and zoned out on TV soaps till about 4 a.m. She told me about a job interview but . . . what's the point? I don't want a new job anyway. Do you think I am really a nutcase? (sighs)

Therapist: Everything seems pointless, some part of you says nothing is going to work? _______ *(She nods.) When you get really down, who can you turn to for support?* _______

May: Turn to? What do you mean? My mom just lectures me—I dread her phone calls (winces)—don't have any friends here really—and my boyfriend is busy all the time, so . . . I cuddle the neighbor's cat sometimes. (giggles) I never really was good at making friends. I was always the odd one out, shy. So. . . .

Exercise 9.14. Empathic Reflection

Now add a simple empathic reflection, slightly on the leading edge of the words the client used. Since the client didn't use a feeling word, it may feel slightly like a conjecture, but it will be the word that comes to you as you attune to the experience of having no one to turn to.

Therapist: Sounds kind of ______________________ (one word is enough.)

May: (shrugs; then nods)

Exercise 9.15. Reflect the Pattern that Protects and Imprisons

Reflect May's reactive pattern. She says that she feels safer to stay alone than to reach out to others for support. How would you reflect this pattern to May? A pattern can include some variety of "The more you/others do_______, the more, you feel______, and the more you feel_________, the more you/others __________." Now provide a summary reflection of her pattern.

____

____

____

____

Following your reflection, May tears, nods, then admits glumly: "Sure, but what can you do? The only time I feel good is when I swim—used to swim a lot—compete even. But couldn't make the finals, so . . . I just want to feel better. At 28 years old, I should be in control of my life."

Exercise 9.16. Review of Basic EFIT Elements in a Beginning Session

1. Patterns of Affect Regulation—Briefly describe how May deals with her vulnerable emotions—her fears, unmet needs, and longings.

   ____

   ____

2. How does her affect regulation at once protect her and also shape a prison or a self-defeating process for her? Describe her attachment dilemma.

   ____

   ____

   ____

3. How would you describe her basic within/between pattern of engagement?

   ____

   ____

4. Model of others: How does she portray others?

____

____

5. Model of self: Identify some emotional handles that reflect themes of her model of self, especially with regards to worthiness and competence.

____

____

Exercise 9.17. Themes of Emotional Disorders

Select one or two of the key elements of emotional disorders listed and identify the patterns and themes that you would want to highlight in May's story.

Key Elements of Emotional Disorders.

- feeling lonely, unlovable, unwanted, and helpless
- sense of loss, a sense of failure, and self-criticism
- intense unacceptable negative emotion that is lacking in clarity
- vigilance for threat that biases perception
- intensifying attributions and fear of fear itself
- avoidance strategies such as suppression

Identify two themes or elements of emotional disorders and give an example from May's life and story.

Key Element 1: ____

Example: ____

____

Key Element 2: ____

Example: ____

____

Practice: Tango Move 2. Emotion Assembly and Deepening

As the therapist mirrored May's present process in Tango Move 1, May felt increasingly validated and understood by the therapist. She found it odd and a little surprising that although the therapist seemed to notice that she avoided others as much as she tried to avoid her own feelings, there was no sense of judgement nor attempts from the therapist to try and get her to change. The therapist seemed to understand that she didn't trust anyone, and yet she found herself beginning to trust the therapist, just a little, and in some very small way began to feel fleeting glimmers of longings for safety with Tim and her mom. The therapist seemed to accept her tendency to pull away from everyone and give up on herself, and this evoked a tiny bit of curiosity in May to explore this stuck place in which she was caught.

Exercise 9.18. Surface, Reactive Emotion

What is May's basic surface emotional response?

____.

Exercise 9.19. Identify the Trigger, Bodily Arousal, and Meaning Made

1. *When* is this reaction is triggered? ______________________________
2. After naming the triggers, can you list her bodily responses when she experiences these triggers?

   ____

   ____

3. What are the meanings she is likely making of these triggers and bodily responses?

   ____

   ____

Exercise 9.20. Using Reflection, Evocative Questions, or Conjectures to Assemble Elements of Emotion

What would you say to May to:

1. Validate and normalize the trigger and her explicit response, for each of the following triggers:

   Example: Trigger—Tim is busy: <u>It makes sense that when Tim is busy, you get frightened he is pulling away from you, and it is so easy then to crumble in depression and loneliness.</u>

   Trigger: Mom gets angry. ____________________________________

   Trigger: Boss complains. ____________________________________

2. Conjecture tentatively about her basic perception (safety/danger).

   ____

   ____

3. Explore her bodily response by asking an evocative question.

   ____

   ____

4. What evocative questions can you ask to explore the meaning (view of self and/or other) that she makes of the experience?

____

____

____

____

5. Name her action tendency. What are her action tendencies in this narrative and in the session?

____

____

May describes the fractured relationship with her mother since she discovered that May and her high school boyfriend had started a sexual relationship when she was 15 years old. "Maybe I shouldn't have cut her out of my life." Her voice tightens, and her jaw tenses as she adds, "But she says the meanest things! Every time my phone rings, I startle for fear it will be her calling. The thought of hearing her voice puts me in a panic, drains all my energy. I go cold and just want to disappear and talk to no one."

Exercise 9.21. Assemble Emotion Into a Coherent Whole

Now help May assemble her emotional experience by providing a summary that organizes her experience by linking danger cue (trigger), bodily response, meaning made, and action impulse. Write a summary reflection that assembles May's emotion.

____

____

____

____

Exercise 9.22. Distill Poignancy

Next, distill the most poignant part of her experience into one statement. Poignancy is what an EFT therapist attunes to in attempt to capture the emotional essence of experience, the part of the message that seems to be most emotionally alive and newly put into words. It is the core attachment experience that *an emotional handle* reveals (see Brubacher, 2018; Johnson, 2020).

____

____

Practice: Tango Move 3. Shaping Encounters

The crux of change in EFT is using newly discovered and expressed emotion to shape new ways of interacting (internally and interpersonally). Encounters in EFIT take place in dyads between the client and therapist, with an imagined other or between two parts of the client. Just as we are first and foremost *relational beings*, it is as necessary to shape *interpersonal change events* with individuals as it is with couples and families.

In the EFT Tango Move 3, the EFT therapist shapes interpersonal encounters to structure corrective emotional experiences that change individuals' key inner and interpersonal dramas. Encounters with different dyads may shift and flow multiple times throughout a session. The primary guide—as to *when* and *with whom* to shape an encounter—is that of attuning to and following the client's emotion as in Tango Move 2. Specifically, while staying close to a client's present moment emotional experiencing, the EFT therapist will choose a dyad in which the emotion is most alive for shaping an encounter in Tango Move 3 and then process the impact of that encounter in Tango Move 4. The dyadic encounters can be set up between the client and therapist, with client and an attachment figure, from client to an abusive or rejecting other or between two parts of self. As described in Chapter 3, encounters follow a basic process of the therapist *shaping the encounter* by creating a context, helping the client to anticipate making contact, and establishing safety followed by making a request for the disclosure and maintaining a clear focus on the specific interpersonal disclosure.

Exercise 9.23. Move 3. Shaping an Encounter With an Imagined Attachment Figure

Following May's distilled message, regarding her panic reaction to her mother, imagine how you might help May shape an encounter with an image of her mother. How might you shape this message?

- Invite her to close her eyes and picture an image of her mother, asking her what she looks like, where she is, what she is wearing, and/or what she is doing.
- How can you repeat May's distilled message of fearing that her mother is out to hurt her and doesn't care about her, to help her anticipate the encounter?

____

____

____

- Then how can you direct May to disclose her experience to this image of her mother?

____

____

____

Given the context of May's relational world, you could choose to invite her to share distilled messages with others in the course of therapy (potentially with you, or with a key other person such as a sudden memory of her father who left when she was 10 years old, or it could be a message between two parts of herself, such as a lonely younger self). The EFT therapist will choose to shape encounters based on which dyad is most alive with emotion or is most blocked emotionally and seeming to interfere in the client's present moment processing or which attachment figure (imagined other or therapist's presence) may be the best resource in this moment.

Consider the example of May's response to her memory of her father leaving. The EFT therapist might shape an encounter based on this pivotal loss. After assembling and deepening her emotions, the therapist says,

> *"You said you can still see dad packing the truck and yourself at 10 years old looking out the dining room window—seeing him drive away, with that knot in your stomach, knowing he was not coming back. Can you picture that dad just now? Can you imagine telling him about the knot in your stomach and how much it still hurts in the core of your being that he drove away that day—that you lost you dad—how it still hurts?"*

Exercise 9.24. Shaping Other Encounters

Following a similar process, we will now practice shaping encounters with May's boyfriend, Tim, between parts of self, and with you as therapist.

1. What might you say to May to shape a message to her boyfriend, Tim? She is missing him desperately, yet in her fear that he is pulling away from her, she has numbed out and has pulled away from him.

   ____

   ____

   ____

   ____

2. Now practice shaping an encounter for May between two parts of self. This could be a message from her "concerned self" who brings her to therapy and risks opening up and the "hidden self" frozen in fear who isolates from others and dismisses her own emotions. After helping her imagine and make contact with these two parts, how can you shape the encounter?

   ____

   ____

   ____

   ____

3. With you as therapist: This encounter requires less formal setting up and imagining. Assume May has just told you that she is afraid you will get tired of listening to her dark, depressing stories, and you simply invite her to repeat that key

disclosure again. (You could do this to heighten her fear—and then to respond to her fear with genuine, empathic presence. Together with May, you could then process this interpersonal interaction of clear expressions and responses.) Write out a simple request for May to repeat this message to you:

____

____

Practice: Tango Move 4. Processing Encounters

In Tango Move 4, processing the encounter, there are two elements to pay attention to in processing a client's experience of a dyadic encounter: first, the experience of *sharing* a newly distilled message and second the experience of *receiving* a clearly shared message. Let us return to processing the encounter between May and her mother.

Exercise 9.25. Process the Experience of the One Disclosing (How was it to share?)

Imagine you are May, and the therapist says, "How this was for you to share this clear message to this image of your mom? How was it to tell her how frightened you are that she doesn't care and that you are convinced she will try to hurt you if she has a chance?" Write out how you suppose May might respond.

____

____

____

____

Exercise 9.26. Process the Experience of the One Receiving the Message (How was it to hear?)

This time, imagine you are May, and the therapist says, "How do you imagine your mother would respond to hear you share your fear of getting hurt by her—how much her words have fractured your soul?" Write out how you suppose May may respond as she speaks from her image of her mother, who has just received May's message.

____

____

____

An EFT therapist will formulate evocative questions to process the impact of each encounter with an imagined other, often taking time to reflect the key message that was just shared. For example, using May's response to Tim, the therapist says, "You just told Tim that you act as if you have given up on your relationship, when inside you are missing him so much—that you long for him to come close to you." Then the therapist asks May, "What was it like inside for you to share this with an image of Tim?"

It is difficult to speak to an imagined other without implicitly anticipating how this disclosure would impact the imagined other. Thus, an EFT therapist will also help the client to process the client's imagined impact and response of the other. The therapist might ask May, "How do you picture Tim responding to your sharing this with him?"

Exercise 9.27. Processing Encounters With Imagined Others

Your task is now to consider how you would process an encounter between May and her father. Drawing on the example with Tim, write out how you might reflect the key message May disclosed to her father about her anguish at seeing him drive away and out of her life. Then invite her to share what it is like inside for her to share this with an image of him.

1. Reflect the key message she shared with her image of her father.

 ____

 ____

2. Follow this by evoking the impact on her of disclosing to the image of her father.

 ____

 ____

3. Evoke from May how she imagines her father might be impacted or respond to her disclosure.

 ____

 ____

 ____

Exercise 9.28. Processing an Encounter Between Client and Therapist

Imagine the encounter is with you, the therapist. How are you likely to disclose the impact on you of her willingness to tell you she is afraid you will get tired of her darkness? And then, how might you check in with May how your disclosure impacts her?

____

____

____

____

Encounter between parts of self: If the *other* was a part of herself, the therapist would invite her to hear from the other part how it was to receive this message. For example, "How was it to hear your responsible-bring-yourself-to-therapy part, telling your frozen, heart-broken 10-year-old self that she sees your pain and wants you to know it is okay to let yourself sob—that of course you are heartbroken at dad's departure—and that of course she wants to know your feelings always matter?"

Tango Move 5. Summarizing, Celebrating, and Integrating

Following an encounter, the therapist will mine the moment, summarizing and celebrating the corrective emotional experience that the client has just created. This helps the client to slow the process and pay attention so as to integrate the shift. For example, regarding the encounter between two parts of self, the therapist says, "Look what you just did! Your frozen-in-fear-and-all-alone self just spoke to the wiser, caring self who brings her to therapy and said, 'I am terrified—terrified I'll always be alone—never good enough for someone to stay with me—always on the end of rejection and being left to fend for myself' and your older, wiser, caring self said so tenderly, 'I know how terrified you are—I see you need more support than you are getting just now—so I am reaching out for help for you. We deserve help, and I'm taking you to therapy—here we'll find someone who can help us—someone who is safe to come to with your fears. I know you're afraid and so alone—and I'll keep bringing you here to this safe place until we can do it on our own . . . until you can see you are good enough for someone to love!' What a powerful team you have inside that is cheering you on, recognizing you need the help of someone else just now!"

Exercise 9.29. Integrating the Impact of the Encounter

Write down how you could similarly celebrate May's encounter with Tim, heightening the impact it is having, giving her time to savor and integrate the process.

____

____

____

____

Stabilization at the End of Stage 1

The change event of Stage 1, stabilization, is completed when clients are aware of their basic pattern—of action impulses and responses to threat or vulnerability that have become the automatic way of coping. They are also aware that this pattern is no longer serving them well—in fact, it has become quite ineffective in their relationships and in life in general. What is shifting for them by the end of Stage 1 is that these rigid, automatic patterns of coping have moved into their awareness; the triggers signaling threat that typically set these patterns in motion have also been discovered and validated. Clients move from self-deprecation and exasperation with themselves about their problematic coping strategies into more of an accepting, empathic position similar to what they have experienced from the therapist. Ineffective patterns of coping are now seen as best attempts at coping with depths of terror or pain that previously had no words. There is a sense of "My struggle really has been this difficult and I got caught in coping this way—not because I am foolish or hopeless—I was doing my best to respond to overwhelmingly, threatening experience."

The client is beginning to see self—like the therapist does—as a vulnerable human being—caught in need of comfort and response, operating automatically—in the moments of threat with little to no awareness of self in need. They are beginning to feel hope in grasping that if *the problem is the pattern*, they can explore what they are doing to cope with unwanted feelings and can discover alternative strategies.

The end of Stage 1 is marked by:

- Improved emotional balance, with access to core underlying emotion.
- Expansion of self into more acceptance and awareness of how *frightening, foreign, and unacceptable emotions* and processing strategies shape a lasting feedback loop.
- Expansion of awareness of key attachment dramas and how they shape self and dances with others.
- Improved exploration—openness, responsiveness, and engagement in session and with the therapist.

As you read the following description of May at the end of Stage 1, note the markers of her stabilization that are underlined.

> *May is feeling more stable. She is having occasional moments of calm and hopefulness. She is recognizing that her core problem is not that she is flawed but that she became caught in an imprisoning pattern of coping with her losses. She sees that in her best attempts to manage her pain over the broken relationship with her mother, the distress of working for a critical boss, and Tim's increasing distancing and seeming lack of interest in her, she got stuck in expecting judgement around every corner and in concluding she must be unlovable, unworthy, and flawed. In Stage 1 stabilization, she came to recognize her pattern of self-protection as the very prison that was holding her back from being seen and heard and from receiving the comfort and understanding from others that she craves. She came to recognize that the fear of being judged and banished from love and connection was the core emotional music driving the patterns in which she was caught. She began to have some access to her fear of being judged and banished. It was the same emotional music playing in the patterns with her estranged dad, with her unreliably responsive mother, with Tim, with her boss, in her inner relationship with herself, and in the ways she minimized the abuse from her ex-boyfriend. Exploring her grief, her fears, and the value she has for each of her current relationships, she began to see alternatives to her rigid self-protective pattern of* the more I mistrust and distance from others and my own emotions, the more dangerous and unavailable they become. *In the secure relationship with the therapist, she became more willing to engage with exploring what felt like foreign, frightening, and unacceptable emotions, and she began to feel safe enough to explore the trauma she had survived.*

Exercise 9.30. Identifying Markers of Stabilization

Now as you read about the case of David at the end of Stage 1, please underline the markers of stabilization, following the earlier example of May. David arrives at the end of Stage 1 with an awareness of his pattern of swinging between automatically turning up the emotional panic alarm to a state of frenzy in which it becomes ineffective to get a human response and turning down any hints of emotional alarm bells to the point where nearly all zest and motivation has been suppressed. He has come to recognize this automatic survival pattern and the underlying pain of isolation and abandonment driving these patterns. The terror of isolation driving his swings between frenzy and numbness is becoming acceptable and familiar in the context of the therapist's repeated validation and acceptance and the coherence he and the therapist have collaboratively made of these patterns and terror.

He experiences through Stage 1 that he is *continuing to do as he has been done to* (Bowlby). For example, he says, "I am dismissing my own needs and longings—don't know what they are really—just as long as I take care of others—as long as there is no conflict or strife—no one has ever really heard my needs—but I'm okay really—kind of lonely—but I shouldn't complain. Oh, there I go—doing it again—dismissing my needs, as though it doesn't matter that I am lonely. My parents were environmental activists—not sure if they actually said it—but it feels like they said, "You're crying because you didn't get invited to the party, and the planet is being destroyed?" I'm noticing how hard it is to trust that you (therapist) really have the patience to listen to all my whining—I feel like I am whining when we take time to look at how small and unimportant I have felt—but I am beginning to see how—this is the problem: No one heard me, and I don't listen to me either."

Check the answer key to compare with what you have underlined as markers of David's stabilization.

In the collaborative discovery process of Stage 1, the pattern of hyper-activating or hypo-activating emotions and longings is framed as a best attempt but a presently ineffective or outdated way of coping. The habitual pattern of ignoring or exaggerating emotions and needs is seen as having been adaptive at one time and no longer to be serving them well. Emotional pain (or hurt) has been identified by social psychologists (Vangelisti, 2009) as a complex emotion, combining anger, sadness, and fear of loss.

Stage 1 stabilization reframes the problem in depression, anxiety, or a particular mood disorder as a habitual way of processing experience. Clients recognize how their interpersonal patterns and view of others as untrustworthy and unresponsive reinforce their internal emotional experience and view of self. They recognize how they are continuing to reinforce these patterns and they gain some access to the core underlying emotions driving their patterns and processes of emotion regulation.

In the stabilization process, clients come to recognize the negative feedback loop: Their ways of viewing and dealing with distress increases and maintains their unwanted emotions, and the distress or unwanted emotions reinforce their ineffective meanings and strategies for coping. They recognize how their inner cycle of processing emotion, by turning it up or tamping it down, mirrors their interpersonal pattern of how they reach or do not reach to others in distress and how others respond or do not respond.

Exercise 9.31. Reviewing the Basic Pattern and Underlying Emotion Driving the Pattern

In the client scenarios of May and David, we can identify the basic repetitive pattern that each client has come to embrace as their real problem. We can also identify core underlying emotions driving each one's pattern. Complete the exercise below for David by following the example given for May.

Example: May's Pattern: The more she mistrusts and distance from others and her own emotions, the more dangerous and unavailable others become.

Underlying core emotion: Her fear of judgement drives her patterns of avoidance.

David's Pattern: ____

Underlying core emotion driving the pattern: ______________________________

Stage 2: Restructuring

Stage 2 of EFIT, as in emotionally focused couple therapy (EFCT), occurs in the safety of a client's recognition that the real problem—the root of their distress is not a personal deficit or a hopeless, helpless reality based in another's treatment of them. When the client experiences that their problem and agency for change are rooted in the repetitive pattern of how they make sense of and react to difficult emotions, they are ready for the deeper exploration of Stage 2. As the automatic survival patterns are validated in Stage 1 and the fear and pain—of rejection, annihilation, or abandonment that continue to fuel these patterns—are evoked, experienced, and expressed, the therapist helps the client explore with increasing depth and emotional engagement the core underlying pain and terror that their coping strategies have kept at a distance. This is the heart of the restructuring process of Stage 2.

In the collaborative discovery process of Stage 1, clients own the patterns of *how they shape their world* (the perceived threats; their automatic physiological fight, flight, or freeze reactions; the meanings they make about self and others in the moments of threat or distress; and their habitual action tendencies). In Stage 2, they explore and engage *new options to reshape their world.* The discovery of new meanings and interaction patterns emerges through a gradual entry into the full experiential depth of unexplored fear and pain. In increasingly alive ways, clients discover in Stage 2 how their habitual strategies for coping with a sense of uncontrollability, unpredictability, and unchangeable existential realities keep the core fear and pain locked away in a metaphorical vault labeled *unacceptable and dangerous.* Gradually, the therapist helps the client to move directly into the intensity of this fear and pain. It becomes manageable and transformative to face and experience heightened fear and pain in the safety of dyadic regulation with the therapist and at times on the relational safety of the imagined presence of a secure attachment figure or a compassionate part of self. A key factor that distinguishes Stage 2 from Stage 1 is that emotion is followed and expanded into greater emotional depths and with more coherence in Stage 2. Fearful and painful emotions are experienced in fresh and new ways. Deliberately choreographed encounters restructure emotional experience and shape new ways for clients to engage with others and their own experience, including the existential dilemmas of life, such as unalterable circumstances and losses.

Deepening in Stage 2: Case of May

Using EFT Tango Move 2 and the interventions of heightening, conjecturing, and reframing along with validating, reflecting, tracking, and evocative responding, the therapist helps May begin the Stage 2 process of deeply exploring her core underlying fear that her coping strategies have kept at a distance.

May has an increasing awareness of how her self-protective patterns of isolation and emotional distancing can trap her in depressive episodes. She recognizes her heavy heart as an emotional signal of her need for connection. She increasingly listens to the emotional music of sadness and loneliness when it first appears—moving her to reach out to Tim and to her growing circle of friends. To her surprise, she does experience some responsivity from them when she reaches out. There remain, however, times when she collapses into depression "before she knows it." Feelings of being alone in the world, unlovable, and unwanted expand like a massive balloon, filling the room and trapping her beneath it. "It's there before I know it—pressing the life out of me—barely room to breathe." Recognizing May's increasing emotional balance, disrupted by collapses into depression, the therapist decides to assemble the process of emotion in her depression and to then deepen the core underlying emotion.

Therapist: It sounds like before you know it, this balloon of depression is weighing down on you—almost like you don't know what brought it on—you almost don't notice Tim's busyness or your heavy heart before the old, familiar, bitter messages fill the room like a massive balloon—saying, "You're alone—no one shares your fears and worries—no one really cares—they're only mean and hurtful—out for themselves." (assembling—bodily arousal and meaning made)

May: That's right—it all happens so quickly!

Therapist: And I wonder if the heavy weight in your heart (previously identified as May's signal for needing to reach out) almost gets ignored as you listen to those old bitter messages take over—expanding to fill the room and pressing the life out of you? (May nods). It must be very difficult indeed to listen with kindness and patience to the heavy weight in your heart—when the balloon filled with old familiar bitterness presses down on you?

May: I totally ignore my heavy heart—true!

Therapist: I remember in our earlier work that that core weight in your heart has always had such important messages! Such pure sadness—longing for comfort—yet fearing rejection or judgement. Your eyes are filling with tears as I say this—do you feel that heavy heart just now? (May nods.) Yeah? Can we stay with the heaviness in your heart? (Pause. May nods.) Notice how heavy it is (pause)—how tight. (pause) Beneath all the pressure of the noisy balloon—you can feel the weight in your heart. —(pause) And what does this heavy heart say? (pause)

May: (shudders) Terror—terror—no one sees—no one cares—all alone—no one to reach to—like I am 10 years old again and all alone!

Therapist: Ah—you stop and listen beyond the pressure of the noisy balloon—and you hear your tender beautiful heart saying, "I am so afraid no one sees me"—and suddenly you are back at 10 years old again—all alone and feeling the deep longing for someone to see how much you need comfort, yeah? (May weeps.) And just listening to the terror in your heavy heart brings you to tears—it is so very, very sad—to feel this much fear and aloneness and not know how or whom to reach to for safety! That is the message of your heavy heart—isn't it?—"I need someone to see me—to notice me and to care—then I can know I am ok." (May takes a big sigh—looks up—nodding.) So, when this heavy balloon of depression sneaks up on you and you can barely breathe, you recognize there is a beautiful aching heart underneath all the pressure and the noise—that longs to be noticed and cared for—that says, "Listen to me—I am still here—I just need to be seen and comforted—I need to know someone is there for me!" Discovering this longing to be connected to someone who loves you opens you to a flood of tears and sadness. This sadness and fear of being unnoticed is alive with a pull to reach out—yes? This sadness and fear is alive, and you breathe deeply through those tears—so different than the weighty balloon that keeps you from breathing—keeps you from feeling. (May nods, smiles, and sighs again.)

Exercise 9.33. Affect Assembly Toward Deepening—Tango Move 2, Stage 2

Drawing from the therapist's Tango Move 2, can you complete the partial list below of the elements of emotion the therapist is assembling with May as she seeks to make sense out of how depression continues to take over at times in spite of her periods of emotional balance? This affect assembly paves the way for increased deepening of her core emotional experience.

Elements of emotion assembly: (Fill in the blanks below.)

a. Cue/immediate perception: Tim's busyness/a danger signal.

b. Bodily arousal: ______________________________

c. Meaning making: Bitter messages, saying, "______________________________

______________________________."

d. Action impulse: Ignores the heavy weight in her heart that tells her she needs to reach out; listens to the bitter messages; floods into tears and sadness.

e. Core, underlying emotion: ______________________________

Exercise 9.34. Emerging Shifts in Views of Self and Other

In Stage 2, as May deepens and engages with a more coherent and expanded emotional experience, her internal working models of self and other are sharply in focus, and some new aspects are beginning to emerge. Model of self usually pertains to a sense of one's lovability, worth, and competence, and model of other is related to the degree to which others appear to be reliable, dependable, and accessible. How would you describe May's core models of self and other? After providing your description of each model, please comment on how these models are beginning to shift with this Stage 2 assembly. *Hint*: *There are some growing awareness of core longings within herself and some responsivity from others at times.*

1. Client's view of self: ______________________________
2. Emerging shifts in this view of self: ______________________________
3. Client's view of other: ______________________________
4. Emerging shifts in this view of other: ______________________________
5. How might a therapist provide a summary that combines her view of self and other with elements of her process of emotion into a coherent whole?

____

____

____

____

____

Exercise 9.35. Identifying EFT Heightening Interventions in Tango Move 2

Key interventions and instances of the therapist's nonverbal RISSSC manner are used to deepen May's core emotion and expand fresh, new experience. The therapist is sure to use a simple, soft tone and a slow pace with repetition. The therapist also invites greater awareness of May's felt experience through evocative responses and empathic conjectures.

Identify instances of the following interventions from the earlier transcript.

1. **Heightening** (with repetitions of imagery):

   ____

2. **Evocative responding, including *evoking by directing her to stay*** *with the bodily felt sensations* of her emotional experience:

   ____

   ____

   ____

3. **Evocative question** to access the message of need in her bodily felt core emotion:

   ____

4. **Empathic conjecture** which actually "seeds attachment" (paints a picture of secure attending to the bodily felt message or longing, while also heightening the heaviness and fear):

   ____

   ____

5. Empathic conjecture to reframe her tears as a core longing?

   ____

   ____

   ____

   ____

Shaping Stage 2. Corrective Emotional Experiences

As emotional experience evolves through EFT Tango Move 2, new action tendencies and new meanings emerge. Core emotion that is elucidated, expanded, validated, and heightened in Move 2 of the EFT Tango is then turned into new expressions in encounters with imaginary key figures in the client's life in EFT Tango Move 3. Corrective emotional experiences are *shaped* (Move 3), *processed* (Move 4), and *integrated* (Move 5) through the EFT Tango.

The underlying attachment fears first accessed in Stage 1 are more accessible and more deeply experienced in Stage 2. These core emotions are explored, expanded, and distilled before interpersonal encounters are shaped to create corrective emotional experiences. Following core emotion is the foundation from which clients are helped to shape new patterns of interacting and new models of self and other, through carefully choreographed dyadic encounters.

Guidelines for Shaping Encounters in EFT Tango Move 3

In the more intensely engaged process of Stage 2, while the therapist attunes, follows, and heightens the client's emotion, different dyads for shaping encounters emerge as being most relevant to the client's present moment experience. Encounters may be in different dyads, including client and therapist, client and an imagined other secure attachment figure, client and a hurtful other who is a source of pain or unresolved trauma, or between newly emerging parts of self within the client. In choosing *with whom to shape an encounter (Tango Move 3)* and *when* to do so, the therapist attends to distilled, deepened emotion to identify

1. The dyad where emotion is most alive
2. The dyad where emotion is most blocked. This could be an attachment figure or an abusive other.
3. The secure attachment figure (imagined other or therapist's presence) that may be the best resource in this vulnerable moment
4. The client's internal reaction towards his or her core fear or core struggle or associated aspect of self (such as the small, abandoned child part of self who made key decisions about self or other or an injured part of self that carries guilt and shame about the injury, or a key element in an existential crisis where one struggles for meaning or purpose). Before shaping an encounter between with two aspects of self, emotion is assembled and distilled so the client can emotionally engage with two coherently distinct aspects of self.
5. The spontaneous emergence of an encounter between therapist and client. When newly accessed emotional experience is expressed between client and therapist, the therapist is likely to slow the process—repeat the moment—and flow organically into Move 4 of the Tango to process the impact of that experience.

The corrective emotional experience is intensified when each person's (real and imagined) experience is evoked, repeated, and savored *in the choreographing of an encounter in Tango Move 3*. As described in Chapter 3, encounters are carefully shaped by creating the context and anticipating contact, making the request, and maintaining focus. The impact of the encounter is deliberately processed in Tango Move 4. Encounters not in imagination but directly between therapist and client are also processed explicitly, providing moments of therapist transparency, interpersonal engagement, and intimacy.

When the imagined other is an "offending other" such as in trauma resolution, the therapist takes extreme care to help the client to hold the *offending other* and not *self*-responsible for the trauma. Typically, when the imagined other is an abusive other, the client needs support to keep the image at a safe distance and supportive permission to choose to block an imagined response from the other. When needs for permanent distance from an abuser are validated, new views of self and other also emerge. That is, *view of self* is redefined as a person of value *and view of other* is distinguished between there being some safe others and some unsafe others. This newly refined coherence of who is safe and who is unsafe is an empowering shift.

Encounters in the Context of the EFT Tango Moves

Following and reshaping clients' emotional experience in EFT Tango Moves 1 and 2 sets the stage for creating corrective emotional experiences in Tango Moves 3 and 4 when clients "explore new ways to engage with their own experience, with others, and with the existential dilemmas of life" (Johnson, 2019, p. 75). All corrective emotional experiences are maximized when validated and integrated in Move 5 of the EFT Tango. Next we explore shaping several Stage 2 encounters, beginning with an exploration of assembling and deepening core emotion as the guide for choosing which encounters to shape and when to flow between encounters with the therapist, between parts of self, and with imagined others.

The therapist attunes to May's core emotional experience to guide her in choosing which dyadic corrective emotional experience to shape. In her core struggle of self-loathing and pushing away the love that is being offered by her boyfriend, Tim, May touches on underlying fears of Tim changing just like her abusive ex-partner had done. While attuning to May's core fears and emerging expressions of emotion, the therapist processes a brief encounter between therapist and client and then shapes an encounter with May and an image of her abusive ex-partner toward whom her emotion seems most blocked yet most intense.

Exercise 9.36. Identifying Interventions

As you read the following transcript, please note the interventions used through the Tango moves. When you find a blank space, fill in the intervention that the therapist just used. Please choose between the following EFT interventions: reflection, validation, evocative question, heightening, and empathic conjecture (in proxy voice).

Tango Move 1: Reflecting Present Process

Therapist: You've talked about the walls you keep up between yourself and Tim—how you can't trust it is safe to let in the one person who wants to be there for you—that you've nearly stopped reaching out for him in the last while—so afraid one day will be his last—that the abuse you survived from your boyfriend before Tim has left you very cautious—not ready to trust anyone again." (tracking and reflecting, validating)

May: I'm just so afraid this relationship with Tim will not last—I didn't realize how afraid I was before the work we've done—I just shrugged him off—so sure I didn't have a chance that he would stay with me—always on the look-out for him to change and stop loving me—like Brody did. Now I am more and more aware of how important he is to me—and I really do not want to lose him, but you can never tell. . . .

Therapist: So afraid of being hurt again, yes? Just not seeming possible to trust him? #1_______________

May: Definitely; people can change on a dime, you know. Suddenly it can all change.

Tango Move 2: Assembling and Deepening

Therapist: Makes sense you are afraid—given what happened with Brody. #2____________. He has had such a strong impact, such a hurtful impact! You invested so much in that relationship . . . only to have him suddenly flip out on you! (tracking and heightening)

May: Two years—yes, and he suddenly went from sweet Brody to a raging maniac! And I'm still jumpy, and I hate it. He had no right to do this! What ever happened to him? (looks down and away)

Therapist: Yeah. Still so jumpy. He frightened you so much—hurt you and left you feeling unsafe to trust anyone—especially a kind man like Tim, yes? And you hate it! Just before you got quiet and looked away, you said, "He had no right to do this to me!" He had no right to hurt me and leave me fearful of trusting anyone ever again! (validating) #3________________.

Tango Move 3: Encounter Between May and Therapist

May discloses newly accessed and heightened emotion to the therapist. This is an encounter between them that the therapist will process momentarily. May shared, "Absolutely"—looking directly at the therapist. "He had no right to go from his kind, sweet self to suddenly raging at me—I know his drug use played a factor—but it was still not ok, and it's left me on edge all the time! He left me with no chance of ever trusting Tim or anyone!"

Tango Move 4: Processing Encounter Between May and Therapist

Therapist: How was it to look directly at me and tell me in this forceful, assertive voice—"He had no right to do this to me!"? You just stated a very powerful message! #4________________, heightening

May: It felt good—I've never really said that before—it felt like a message that came from my toes!

Therapist: Wow—it did feel like a powerful message to me too! Your feet flat on the floor and speaking a powerful message—feels good to state that so clearly—to recognize and then hear your own deep voice stating he had no right to do this to you—to hurt you and frighten you even to this day! (therapist self-disclosure, validating) #5____________

Again, the therapist is guided by attuning to May and following her emotional experiencing as it deepens and clarifies. After heightening and integrating the impact of May's clear message to the therapist, the therapist decides to create an encounter for May to risk disclosing this emerging clarity to an image of her abusive ex-boyfriend. This will give May an opportunity to further consolidate her emerging emotional shift from fear to core assertiveness and increasing coherence of the trauma she survived.

Tango Move 3: Shaping a Safe Encounter With an Abusive Other

Here is an example of the therapist shaping an imaginal encounter with Brody, who acted abusively toward May in a previous dating relationship.

Therapist: Can you find a safe way to picture Brody right now? Perhaps picture your dog beside you here and know that I am right here with you and imagine Brody as far away in the distance as you need him to be—and can you image telling him from this deep, solid place—with a voice from your toes—"You had no right to do this to me!—no right to hurt you me like you did—no right to punch that hole in my wall and leave me feeling damaged and frightened even to this day!" Can you imagine speaking to an image of Brody at a safe distance from you? (evocative questions, heightening needs for safety and sources of safety)

May: I see him—way over there—like as far as the other end of the waiting room, and he looks pathetic really—like he doesn't want to listen.

Therapist: How is it to see him looking like that? He is standing there—and you about to speak to him from a solid, angry place—to tell him how he hurt you and how it was very, very wrong, and you are tired of carrying the wounds of his abuse? (evocative question to anticipate contact, #6______________)

May: Very scary—but I gotta do it! I've rarely let myself see how much he hurt me—but he did!! He did!!

Therapist: That is right—he hurt you so badly! You've become so skilled at numbing out when the pain began, and just now you are letting yourself feel the pain—feeling the pain and the injustice of what he did and as scary as it is you are almost ready to tell him—"Brody—this was all wrong! I did not deserve this!" (heightening, #7___________)

Therapist: What happens inside when you picture this image of Brody and you consider telling him how wrong he was? (heightening May's experience of the enactment, #8________________________)

May: I feel really tense. My stomach is one big knot.

Therapist: Ahh . . . really tense—stomach in a knot and—it's almost like your chest opened a little. You took a breath, just seeing there he is. Yeah? Yeah. Can you feel that deep breath? Can you feel the strength in your toes? (reflecting bodily arousal, #9__________________, evocative response to stay with bodily experience)

May: Yup.

Therapist: Picture yourself saying, "Brody, what you did was so wrong; there is no way that was ever okay what you did to me?" (long pause) <u>Directing encounter</u>. *"My voice keeps getting choked off from me. I'm trying to find a way to speak to this image of Brody—to say it was so wrong!" (heightening, #10____________________)*

May: (finding her voice and her courage). It was wrong, Brody—you had no right to hurt me like you did. . . . You've left me frightened and unsafe in the world—but I'm taking back my right to be here. I deserve better, and I deserve to feel safe!

Tango Move 4: Processing Impact of the Encounter

The therapist heightens, repeats, and processes with May how it feels to make these courageous statements to an image of Brody. May's demeanor changes. Her breath slows down, and she smiles.

May: (to the image of Brody) You can leave now! I don't want to see you again.

Therapist: How are you, May? (evocative question)

May: I never knew I could do that—I feel so powerful—in a peaceful sort of way. The best part was telling him he could leave now—I didn't want him there anymore. I was done—said all I needed to say. I do deserve better—that is the message I feel from you all the time—that I do deserve to be treated well and it was so great to say that out loud! And I could feel Tim smiling on me. This is his scarf. She swirls another loop around her neck.). It smells like him, and it keeps me safe.

EFT Tango Move 5: Integrating

Therapist: Almost like you are starting to feel the warmth of Tim's safety just now—"just maybe he is someone I can trust?" #11_______________, #12_______________

This transcript illustrates how an EFT therapist follows the moves of the EFT Tango to shape corrective emotional experiences. Present-moment emotion is assembled and deepened. The newly distilled emotion is shaped into an encounter with a relevant other.

In this example, the relevant encounters included an encounter with the therapist and then with an imagined abusive other from May's past. The following transcript provides you with an opportunity to assemble and deepen emotion—and to let this process guide you in deciding which encounter to shape.

May: I see myself, 10 years old, looking out the window—dad packing the truck and driving away and not even turning back to wave at me. I just don't think it was ever the same after that.

Therapist: (repeating the cue to deepen May's emotional experience) Your dad driving away and not even turning back to wave—changed your life forever!

May: (wincing in pain, blurts out) My father is not going to hurt me anymore—I realize that—but I feel guilty for entirely cutting him out of my life. I'm sure he feels more pain than I do.

The therapist repeated the cue to promote a deeper experience and that triggered May to wince in pain (bodily arousal) at the same time as she dismissed her loss and guilt, focusing instead on her dad's pain.

Exercise 9.37. Reflecting Present Process, Including Action Tendency

Practice taking the next step of assembling May's emotion in this moment. Provide a reflection statement that links the cue (e.g., the image of her dad driving away) with her action tendency of dismissing her pain by focusing on her dad's pain. Keep in mind you are working to help her feel her pain while at the same time to notice what she does with it.

____

____

____

Deepening May's experience through linking the cue with her tendency to dismiss her own pain and lingering with the image of May's life never being the same after that pivotal moment of dad's departure, the therapist further assembles May's emotion by evoking the meaning she made and continues to make of this event.

Exercise 9.38. Evoking the Meaning

Choose the best response to evoke and deepen May's experience of the meaning she continues to make of this pivotal moment.

a. What does that moment of dad's departure say to you today?
b. Why do you think your dad left without saying good-bye?
c. Your life changed forever that day—so sad—nothing could make up for that tremendous loss!

The therapist uses the response that most effectively helps May to put words to the meaning she made in the moment of her dad's departure. In articulating the meaning she made, May recognizes that she continues to feel a similar anguish today. In expressing this, she shifts to an even deeper pain—a sense of feeling abandoned by her mother in that indelible moment of her dad's leaving.

May: His driving away—with no wave—it said that he didn't think I was important—not worth his staying. But worse than that—Mom had no time to see me—she wasn't there for my pain—her pain took up all the space!

EFT Tango Move 3: Encounter With the Therapist

As May reflects more on her pain, she slips back into her automatic pattern of dismissing her own pain and suddenly notices what she is doing.

May: This leaves me questioning—did I do the right thing—cutting him out of my life even when he wanted me to let him back in? Does it really matter anymore how much it hurt way back then? (In spite of momentarily dismissing her present moment experience, May has stabilized and can pause and stop the old pattern and validate her experience.) But hey—(speaking directly to the therapist, looking directly in the therapist's eyes) I know I tend to move away too quickly from my own pain, and it did hurt a lot! It killed me!

Exercise 9.39. Encounter With the Therapist

Which of the following describes what happened in this moment?

a. May spontaneously enacted a new congruent message in an encounter with the therapist.
b. May demonstrated her new ability to step out of her familiar pattern of dismissing her own pain and to validate her core emotion.
c. May's new experience of recognizing the depth of previously blocked emotion is likely heightened as an empowering moment in the safety of the therapeutic relationship.
d. All of the above.

EFT Tango Move 4: Processing the encounter with the therapist of a new, congruently expressed message. Note how the therapist draws attention to May's agency in the face of her pain.

Therapist: How is it inside for you to have caught yourself pushing your pain aside and to have told me that in fact it did hurt a lot when dad left without even turning to wave at you, leaving you totally alone with a devastated mom who had no comfort to offer and a dreadful message in your head that you weren't worth his staying?

May: It feels great! I am tired of pushing my pain away! You get it—it makes total sense that he broke my heart. And my mother did nothing. She wept in the corner, and I was all alone!

EFT Tango Move 5: Reflection and Heightening to Integrate

Therapist: What an important step—to notice that you don't need to ignore your pain any longer! Telling me directly how much you were crushed by this experience is powerful indeed! Finally, you are free to feel the ache of 10-year-old May losing your dad and finding your mom unavailable to comfort you.

Exercise 9.40. Summarizing and Validating

In your own words, how could you further summarize and validate the emerging shift May is creating? How can you integrate and validate that in the safe context of the therapeutic relationship, May is beginning to allow her *frightening, alien, and unacceptable* feelings to matter and to be heard? How can you heighten that she may be starting to trust the core messages and needs in these underlying emotions?

____

____

____

____

____

Exercise to Choose which Encounter to Shape Next

The therapist, attuning to May's experience, is attempting to get a felt sense of where the emotion is most alive—to whom May needs most of all to express her newly accessed and validated emotional experience. If you were the therapist, which possible encounter would you shape? Circle the number and describe why you selected this encounter.

1. For May to express to an image of her father how much she still hurts when she remembers that day that changed her life.
2. For May to speak from her adult self to the 10-year-old self whose world was shattered when she lost her father and her mother was too devastated to comfort her.
3. For May to speak with an image of her mother who failed to give her the comfort she needed.

Write down your reason for choosing which encounter you would shape next.

____

____

____

There is no right or wrong answer here. Your decision simply needs to fit with your sense of where the emotion is most alive or is most in need of expression and then to continue to follow the moves of the EFT Tango to shape, process, and integrate that encounter. In their work together, the therapist will do each of those encounters with May. What follows are encounters, chosen as the therapist follows May's emotion: first, an encounter with an image of her mother, then an encounter between her adult self and her 10-year-old self, and finally, an opportunity for you to shape an encounter with an image of her father.

Shaping an Encounter With an Imagined Attachment Figure

In EFIT, the therapist follows the emotional charge. To the therapist, it appears that the most accessible and intense emotion for May in the present moment is her resentment to her mother for being unavailable for comfort during that moment of traumatic loss. To this day, May acknowledges that she continually blames her mother for not offering her enough support. The therapist decides to follow the emotion and to choreograph an encounter with an image of May's mother.

Exercise 9.41. Tango Move 2—Assembling Emotional Experience Toward an Attachment Figure

Consider how you would assemble May's emotional experience toward her mother, beginning with her deepening awareness that underneath her typical present-day criticism of her mother is a deep injury, which occurred when her dad left and her mom failed to see her pain. May to this day appears to minimize this injury and her related struggles. How might you use the following emotional handles, images, and attachment themes to help May begin to assemble her experience toward her mother?

May's emotional experience: "I feel invisible; I look past my pain; I don't matter; I am a crater of nothingness; I cry frantically; I feel stone cold."

Write a summary statement that you would reflect back to May regarding her core feelings towards her mother.

____

____

____

____

Anticipating and Directing the Encounter in Move 3

To help May anticipate contact with her mother in the scene at 10 years old, and to heighten May's core pain, the therapist could repeat the cue, using the RISSSC manner to heighten core emotion. That is, using **r**epetition, **i**mages, a **s**oft tone, **s**low pace, **s**imple (and specific) language and the **c**lient's words: All alone at 10 years old, heartbroken your dad was leaving and terrified you would never see him again, and mother in the corner weeping, seeming not to even see you—was like falling into a crater of nothingness a crater than echoed, "You don't really matter here!"

The therapist then asks May what she'd like to tell her mother in that scene and invites her to express how difficult it was, what she blames her mother for, and to express her sadness and her fear.

Therapist: What did you say to yourself that day? What did you decide about who you are in your mother's eyes?

May: She was so cold. Like having a mother who looked right past you while your heart bleeds all over the floor. I would want her to know that to this day, I think she doesn't care when I am hurting or afraid. I just don't understand why she didn't care more about her own daughter! (In saying this, she flips into anger and weeps bitterly.)

Exercise 9.42. Directing the Encounter in Move 3

Select the response below that most clearly directs May to disclose this to an image of her mother, from her 10-year-old, angry, heartbroken self.

a. "Can you give your 10-year-old self a chance to share this anger and these tears with an image of your mother? Can you tell her, 'You looked right past me while my heart bled all over the floor—like you really didn't see or care about me!'?"
b. "Your mother needs to know about this. Do you think she realizes that when you get angry with her today, you are still hurting from your 10-year-old experience?"
c. "You had no other meaning to make that day—mother weeping for her own loss while you as a child were left alone with your own anguish—that was unacceptable—and you had no option but to conclude you were invisible to her—that she didn't care."

EFT Tango Move 4—Processing an Encounter With an Imagined Attachment Figure

Following May's expression to an image of her mother, the therapist processes the encounter.

First the therapist explores the encounter *from May's perspective*. She checks with May, "As 10-year-old May, how was it to tell this imagined mother how she abandoned you when you desperately needed her?"

Next, the therapist processes the encounter from the perspective of May's imagined mother, who has just heard May's disclosure of pain—her anger, her grief, and the terrifying meaning she made—that her mother didn't find her worthy of caring for. The therapist now wants to engage May in putting words to the response she imagines her mother would make in this moment.

Exercise 9.43. Move 4—Processing an Encounter (Imagined Attachment Figure)

Which of the following responses would help May *deepen her experience of how she imagines her mother's response* in this moment of encounter? All of the options may be helpful, but only one evokes May's imagination of how her mother will respond. Choose one.

a. "It must have taken a lot of courage to tell your mother how much she let you down that day—and how you still resent her for that big mistake!"
b. "What do you imagine this image of mother would say to 10-year-old May telling her how heartbroken and abandoned she felt, not just by dad but by her mother as well?"
c. "Your mother is likely to be very touched by your words. I'm sure she will feel deep regret and be very appreciative you have finally told her this! How does it feel to take in this new story of a mother who has always loved you?"

An EFT therapist must be prepared for a client to experience a less than positive imagined response while processing the encounter in Tango Move 4. Here the therapist must be ready to work with an imagined figure who is nonresponsive or disappointing. If May imagines her mother's response to be defensive or disappointing, the therapist will help her to stay engaged and *to respond again* as in EFT Tango Move 3 to her image of her mother with an additional engaged message. Remembering that pain is a complex emotion of anger, sadness, and fear of loss, the therapist attunes, reflects, and heightens each aspect as they arise for May and encourages her to express them clearly to this image of her mother.

Anger and fear. Next are two responses a therapist could make to heighten and engage May in her present moment experience, first of anger and then of fear, and to shape further congruent encounters with an image of her mother. The second example uses proxy voice to shape the encounter. Either format works to anticipate contact and focus on the distilled core emotion.

- "You are still angry—yes! Very angry that she ignored your panic and pain. Tell her, please, about how you still blame her for this!" (matching the tone of May's indignation)
- "It must be frightening to be angry with her. Can you tell her, please, 'I am too afraid you will stop loving me if I blame you for ignoring me when dad left?'"

Sadness and loss. When a person risks expressing core emotion to an attachment figure, grief that this was not previously attended to frequently emerges. How might you validate and heighten May's grief and encourage her to share it with an image of mom?

Exercise 9.44. Move 3—Shaping Additional Encounters With an Attachment Figure

Write down how you might validate and heighten May's grief and encourage her to share it with an image of her mom.

When May expresses readiness to hear from her image of mother again, the therapist invites another imagined response and checks with May how it is to receive the reply from her *imagined mother* and gives May an opportunity to respond. This follows with the therapist *prompting a reach* to an imagined attachment figure. While May is emotionally engaged in the experience of her 10-year-old self, the therapist invites her to explore what she needs from this image of her mom and prompts her to make a request to her mother—to ask for what she needs. Core emotion tells us what we need.

Exercise 9.45. Prompting a Reach to an Imagined Attachment Figure

Before prompting a reach, the therapist helps May to access the need embedded in her emotion. Select the response that best captures May's underlying attachment fear and anguish and invites her to listen to what the emotion tells her she needs. Only one of the responses below heightens May's fear and focuses her on listening to the need embedded in her core fear.

a. "You feel that aching in your heart just now—that mom seemed not to notice you in pain. Tell her about the broken, aching place—and ask her if she felt that brokenness too when he left."
b. "So afraid—so afraid that if she sees your heartbreak, she may just shrug you off—it feels so risky to ask. What does that frightened place need from her just now?"
c. "So heartbroken. Can you ask her to tell you what if was like for her when your dad left? Was she afraid she couldn't be a good parent?"

Exercise 9.46. Your Conjecture about May's Need Embedded in her Fear

As you attune to May's experience, what do you imagine her request may be?

After eliciting this attachment-related affect, the therapist turns to evoking the client's needs embedded in core fear. As in the blamer softening change event of EFCT, it can be useful to heighten the vulnerability a client is experiencing and from that vulnerable emotion to prompt the client to discover what they need. When the imagined other doesn't respond positively, it further refines the client's emotional reality. In the case of May, as she risked attending to her core emotion, listened to what she needed from her image of her mother, and then expressed that need to her imagined mother, she received a felt sense of mattering while at the same time sensing her mother's real-life limitations in responding.

Some clients experience imagined others to be dismissive, in denial, or simply non-responsive. In such cases, they may liberate themselves from pursuing love and validation from a non-responsive other through the process of fully experiencing and integrating the impact of imagined non-responsivity or hurtfulness. A different client, Casey, processed painful judgement and physical abuse at the hands of her father, who is currently alive and experiencing early-onset dementia. Deepened emotion, expressed in encounters with an image of her father, helped her to face fears, core loss, and grief and to find an assertive voice to express how very deeply he had injured her and how wrong his actions were. The liberation she experienced through this process of fully processing her emotions and finding a voice to express them to an image of the one who had injured her was felt as a loosening of muscles through her entire body. In this process, she clarified views of self and other—distinguishing that while *some* others, like her father, are unsafe or unreliable and she has no desire to hear a response from them, she also discovered in the context of the safe therapeutic relationship that some others are indeed safe and reliable. Depression gradually lifted, and she found long-lost energy and motivation.

Many EFT interventions are useful in shaping and processing Stage 2 corrective emotional experiences. These often include validation, reflection, and repetition for staying with and heightening emotional experience. Conjectures are also used—always within the attachment frame, with tentativeness and readiness to be corrected. What is important is to follow the client's emotion as closely, respectfully, and empathically as possible, trusting that following the process of emotion will lead toward transformation.

In EFT Tango Move 5, the therapist works to consolidate and integrate the corrective emotional experience. The EFT therapist validates and integrates the shifts that occur as clients disclose distilled, emotionally alive core message to *imagined others, between parts of self, and with the therapist.* Empathic attunement for clients' present moment experience is what matters most of all. It is what guides the therapist in heightening, summarizing, and celebrating whatever shifts and coherence the client creates through the corrective emotional experience. Key features of consolidating and integrating in EFT Tango Move 5 are to provide an explicit, alive summary that heightens the work the client has just done, validating and celebrating the shift they have created.

Exercise 9.47. Integrating and Validating in EFT Tango Move 5

In Tango Move 5, the EFT therapist helped May to take in and process the shifts she created, particularly in this example of addressing and hearing from her *imagined mother.* Only one of the following examples of EFT Tango Move 5 does NOT serve to integrate and validate May's corrective emotional experience. Select the response below that **fails to integrate and validate** May's corrective emotional experience and identify what it is lacking.

a. "Do you understand it better now? Your mother had her own grief to deal with. It is not that you were not deserving. It was all she could give you then. If you see the incident from her perspective, you can still know that you are worthy and loveable."

b. "You heard your imagined mother say to you that it is okay for you to be angry at her—that she totally gets it. She acknowledged that in fact, she did miss noticing you! She expressed that she is so sorry she didn't see your pain. You faced your fear and risked sharing your tears of anger and fear with your imagined mother, and it shifted your sense of the relationship between you! Asking her to assure you she cares for you pulled for the most compassionate tears you've ever felt from your mother, opening you to feel stronger and more lovable and worthy!"

c. "You just created an amazing shift inside! You risked reaching to an image of your mother, and she responded. Some of her responses were hurtful, but you persisted. You told her your 10-year-old self needed her to mother you, and in the end, you felt a very calming, soothing sense that she heard you and reached back to you with love and remorse. This shift leaves you feeling stronger—able to tolerate the reality—even if she doesn't express this to you in real life."

d. "You gathered so much courage to tell this image of your mother that you feared there was no room in her heart to hear you pain and anger and initially she responded like you feared—she shrugged and said she has no more to give! But you risked again and said, 'That's not ok, mom; you're the mom, and I need you to see my pain!' And she heard you and she admitted, 'It's true, I let you down big time. I am so sorry! You deserved so much more!' She heard you and responded to you. And you feel worthy and certain of her love."

Following this encounter with an image of her mother, May is getting a sense for the first time that her mother may actually understand how much she did let her down and failed to support her when she most of all needed her. She senses that her mother actually cares about her pain, and she is flooded with another wave of grief and compassion for her shaky little 10-year-old self who continues to feel so unworthy. The therapist hears the emotional charge here to be the feelings of compassion towards her younger self and seizes the opportunity to heighten and consolidate that emerging compassion by shaping an encounter between parts of self.

Exercise 9.48. Shaping an Encounter Between Parts of Self—Adult May and 10-Year-Old May

Choose which of the following statements or questions would be most effective to choreograph an encounter between May's adult self and her 10-year-old devastated self? *Hint: They are all EFT-appropriate responses, but only one specifically serves to shape an emotionally engaged encounter (EFT Tango Move 3).*

a. "You were left totally alone with no one to care for you! No one to notice your devastation and sheer abandonment that dad drove off without even waving good-bye! What a heart-wrenching scene!"

b. "Can you picture you 10-year-old self? What does she look like? Where is she is standing? What expression do you see on her face? Can you feel what it is like to look from your adult self to this young, devastated girl?"

c. "I can understand that if your father drove away without even saying good-bye, you must have been heartbroken. And you so much needed at least to have your mother notice your heartbreak and to offer you comfort. You must still need her to understand today how she let you down!"

d. "Can you tell the 10-year-old part of yourself that you see her pain?"

In response, May replies, "I can see her—standing at the window—in jeans and her favorite yellow sweater—she's frozen stiff. No tears. Just cold." The therapist then invites May to find a message to express to her younger self, saying: "What do you want to say to her from your tender heart today?"

After May expresses compassion, validation, grief, and love to her 10-year-old self, the therapist validates, heightens, and reflects her message and invites May to share how it felt to finally tell 10-year-old May how sorry she is that she had to live through this (Tango Move 4). May responds, "I am so happy to tell her this—it feels amazing to be able to reach her and let her know she absolutely deserved all that care and comfort from mom and dad that she so desperately wanted—but I am so sad, too, that she never got it when she needed it!"

Exercise 9.49. Processing With the Receiving Other in Tango Move 4

(The second part of Tango Move 4) The therapist invites May to speak *from* the 10-year-old self and share what it was like to hear this validation, compassion, and love from her adult self today. How do you imagine 10-year-old May may respond?

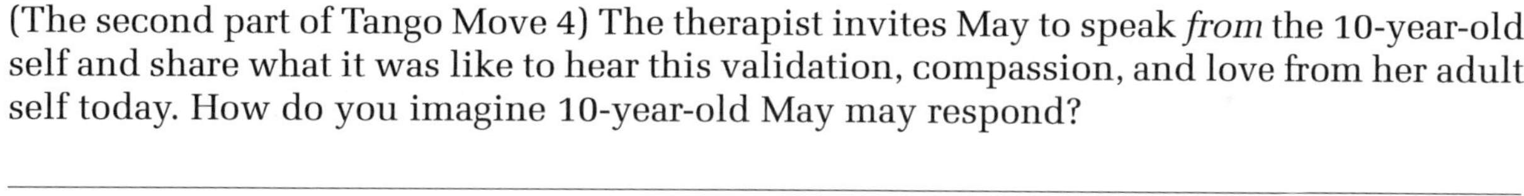

Following several exchanges back and forth between 10-year-old May and adult May, the therapist integrates and celebrates the corrective emotional experiences that she helped May to shape (Tango Move 5).

Exercise 9.50. Integrating and Summarizing—EFT Tango Move 5

Choose one of the following therapist responses that best summarizes and integrates what May has just done.

a. The therapist tells May to continue speaking to this devastated part of herself with this same love and compassion whenever she gets depressed, explaining that this self-compassion is a strong protection against depression.
b. The therapist praises May for her self-compassion and asks her where she found the insight within herself to let the 10-year-old self know that she cares for her.
c. The therapist validates how May engaged with her experience in a new way. The therapist also heightens how May's validation of her sadness and anger toward her dad opened her to discover some longings to consider reconnecting with him—not out of guilt but out of curiosity to know this man she lost.
d. The therapist explains how being able to confront her unexpressed emotions to herself will help her find greater assertiveness for her own needs in future relationships.

An encounter with an absent attachment figure

When the greatest emotional charge or block for May appears to be related to the abandonment, unresolved grief, and longings for a relationship with her father, the therapist will shape an encounter focused on this absent attachment figure. You may wish to experiment by writing or speaking aloud how you would follow the EFT Tango Moves described earlier to choreograph an encounter for May to speak to an image of her father—to share the pain she continues to live with, remembering the day he drove away and changed her life forever; how she is only now beginning to realize she longs to share the pain—her sadness, anger, and fear that perhaps she just wasn't worthy in his eyes; she may also want to examine some emerging curiosity about who he is.

To choreograph an encounter similar to that with an image of May's mother, you could use the guide provided next to shape a corrective emotional experience in an engaged encounter between May and her imagined father. You are invited to experiment with this in your own writing or with a partner—one of you as the choreographer and the other in the role of "May". No "correct" answers are provided in the answer key. This is for your experimentation. Enjoy the exploration as you help it to evolve!

Guidelines for Your Exploration of May's Encounter With an Image of Her Father

EFT Tango Move 1—Reflect the present process between May and an image of her dad. Reflect longings or curiosity to know her father that may be starting to emerge as she maintains her pattern of keeping him out of her life and also faces unresolved hurt—anger, sadness, and fear—around his abrupt departure from her life. (The more she keeps him out, the more she is curious about....)

EFT Tango Move 2—Assemble her complexity of emotions—emptiness, a vacuum, no father to lean on, meanings she makes, such as, "What's wrong with me that you could shut me out of your life?," anger, bodily response of numbness, action tendencies to cut him out of her life and to get distracted from her own core emotions by feeling guilt and pity for him. Write a summary reflection that puts her elements of emotion—trigger/perception, bodily arousal, meaning making, and action impulse into a coherent whole, including the underlying core attachment fear. Distill and deepen it into a clear message to share with an image of her father.

EFT Tango Move 3—Choreograph an encounter with an imagined other (her father).

a. Anticipate contact with an image of her dad. How will you help her to picture him? How will you help May to bring an imagined sense of his presence alive?
b. Shape and repeat the key message you want her to share with him. What specific message will you ask her to share with him?
c. Direct her to share it with him, keeping her focused if she exits. How will you direct her to share the message?

EFT Tango Move 4—Processing the encounter. First evoke from May's perspective what it was like to share this with an image of her father. Second, evoke from May what she imagines the father's response would be when asked what it was like to hear his daughter say this to him.

Repeat EFT Tango Move 3—Choreograph May's imagined response from this image of her father. Invite her to imagine how he will respond. You can invite her to speak his response out loud, taking the imagined voice of "Dad" or "Colin" (his name).

You may also choose to repeat Tango Move 4—Processing these encounters—Eliciting what it was like as May's father to tell May what was happening for him that he was able to step out of her life as he did and asking May what it was like hearing from this image of her father. (This is not as an excuse but to help this image of her father to be impacted by his abandonment of his daughter.)

EFT Tango Move 5—Finally, summarize and integrate the key elements of the encounter. Savor the corrective emotional experience you will have helped May to create. Heighten the newly congruent form of contact with this image of her father. Explore Tango Move 5 to heighten, summarize, validate, and integrate this new interpersonal engagement and expression.

If you did this exploration with a partner, take time as well to give each other feedback on the experience. For example, as May you might share about the moments you felt most deeply understood by your partner and the moments some new emotional experience emerged. As the choreographer, you may share about moments you felt most closely attuned to "May" and moments you found most challenging to be taking the lead through this process. A more extended case in video format, similar to the case of May, can be found as an EFIT training video at https://steppingintoeft.com/

Consolidation in Stage 3

The essential elements of Stage 3 consolidation are to consolidate and integrate the changes the client has made through the process of therapy. In Stage 3, the therapist helps clients to form a coherent narrative of how they moved from distress, depression, and anxiety to their new sense of security and agency.

May has moved from depression, exhaustion, and isolation to resuming her engagement in swimming meets, reaching out to her boyfriend Tim, re-establishing a positive relationship with her mother, and returning to university to complete her education degree and her goal of teaching children on the autistic spectrum. She has shifted her automatic pattern of dismissing her own emotions or longings for connection to recognizing them and using her emotions to direct her actions. When she feels anxious about a term paper or upcoming exam, she reaches out to her professors and fellow students to discuss her concerns. When she needs some comfort or reassurance, she reaches out to Tim and at times also connects with her mother. Depression has been replaced by the secure bond she feels with Tim, with several girlfriends, and the growing connections she and Tim share with several other couples and their children. She recognizes her dad's limitations and no longer feels personally guilty or ashamed for who he is. She knows she is valued by her parents and that she did deserve more love and care than they were able to give her as a child. She is proud of herself for being in a safe relationship with both of them, in spite of their limitations and her father's remaining distance.

The therapist's role in Stage 3 is primarily to shine a light on the client's newfound capacity to pay attention to his or her own emotion as a reliable guide to their needs, wants, and actions. The therapist will evoke the client's reflections on how the new working models of self and other that the client has discovered through therapy are extending and integrating across everyday life. The therapist will validate and heighten the client's new sense of competence and value.

To evoke May's reflections on the discoveries and changes she has made through therapy, the therapist reflects an apparent shift and uses that example to evoke more observations from May about her experience of change. "Before, most others were 'menacing figures' who you shied away from out of fear of their judgement. Today as you describe your meeting with your practicum advisor, I am hearing you describe a very different way of handling yourself. It sounds like you really felt you had a right to be there—that you had a voice—and felt confident you had something to offer! Is that right?" After hearing confirmation from May and heightening this shift, the therapist asks, "Can you tell me more about how you experience yourself and others differently now?" One of May's touching images is having moved from the garbage dump, to standing on a pedestal as a "golden child, worthy of love"—echoes of the new self-worth and confidence, gained from the resolution of her of the abuse she survived and the relationship bonds she is forming with Tim, her mother, and somewhat with her father.

Exercise 9.51. Interventions to Evoke Stage 3 Reflections

See what evocative questions you can create to evoke more reflections from May on the new sense of agency and competence that has evolved for her through her therapeutic journey. You may wish to prompt her to focus on new solutions she may be discovering, new ways she deals with difficult emotions, and metaphors or rituals that mark the changes she is experiencing. You may also evoke her picture of the future as she continues on this path.

____

____

____

____

____

Exercise 9.52. Validating and Integrating Change

In Stage 3, the therapist summarizes May's therapeutic narrative to validate and integrate the changes she has made. This is much like EFT Tango Move 5—integrating and validating the entire therapeutic journey. Please identify the following elements in the transcript by placing the corresponding letters after each excerpt that best illustrates a change. Some are illustrated more than once.

a. Changes in client's patterns of emotion regulation.
b. Changes in client's meaning frames.
c. Changes in how client engages in relationship.
d. Changes in view of self.
e. Changes in view of other.
f. Potential view of therapist as an attachment figure.

1. "I am so touched by the journey you have taken! You've come from a place where you barely had words for your experience other than the heavy black cloud that weighed down on you and you had no ways of getting out from under it. You tried more and more to deal with the darkness on your own by isolating more and more. And then you began to listen to weight in your heart and to the

hidden longings to feel safe and loved. You've followed your newly discovered longings to reach out more to others. And you've discovered you are valued and wanted. You've reached out consistently to Tim and to friends." ___

2. "After coming to a resolution of that painful relationship with Brody, you came in touch with a new sense of your own worth" ___
3. "You have also discovered people in your life with whom you could begin risking and trusting." ___
4. "You've started speaking much more assertively and clearly to your friends and family. You shaped a new relationship with your mom and stepdad—grieving some losses of how they are not all you want them to be—but you found some ways to make that relationship a two-way supportive one where you feel safe and respected." ___
5. "Sadly, you discovered your father is not open to staying in connection with you. That was very heartbreaking, yet you've grieved that loss, found ways to validate your experience and know you are making the best choices of where to seek reliable and available support in your life today." ___ and ___
6. "I feel so proud of the crowd of people you have gathered to stand in the background as your cheerleaders now. Even as we are terminating our therapy—I want you to know that I admire your work and believe in your capacity to keep expanding on all these changes you're making. I am cheering for you, too!" ___

SUMMARY

The chapter takes you through the EFT process of change with individuals who are facing anxiety, depression, traumatic reactions, relationship distress and unchangeable circumstances of life. This general process of change begins with stabilizing strategies of engagement with emotions, with self, and with others. It then moves toward restructuring these strategies by engaging more fully with emotional experience in order to reprocess emotional experience, which thereby creates new meanings and new ways for engaging in life. The EFT Tango is a map for therapists to mirror and reflect present moment experience, to then assemble and deepen difficult emotion, toward shaping corrective emotional experiences.

You had opportunities through this chapter to experience that as *relational beings*, the corrective emotional experiences that we shape are necessarily *interpersonal* events. The interpersonal encounters are between client and therapist, between client and an attachment figure, from client to a hurtful or unresponsive other, or between parts of self within the client. The change events that we shape in EFIT are interpersonal encounters that change individuals' key inner and interpersonal dramas.

The client case examples as well as the personal reflection exercises (www.routledge.com/9780367483425), available online, highlight two key factors about EFIT: First, the primary goal is not to "fix a problem" but to create a genuine encounter—a caring, accepting presence—willing to walk in and through the dark and painful places with another. This makes it possible for the one experiencing distress to process the experience more fully rather than blocking it by panicking or numbing it out. Fully processing experience within a genuine encounter is in itself a transformative process. Second, by focusing on the process *within* the content of one's distress, EFIT helps individuals to discover in an alive, explicit, immediate way how it is their manner of regulating emotion that shapes their suffering and that lasting change is created by discovering and fully engaging previously disowned core emotion in a safe interpersonal context.

The change process of EFIT is relevant at a personal level for therapists and clients alike, when facing personal struggles, and when facing massive existential issues like the 2020–2021 pandemic. The sense of perceived danger and uncontrollability that characterizes emotional disorders (Barlow et al., 2010) is also a realistic response during the pandemic, when urgent needs for support from others were more apparent than ever! As Bowlby's attachment theory reminds us, emotional disorders occur when a healthy response becomes a rigid, automatic response regardless of the context or its having become outdated and unneeded. EFIT provides an effective model to validate present moment coping, to explore the underlying disowned emotions driving internal and interpersonal patterns, and to move fully into those emotions to restructure more secure strategies for regulating emotion. The change made possible through EFIT is not oriented toward changing external issues that are beyond one's control. Change in EFIT is about shaping secure attachment strategies for engaging with others and with one's inner emotional experience.

Stage 1 of EFIT offers a level 1 healing process of change—a discovery that problems and agency for change are rooted in the repetitive patterns of how one makes sense of and reacts to difficult emotions. In the collaborative discovery process of Stage 1, individuals own the patterns of how they shape their world and discover the core attachment emotions driving these patterns. In Stage 2, they explore and engage new options for reshaping their world. The process of safely and fully engaging with core pain, fears, and attachment vulnerabilities pulls individuals into new ways of shaping their world. Level 2 change comes through connection with another while fully reprocessing emotion. Internal working models of self and other can shift through EFIT even when a relevant other is non-responsive or in denial of injuries they have caused. Individuals can restore broken bonds and experience others who are no longer available to them in real life, as powerful resources. In Stage 3 of EFIT, the shifts in models of self and other are summarized, validated, and celebrated, along with the new meanings and behaviors that emerge from the newly reprocessed emotional experience. As you face your life challenges, you are invited to reflect on the EFIT discoveries you have made working through this chapter. Consolidating and celebrating these learnings may be the most effective way to consolidate the pathways towards *emotional fitness* made possible through EFIT—a path toward accessing and trusting emotion as a guide.

Cases in this chapter are composite cases of numerous clients blended together. Videos similar to material given for May, particularly in Stage 2 can be seen in a 14 hour therapy series with one client working with Lorrie L. Brubacher from beginning to end of therapy, available at https://steppingintoeft.com/. Several other EFIT sessions with clients processing trauma, grief, depression, and addictive patterns are also available at that website.

ANSWERS AND SUGGESTED RESPONSES

Exercise 9.1. Move 1—Mirror the Present Process

Answer: **C.** is a present moment reflection of the behavioral aspect of *how* he copes. The therapist hones in on his fragmented story and how "hyper" he seems in the moment. A. although offering some empathy and validation, is focused on insight and explanation, and B. is didactic teaching a behavioral skill and giving reassurance.

Exercise 9.2. Move 2—Affect Assembly and Deepening

Answer: **B**. This focuses first on the trigger (losing in court) and his action tendency of pushing, speeding up behavior, and then links that trigger and action tendency to his perceived danger of losing (the meaning he makes) and a felt sense of emptiness and dizziness. A. is empathic but focused on searching for insights. C. provides an explanation and a cognitive reframe (e.g., looking at himself in a more positive light).

Exercise 9.3. Move 3—Shaping an Encounter Possible Responses:

1. In an encounter with the therapist, Stephen is likely to discover more explicitly, his pattern of automatically dismissing others' positive feedback—how positive feedback invariably triggers embarrassment or shame.
2. In his encounter between two parts of self, he is likely to discover more of his longing for comfort and more of the rigid pressure and harshness he feels. He may also discover how afraid he is to stop pushing himself—finding compassion for his tired self or a deeper awareness of his exhaustion and longings.
3. In his encounter with an image of his mother, when he actually takes the risk to express the anger he has been avoiding to an actual image of his mom, Stephen discovers that underlying his anger is deep sadness and longing to be seen as good enough in her eyes.

Exercise 9.4. Move 4—Processing an Encounter

Answer: B. This begins with an evocative question his present moment experience, combined with reflecting what he did. This invites him to reflect on the impact of discovering his unexpressed pain and longings, while expressing his resentment to an image of his mother. A. is didactic and moves away from his present moment experience. C. provides an historical explanation that does not bring his present experience more alive.

Exercise 9.5. Move 5—Integrating and Validating

Answer: A. This does the most to explicitly validate and integrate the core themes of Stephen's in-session courage and expression of newly emerging emotion. b. and c. both lack focus on integrating emerging core themes. d. is primarily didactic.

Exercise 9.6. Formulating a Reflective Summary

Key words to have included in your reflections may include

1. Sense of self: I'm a loser—not chosen—not enough—must push and stay hyped, or I'll be nothing.
2. Ways of dealing with emotion: He touches on difficult emotion then shifts—pressures himself to avoid inner feelings; works hard to perform but no performance is enough; rest is only temporary. The image of being caught on a *treadmill* is useful.

3. Ways of connecting with attachment figure: He demands or becomes angry and pushes his wife away—doubts her choice of him so pressures himself and her.
4. Core, underlying emotions: Exhaustion/tired—empty /helpless—freaked out/ afraid of rejection.

Exercise 9.7. Attuning and Exploring in Beginning Sessions

Key elements to attune to in early sessions:

1. Client's manner of engaging with the therapist and with others:
   - Talks rapidly and nonchalantly.
   - Others never gave me room to feel.
   - Sarcastic sneer.
   - We were strong—nothing would get us down.
   - Nervous chuckles, clutching belly.
   - Dismiss—help me move on.
   - Silly to dwell on being terrified.
2. Patterns (repetitive internal/interpersonal cycles) of affect regulation:
   - Dad dismissed her fears and pain like she does now.
   - No room for silliness/fear of job hunting—gather courage be strong like dad taught me to be.
3. How client deals with vulnerabilities (getting overwhelmed, minimizing):
   - Clutching her belly.
   - I feel nothing.
   - Chuckles.
   - Mostly numb.
   - Act strong.
4. Signs of dominant models of self (Am I lovable and competent?) and of others (Are they reliable, trustworthy, and responsive?):
   - I'm none of what mom was: confident, assured, beautiful, successful.
   - I'm alone, depressed, unmotivated.
   - There was never room to feel; others never gave me room to feel.
   - Had to be responsible ever since mom died.
   - We are strong—nothing gets us down.
   - Must have been shattered to lose my mom—but who knows?
5. Achievements, moments of competence or personal worth:
   - Did well in MBA.
   - Was a great older sister to her younger sisters.

Exercise 9.8. Identifying the Repetitive Cycle

Suggested Response: Her emotions were minimized by her dad when her mom died, and she minimizes and dismisses her own emotions. She dismisses the therapist before pausing to let the therapist respond. She was dismissed by others, and she dismisses self and others. She is avoidant of self/her own emotional experience and moves on quickly to keep others such as therapist from coming too close.

Exercise 9.9. Finding Emotional Handles

Suggested Response: Bodily response of clutching her belly as she speaks of deep loss. Feel nothing. I'm alone. Be responsible. Be strong. Must have been shattered to lose my mom. Who knows? Move on. Used to be proud. No room for silliness.

Exercise 9.10. Identify Emotional Handles and Signs of Bodily Arousal

Emotional handles: Depressed; down; no energy; I do worry; maybe he is getting ready to move on; sleeping a lot, watching TV and eating bad stuff; I'm fine really.
Signs of bodily arousal: giggles, winces, flips hand in air, shrugs, tears.

Exercise 9.11. Empathic Reflection of Present Process

1. <u>Present triggers:</u> boyfriend is so busy, seems ready to move on; loss of job.
2. <u>Action tendencies:</u> brings you to tears and you brush it off; minimize the fear, say, "I'm fine"; act nonchalant.
3. <u>Emotional response:</u> tired, depressed, barely any energy for anything, and very worried.

Exercise 9.12. Validate by Linking Trigger and Action Impulse

I hear the struggle—fearing your job could be on the line—Tim saying he is busy with his job—mom being harsh—these are difficult things (triggers)—of course they hurt so much (emotional distress) that you find yourself (1) sinking into oblivion—(2) numbing the pain and fear with sleep, TV, and junk food. (3) Shrugging off the pain and (4) not reaching out to anyone (four action impulses).

Exercise 9.13. Finding Interventions

It's hard to know how to believe you can move forward in your life? <u>3. Reflection and a slight reframe that orients towards a goal/longing</u>.

Everything seems pointless; some part of you says nothing is going to work? <u>2. Validating experience</u>.

When you get really down—who can you turn to for support? <u>1. Evocative question with an attachment image</u>.

Exercise 9.14. Empathic Reflection

Answer: lonely (empathic reflection, slightly on the leading edge of the words the client used).

Exercise 9.15. The Pattern that Protects and Imprisons

It feels safer to stay alone—than to risk reaching to anyone for support. You feel like the odd one—never able to get it right—unable to make friends—so you keep everyone at a distance—all alone—and lonely! The more you keep others at a distance, the more lonely and depressed you feel—and the more lonely and depressed you feel—the less safe and approachable others seem—and the more you keep them at a distance.

Exercise 9.16. Review of Basic EFIT Elements in a Beginning Session

1. Pattern of affect regulation: May deals with her vulnerable emotions—fears, unmet needs, and longings—by distancing, avoiding, minimizing, and numbing with distractions.
2. How her affect regulation protects and also shapes a prison: The more she dismisses her own emotions and withdraws to protect herself, the more unavailable and dangerous others seem and the more inaccessible and frightening her own emotions are.
3. Within/between pattern: Avoids own emotions/avoids reaching to others; distants from inner experience/isolates from others who will hurt her and let her down
4. Model of others: Angry, hurtful, unavailable, uncaring, unreliable.
5. Model of self: Odd one, nutcase, never get it right, never good at making friends

Exercise 9.17. Themes of Emotional Disorders

Perceived Danger—Can't trust others; have no control boss is complaining.

Depression—Lonely, unlovable, unwanted, helpless, fearing, loss, sense of failure, self-criticism.

Anxiety—Lacking clarity, intense negative emotion, vigilance, avoidance, emotion feared cues negative attributions.

Overall numbing, sense of danger, helplessness, restricted sense of choice and agency

Exercise 9.18. Surface, Reactive Emotion

Hopeless/dismissive/sad when the therapist says she sounds lonely; tears when she speaks about Tim being busy.

Exercise 9.19. Identify Trigger, Bodily Arousal, Meaning Made

1. When there is no one to go to—mom gets angry; Tim is busy; boss complains.
2. Tears or numbness, or distracting chuckles.
3. Mom doesn't care; she will hurt me; Tim doesn't care; he is moving on.

Exercise 9.20: Using Reflection, Evocative Questions, or Conjectures for Elements of Emotion

1. Validate and normalize triggers and her explicit responses:

   Trigger: Mom gets angry: I understand—when your mom gets angry with you, you find yourself pulling away from her and ignoring even her suggestions of a job you could apply for.

Trigger: Boss complains: It makes sense that when you relive, you give up on yourself—and don't even have the energy to try again.

2. Tentative conjecture about her basic perception (safety/danger):

   It sounds like these are dangerous moments—"Oh, oh!"—everything feels on edge, yes?

3. Evoking her bodily response:

   Where in your body do you feel that uh-oh, dangerous moment?

4. Evoking the meaning she makes of the triggers:

   What does Tim's busyness say to you? What meaning do you make when you and your mom get in a fight? What do your boss' complaints say to you about yourself? What do they say to you about others?

5. Naming her action tendencies:

   To crumble in depression, to give up on others and on herself, and to withdraw.

Exercise 9.21. Assemble Emotion Into a Coherent Whole

Suggested Response. "You recognize how each time you hear your phone ring (CUE), you are immediately flooded with that rush of panic (BODILY AROUSAL) that it will be your mom calling. You notice your body freeze (BODILY AROUSAL) with those dreadful thoughts, "She just doesn't care. She's out to hurt me again! Why can't it be Tim calling like he used to instead of her?" (MEANING CREATION) and you just want to collapse and pull a blanket over you and go to sleep (ACTION TENDENCY). When you get that panicky feeling that your mom is out to hurt you again (HINT of CORE FEAR linked to MEANING CREATION), you just want to disappear, go silent, and talk to no one. There is no one you feel safe to reach to in those moments" (CONJECTURE, SEEDING SECURE ATTACHMENT).

Exercise 9.22. Distill Poignancy

You panic that she is out to hurt you—and freeze with painful thoughts that she doesn't care. What a terrifying moment—that you are in danger and there is no safe other to go to and the safest thing to do is freeze and disappear.

Exercise 9.23. Move 3—Shaping an Encounter With an Imagined Attachment Figure

Repeating May's distilled message: I'd like you to picture this image of your mother and to imagine telling her this important message. Imagine telling her, "It's true, mom, I freeze with painful thoughts that you don't care—and panic that you are out to hurt me—to call me disgusting names. I'm terrified—in danger—and there is no safe other to go to. You are not safe—and the safest thing to do is freeze and disappear. Even though I long for you to care, I pull away from you to be safe."

Directing May to disclose the message to an image of her mother: Can you tell her, please—tell her, "I do pull away even though I long for you—I am so afraid you don't care—that you will hurt me"?

Exercise 9.24. Shaping Other Encounters

1. Shaping an encounter with May's boyfriend, Tim: Can you imagine telling Tim, "I am missing you so much—feeling alone and lost without you. I act like I've already given up on us—I've stopped reaching out to you—so afraid you're tired of me, but secretly I hope you'll reach to me—I'm just too afraid to risk anymore pain, so I numb out and pull away"?
2. Shaping an encounter between "the concerned self" who brings her to therapy and risks opening up and "the hidden self," frozen in fear: Can you tell your hidden self, frozen in fear, "I get how scared you are—that you feel just like the ten year old self standing at the window when dad drove away, and mom was too depressed to notice you—frozen, unable to move—I get the panic—of course you froze then—there was nothing else you could do then. There was no one to hear your cries, but I am here now—I hear how alone and afraid you must feel."
3. Therapist (with a look of tenderness and care): Can you tell me again about being afraid that I will get tired of listening to your darkness?

Exercise 9.25. Process the Experience of the One Disclosing

May might respond: "It was so difficult but quite a relief all at the same time! I could barely get the words out at first—and then it was so amazing that she was actually listening to me without interrupting. It is such a relief to tell her how much I have feared her hurtful words—how they have made me feel so bad! Having her listen to me made me feel stronger—no matter what she says back!

Exercise 9.26. Process the Experience of the One Receiving the Message

Speaking from her image of her mother, May says, "I'm shocked! I never knew she was afraid of me! She has no reason to be! Of course I care about her. She can fight as good as I can, and she fights back—I had no idea she was ever afraid—I just thought she hates me. I actually feel bad to see her so small and weepy. I want her to know I do care! I just don't know how to show it when she's angry or refuses to let me near!

Exercise 9.27. Processing Encounters With Imagined Others

1. Reflection of the key message May shared with her image of her father: You just turned and shared so bravely with this image of your dad that there is a knot in your stomach that still hurts, remembering the day he drove away—that there is still an ache in the core of your being that feels you lost him forever that day.
2. To evoke the impact on her of disclosing: What is happening inside of you as you share this with this image of him?
3. To evoke what she imagines is the impact on/response from her *imagined dad* to her disclosure: How do you sense your dad is responding to hearing you tell him about the knot in your stomach—from when you were 10 years old—that still aches, feeling you lost him the day he drove away?

Exercise 9.28. Processing an Encounter Between Client and Therapist

You might say: When you turn and tell me that you fear I will get tired of your darkness, my heart aches. I see such beauty in who you are as a person, and I am honored to hold the darkness with you. And I am touched that you trust me enough to share it with me. Can you tell me what it is like that I have shared this with you?

Exercise 9.29. Integrating the Impact of the Encounter

To celebrate May's encounter with an image of Tim: Look what you just did! You told an image of Tim that you secretly do long for more connection with him—that in your fear that he may be pulling away from you, you act like you're not interested in him. You sensed that he actually heard you—and you felt stronger simply hearing yourself put those words out loud!

Exercise 9.30. Identifying Markers of Stabilization

David:

- An awareness of his pattern—come to recognize this automatic survival pattern.
- Aware of the underlying pain of isolation and abandonment driving these patterns.
- The terror of isolation driving his swings between frenzy and numbness is becoming acceptable and familiar.
- Coherence made of these patterns and terror.
- *Continuing to do as he has been done to*—dismissing my own needs and longings . . . as though it doesn't matter that I am lonely.
- Beginning to see how—this is the problem: "No one heard me, and I don't listen to me either."

Exercise 9.31. Reviewing the Basic Pattern and Underlying Emotion Driving the Pattern

- **David**—the more he spins between frenzied hyperactivating to get people to respond to him, the more others turn away, the more he numbs out and dismisses all his longings and needs, and the more isolated he becomes.
- **Underlying core emotion driving the pattern**: The pattern of swinging between frenzy and numbness is driven by his fear of isolation and abandonment.

Exercise 9.33. Affect Assembly Towards Deepening—Tango Move 2, Stage 2

a. **Cue/Immediate Perception:** Tim's busyness/danger signal.

b. **Bodily Arousal:** Heavy heart; suffocating; eyes filling with tears.

c. **Meaning Making:** Bitter messages: "You're alone—no one shares your fears and worries—no one really cares—they're only mean and hurtful—out for themselves."

d. **Action impulse:** Ignores the heavy weight in her heart that tells her she needs to reach out; listens to the bitter messages; floods into tears and sadness.
e. **Core, Underlying Emotion:** terror—fears of rejection, invisibility, abandonment, disconnection. May has come to recognize her heavy heart signals her need for connection.

Exercise 9.34. Emerging Shifts in Views of Self and Other

1. **Client's View of Self:** unlovable, unseen, unimportant.
2. **Emerging Shift:** May is beginning to see herself as sad and alone and worthy of receiving soothing connection.
3. **Client's View of Other:** unreliable, unresponsive.
4. **Emerging Shift:** May's view of other is beginning to see that the therapist and Tim and some friends are responsive.
5. **Framing Coherent Whole:** So when this heavy balloon of depression sneaks up on you and you can barely breathe, you recognize there is a beautiful aching heart underneath all the pressure and the noise—that longs to be noticed and cared for—that says, "Listen to me—I am still here—I just need to be seen and comforted—I need to know someone is there for me!" Discovering this longing to be connected to someone who loves you opens you to a flood of tears and sadness. This sadness and fear of being unnoticed is alive with a pull to reach out—yes? You breathe deeply through those tears—so different than the weighty balloon that keeps you from breathing—keeps you from feeling.

Exercise 9.35. Identifying EFT Heightening Interventions in Tango Move 2

1. **Heightening** (with repetitions of imagery). Those old bitter messages expand to fill the room and press the life out of you, that familiar bitterness presses down on you
2. **Evocative responding** (directing to stay with the bodily felt sensations of her emotional experience). "Your eyes are filling with tears as I say this—do you feel that heavy heart just now? Can we stay with the heaviness in your heart? (pause—May nods) Notice how heavy it is (pause)—how tight—(pause). Beneath all the pressure of the noisy balloon—you can feel the weight in your heart—(pause). **Evocative question** to access the message of need in her bodily felt core emotion: "And what does this heavy heart say?"
3. **Evocative responding.** Old messages take over expanding to fill the room and pressing the life out of you (evocative by use of imagery)—when the balloon filled with old familiar bitterness presses down on you? (evocative by use of imagery)—Your eyes are filling with tears as I say this—do you feel that heavy heart just now?
4. **Empathic Conjecture**, which actually "seeds attachment": "It must be very difficult indeed to listen with kindness and patience to the heavy weight in your heart."

5. **Empathic Conjecture** to reframe her tears as a core longing to be seen and cared for to know she is ok: "You breathe deeply through your tears—that is so different from the weighty balloon that keeps you from breathing—keeps you from feeling. Listening to the terror in your heavy heart brings you to tears—it is so very, very sad—to feel this much fear and aloneness and not know how or whom to reach to for safety! That is the message of your heavy heart—isn't it?—"I need someone to see me—to notice me and to care—then I can know I am ok." (May nods, smiles, and sighs again.)

Exercise 9.36. Identifying Interventions

1. Reflection, **2**. Validation, **3**. Heightening, **4**. Evocative Question, **5**. Heightening, **6**. Heightening, **7**. Validation, **8**. Evocative Question, **9**. Heightening, **10**. Empathic Conjecture (proxy voice), **11**. Reflection, **12**. Empathic Conjecture (Proxy Voice)

Exercise 9.37. Reflecting Present Process, Including Action Tendency

Answer: You describe a most painful turning point memory of yourself as a 10-year-old girl seeing dad pack the truck and drive out of your life—pain flashes across your face for a moment—and you quickly brush it off and feel bad—guilty, responsible almost—for you dad's pain that you've never let him back into your life in spite of his attempts.

Exercise 9.38. Evoking the Meaning

Answer: A. Only a invites May to put words to the meaning she made then and continues to feel today about her dad's leaving. **B** turns the focus onto her dad and to speculating about his experience. **C** is an empathic reflection but doesn't evoke the meaning this moment carries for her.

Exercise 9.39. Encounter With the Therapist

Answer: D. All of the above

Exercise 9.40. Summarizing and Validating

Your summary and validation of the shift May is creating could include some of the following: You just stepped out of your typical pattern of dismissing your own experience! It has been almost foreign for you to acknowledge how crushed you were the day dad drove away. As you've trusted this space here with me to-day enough to taste that pain—you are experiencing how very real that pain is—and how real it still is today. You are discovering how, to cope with the ache of dad's departure, you concluded you weren't worth his staying! It's almost a celebration to recognize, "I do still hurt! I hurt for him leaving me, I hurt with feeling it somehow meant that I wasn't worth his staying, and I am beginning to feel angry at my mom for leaving me to grieve that loss alone!"

Exercise for choosing which encounter to shape next—reader's choice to engage; no correct answer

Exercise 9.41. Tango Move 2—Assembling Emotional Experience Towards an Attachment Figure

You feel so hurt and angry with your mom. It was like falling into a crater of nothingness—that when your world was crashing, you seemed invisible to her—felt like you didn't matter. You still feel how stone cold you went that day as you saw your mother crying frantically and seeming to look right past your pain.

Exercise 9.42. Directing the Encounter in Move 3

Only **A.** is a clear, direction to prompt the 10-year-old May to express her alive message to her imagined mother. Both **B.** (focuses on her mother) and **C.** (validates May's experience) distract from the encounter the therapist was building toward—the actual expression from May to her imagined mother.

Exercise 9.43. Move 4—Processing an Encounter (Imagined Attachment Figure)

B. is the only response that invites May to describe how she imagines her mother to be responding to her disclosure. **A.** does not evoke her imagination of how mom will respond. **C.** speaks for the mother, but it may not be May's experience.

Exercise 9.44. Move 3—Shaping Additional Encounters With an Attachment Figure

A response that could validate and heighten her grief and loss and encourage her to share it: You ache deep in your heart that your mom failed to see your deep heartache of grief and sadness! Can you tell her about the well of sadness in your heart that no one saw?

Exercise 9.45. Prompting a Reach to an Imagined Attachment Figure

Only **B.** invites May to listen to the need embedded in her core emotion of fear and pain. **A.** and **C.** are both insight-related questions to ask her mother.

Exercise 9.46. Your Conjecture about May's Need Embedded in her Fear

Possible answer: "I need to know my pain matters to you—to know that I matter to you!"

Exercise 9.47. Integrating and Validating in EFT Tango Move 5.

Answer: A. focuses on insight into her mother and does not heighten, integrate, or summarize May's experience.

Exercise 9.48. Shaping an Encounter between Parts of Self—Adult May and 10-Year-Old May

Answer: B. This is the only response that shapes an encounter from her adult self to her 10-year-old self by explicitly helping her to access her adult self picturing an image of the 10-year-old. While **A.** validates and heightens her abandonment panic when her dad drove away and **C.** validates her devastation at her dad leaving and heightens her need for understanding and response from mom, neither response focuses on her childhood self. **D.** focuses only on the 10-year-old.

Exercise 9.49. Processing With the Receiving Other in Tango Move 4

In response, the 10-year old May may say some of the following: I just want to weep and soak it in—so amazing to feel that that experience was not normal—just never felt that sort of compassion and validation for me—it warms me—I don't feel frozen stiff like I did then—I feel like I'm not alone there any more—my adult self is holding me and keeping me warm and making it ok to crumble and to be angry him for leaving like he did! I feel like I am actually a bit curious to hear from him and have a chance to talk with him . . . and to get to know who he is.

Exercise 9.50. Integrating and Summarizing—EFT Tango Move 5

Answer: **C.** summarizes, integrates, and celebrates the corrective emotional experience May has just created, validating it is opening more options for May. a is a behavioral and didactic response, while b offers praise and insight.

Exercise 9.51. Interventions to Evoke Stage 3 Reflections

You may have suggested some evocative questions and prompts such as the following:

- Tell me more about the ways you are reaching out.
- When fears and anxieties arise, what do they say to you?
- What are the news ways you are responding when you feel unsure?
- Can you describe some of the new patterns of reaching and responding that you are building?
- What are your signals now that you are needing something from another—and how do you reach for that?
- A golden child worthy of love—Wow! That is an exciting image How do you see this golden child is going to shape her future? Who is she going to include in building this life?
- What are some of the ways you want to celebrate this move from out of the garbage dump to golden sunlight of connectedness?

Exercise 9.52. Validating and Integrating Change

1. **A.** Changes in client's patterns of emotion regulation.
2. **D.** Change in view of self.
3. **E.** Change in view of other.
4. **C.** Changes in how client engages in relationship.
5. **A, B.** Changes in client's patterns of emotion regulation and changes in client's meaning frames.
6. **F.** Potential view of therapist as an attachment figure.

10

HEALING THE ECHOES OF TRAUMA THROUGH EFIT

The research and clinical literature are consistent in suggesting that various forms of interpersonal and other trauma (e.g., abuse, neglect, victimization, military exposure, first responder operational stress) have a propensity to impact what is a fundamental aspect of human functioning—the way in which individuals engage with themselves and others, and with their emotional lives. With its foundation in attachment science, emotionally focused therapy (EFT) (Johnson, 2002, 2019) is well suited for working with the echoes of trauma. Attachment theory provides a theoretical base for understanding the impacts of trauma, and EFT offers a clear framework and on-target interventions to deal with the emotional dysregulation that is central to the aftermath of trauma, along with the encumbering model-of-self and -other deficits that perpetuate those impacts, both personally and relationally. Against the backdrop of earlier chapters, this chapter reviews the impact of trauma from an attachment perspective, including key considerations that bear upon clinical assessment, case conceptualization, and treatment planning with individual therapy clients. Case examples and exercises are included to elucidate essential components of EFT practice with individuals who are facing the aftermath of trauma.

TRAUMA'S IMPACT: AN ATTACHMENT PERSPECTIVE

Attachment theory offers us a clear view of health, as well as a map for understanding how trauma, loss, and abuse can impact and thwart healthy development. Bowlby argued that under optimal conditions, when children's bids for contact and support are consistently and effectively responded to by their primary caregivers, these children will tend to form positive *internal working models* of both self (lovable and worthy) and others (trustworthy and available) that soothe distress and promote healthy exploration and development. Such experiences promote the formation of a generally secure attachment pattern, and times of stress and uncertainty provide valuable opportunities to develop affect regulation skills through a variety of means, including trial and error (exploring from their secure base) or learning and adopting effective strategies modeled by adult attachment figures. As the developing secure child's internal coping repertoires become more sophisticated, discomfort tends to become less destabilizing, higher levels of stress can be tolerated, and more challenging and complex interactions can be pursued, with the ultimate outcome being an enhancement of affect regulation skills and capacity, as well as increased confidence and a positive, growing, and coherent model of self. In short, Bowlby depicted healthy working models of self and other as flexible, adaptive protocols that are subject to

DOI: 10.4324/9781003039457-13

ongoing revision and change considering new meaningful emotional and relational experiences. This developmental perspective suggests that health is the ability to constantly adapt and grow, to be open and aware, and to embrace and learn from new experiences. The self then is ever evolving toward more depth, complexity, and coherence.

Conversely, in less optimal conditions, including intrafamilial abuse and/or trauma, children are prone to develop more insecure attachment styles and strategies, characterized along two dimensions, anxiety and avoidance (Simpson & Overall, 2014). When the prototypical response to the central human attachment question "Are you there for me when I need you?" is a resounding no or more often when such responses are inconsistent or unreliable, children will tend to either protectively resort to various avoidance strategies such as dissociation, numbing, detaching, or intensifying their pursuits for closeness through anxious clinging (Johnson, 2002). In either case, a child's affect regulation skills are less likely to develop effectively in the context of a reliance on more protective strategies such as dissociation, distraction, or other forms of avoidance to fend off intolerable distress and to the detriment of successfully navigating through other demands and developmental tasks of childhood such as gaining an education, relating with peers, and developing a coherent identity (Lanktree & Briere, 2017).

In the absence of intervention or any potentially buffering impact of a felt sense of security with others outside the home (e.g., the refuge of a neighbor, coach, teacher) or sense of competence in specific areas (e.g., sports, academics), these children are at significant risk for a host of emotional and interpersonal difficulties. Indeed, at the outset of treatment, individuals with trauma histories often cite a host of diagnoses that have been applied over the years. These range from addictions (e.g., alcohol use disorder) to various mood (e.g., major depressive disorder), trauma- and stressor-related (e.g., post-traumatic stress disorder) and anxiety disorders (e.g., panic disorder), as well as personality (e.g., borderline personality disorder) and dissociative disorders (e.g., dissociative identity disorder). Seen through an attachment lens, these various and often comorbid disorders can be understood as reflecting different manifestations of restricted capacity to regulate emotion during times of stress or threat, as well as different displays of interpersonal mistrust (i.e., model of other) and/or self-capacity (i.e., model of self, e.g., positive or negative, cohesive/integrated or incohesive). As will be described in greater detail in this chapter, the emotionally focused individual therapy (EFIT) therapist attends to such information but looks past diagnosis, more deeply at the individual—the whole person in context—and closely tracks strategies for regulating emotion, as well as the individual's models of self and others.

Exercise 10.1. Trauma Through an Attachment Lens

With a focus on viewing clients' presentations through an attachment lens rather than emphasizing clinical diagnoses or disorders, the EFT therapist pays close attention to three key areas as they relate to their intrapersonal or "within" experience and their interpersonal or "between" functioning. Name these three areas.

1. ____

2. ____

3. ____

Exercise 10.2. Affect Regulation

With respect to affect regulation strategies or patterns, studies show that attachment strategies tend to fall along two dimensions:

1. ______________________________

2. ______________________________

Now reflect on how you have seen these attachment strategies or patterns (e.g., avoidance as characterized by numbing or detachment and/or anxiety as seen in hurried speech or frenetic behaviors) impact your clients' experiences and work in session. Identify a client and their attachment strategy; then consider how it impacts the in-session process. Briefly delineate this client's strategy and how it shows up in session and its impact on you and your response.

____

____

____

____

____

Share your responses: Expand your experience by sharing your answers with a colleague and explore the similarities and differences in your experiences.

We turn now to an overview of some key guiding principles with respect to assessment, case formulation, and treatment planning when the impacts of trauma are central to the initial presentation of the client.

ASSESSMENT IN EFIT

Viewed through the lens of attachment, the focus of the EFIT therapist at the outset of treatment is to gain an initial picture and felt understanding of how clients' current circumstances and histories have shaped and continue to influence central aspects of their present self and social and emotional functioning. As the therapist begins to create a "safe haven alliance" with the client, it is with this developmental perspective and image of health in mind and a view to understanding the pivotal relational experiences that have promoted growth and resilience, as well as those that have restricted and constrained individuals' natural propensity to grow. The image of health offered by attachment science, a felt sense of secure connection with self and others typified by emotional balance and cognitive flexibility, offers the therapist a benchmark by which to compare the client's present functioning. With this image of health in mind, the key goal of assessment in EFIT is to begin to understand clients' vulnerabilities and strengths and to identify the key factors and pivotal emotional and relational experiences that have restricted growth, and conversely those that have promoted resilience.

The EFIT therapist focuses not on disorders or diagnoses but instead on the core vulnerabilities that keep people stuck and prevent them from living fully. Although information about previous diagnosis and treatment provides useful information in the assessment phase of Stage 1 of EFIT, the goal of assessment is not to define and categorize mental health issues and problems in formal diagnostic systems, such as the various reiterations of the Diagnostic and Statistical Manual of Mental Disorders, Fifth Edition (DSM). Attachment and EFT are fundamentally non-pathologizing. Bowlby himself suggested that, in general, "clinical conditions are best understood as disordered versions of what is otherwise a healthy response" (1980, p. 245). Withdrawal and immobilization can be a functional response to impossible or dangerous situations in which vulnerability is overwhelming (Porges, 2011), such as finding oneself dependent on a dangerous and unpredictable attachment figure. Easily triggered anger and hypervigilance are likewise functional when the alternative appears to be that one is inevitably dismissed or deserted. Blocks to growth occur when such responses become generalized, global, automatic, and reflexive. The EFIT therapist is interested in how a particular client's natural propensity to grow and adapt has become constricted and iatrogenic.

The EFIT therapist focuses on the underlying structure of the client's lived emotional experience. Bowlby indicated that constructs such as depression could be defined more specifically in terms of key elements. He observed, for example, that depressed individuals commonly describe themselves and their lived experience in terms of four adjectives, namely lonely, unlovable, unwanted and helpless (see also Johnson, 2019 for a more comprehensive review). David Barlow's unified protocol model for emotional disorders similarly looks beyond traditional diagnostic nomenclature and recognizes the overlap between various disorders such as anxiety and depression, as well as their common structure such that anxiety and depression can be combined into one joint category, namely *negative emotional disorder* (Barlow et al., 2011). He, too, identifies common elements of various disorders such as anxiety (e.g., hypervigilance, avoidant strategies, heightened sense of threat or danger) and depression (e.g., vigilance to failure, self-criticism, social withdrawal, sense of hopelessness and loss of motivation). These core elements also are common to trauma- and stressor-related disorders, along with elements such as intrusive and other symptoms (e.g., flashbacks, nightmares, dissociation). All emotional disorders can be characterized by frequent and intense negative emotion. This emotion is also experienced with less coherence and clarity and seen as unacceptable to the client *frightening, alien, and unacceptable emotion*. In general, a sense of the uncontrollability of life and vigilance for threat are common core features of an emotional disorder.

Avoidance is a common coping response found in people with emotional disorders both in terms of awareness and in terms of engagement in life experiences. Avoidance as a remedy maintains the disorder and blocks further development and growth. Developmentally, symptoms such as withdrawal, numbing, avoidance, hypervigilance, shame, and self-loathing are a common sequelae of trauma evident in a client's presenting problems and impacting their developmental trajectory. As such the EFIT therapist is interested in when the trauma occurred (at what age), how long it lasted, whether there was more than one traumatic event, and whether there was anyone to rely on at that time. In sum, the therapist assesses for trauma's developmental impacts and potentially moderating influences (e.g., at least one secure attachment or available and responsive source of social support).

Exercise 10.3. Attachment Resource

Name the key attachment resource that buffers against trauma's potentially deleterious impact.

____

In EFIT assessment, the therapist identifies various historical and contemporaneous factors that are likely to impact their clients' clinical presentations. This is the case for a first responder exposed to years of cumulative trauma, a soldier fresh from combat, an individual with a chronically ill partner, and an individual with a childhood history of abuse, loss, or trauma. For example, the presentation of a first responder exposed to years of cumulative trauma compounded by childhood trauma and current social isolation might look very different than that of a first responder exposed to years of trauma in the context of a positive childhood history and significant current marital, social, and organizational support. On this important assessment-related topic, arguments have been made over the years for the inclusion of a separate diagnostic category (e.g., complex post-traumatic stress disorder) with the goal of capturing the differences between what various clinicians and researchers have termed complex compared with simple trauma (e.g., Lanktree & Briere, 2017; Herman, 1992; van der Kolk, 2015).

Trauma-Related Assessment Questions

Questions for the EFIT clinician to consider regarding traumatic exposure may include

- Type of Trauma Endured: Natural disaster, interpersonal, familial, previously trusted other
- Incident Details: Age at onset, duration, relationship to the perpetrator (e.g., trusted family member)
- Level of Exposure: Single incident vs. multiple; proximity of exposure (physically and/or emotionally)
- Response: Was there someone to turn to for support? Was the abuse reported, and was support provided? Did the client engage in treatment?
- Resiliency Factors: Social support, positive self-concept, optimism and hope, security of attachment, including that of an intimate partner
- Resolution: Has the trauma been resolved?

Coping remains a fundamental yet paramount concern. The therapist assesses the degree to which a client's coping strategy might now inform their current habitual affect regulation strategies often seen in hyperarousal (e.g., anxious, jittery, fast-paced speech), hypoarousal (e.g., numbing, dissociation, shutting down), or some combination of the two. Attachment strategies characterized by anxiety, avoidance, or a mixed combination, on the other hand, might be more or less restrictive depending on the client's capacity to adapt. As viewed on a continuum, clients' reactions might range from being highly automatic, rigid, and reflexive (akin to a "narrow window of tolerance") to more flexible and adaptive. In cases in which healthy development was thwarted by trauma early on (e.g., chronic childhood abuse in the absence of any secure connection or support), more rigid and negative models of self and other would be anticipated, as well as more automatic and reflexive affect regulation strategies. Viewed through a compassionate, survival-focused attachment lens, the client's experience and behavior will ultimately be revealed to be "reasonable." Simply put, our clients have good reasons for their responses even when they are ineffective or unhelpful.

No matter what the presentation, the purported dysfunctionality, or the nature or number of diagnoses, the therapist always actively searches for and articulates the client's *strengths*. In some cases, it is a huge testament to a client's courage just to have survived, struggled on, and sought out help. The therapist's non-pathologizing stance is often the first step in promoting clients' abilities to accept themselves and truly explore how their courage and struggle has shaped their world. Entering into a clients' world, the therapist focuses on areas and concerns important to the client, including key concerns about self, relationships with others, how they construct their inner emotional worlds, and the existential dilemmas that naturally emerge.

To summarize, global constructs such as diagnosis and disorders provide the EFIT therapist with an initial framework for understanding clients. As the therapist delves deeper, with a view to looking past such constructs and at their core elements and features (e.g., hypervigilance, sad mood, heightened anxiety, self-criticism, social withdrawal), clues are identified as to what is most important to the EFIT therapist. That is, how do clients view themselves and others? How do their strategies for coping with painful experiences prevent them from living fully? How rigid (or flexible) are these strategies? It is here that the therapist tunes in and finds focus. More surface/secondary data such as diagnoses and disorders, the overall "symptom picture," are important and useful—necessary but not sufficient. From an EFIT point of view, the therapist needs to look deeper, through an attachment lens, at clients' models of self and other and habitual ways of managing emotion to gain the rich understanding necessary for case formulation, on-target and effective intervention.

Personal Reflection

Individuals with a history of trauma are at risk for a host of psychological difficulties, but not all individuals with a history of trauma develop such difficulties. Identify some of the common co-occurring psychological difficulties that you have seen in your work with individuals in whom trauma has played a significant role.

____

____

____

____

____

Tuning in With CARE

Against this attachment backdrop, we introduce a more comprehensive guiding framework to help therapists "tune into" and stay attuned to their clients working through trauma-related concerns. The CARE model (Johnson & Campbell, 2021) when applied in the earliest stages of EFIT assessment remains relevant throughout treatment. As therapists begin to get a felt sense of and initial understanding of their clients, they aim to stay carefully attuned to four main channels: **c**ontext, **a**ttachment, **r**elationship, **e**motion (easily recalled with the acronym CARE).

- Context: As curious and open listeners, experiential therapists seek to immerse themselves in a client's present and past context. This requires giving attention to various facets, including identity (e.g., race, ethnicity, spirituality, religion, gender, sexuality), environment (e.g., socioeconomic, work/organizational, neighborhood), and experiences (e.g., racism, sexism, discrimination). The therapist gains a view of their client's narrative, both past and present, which best represents the client's overall experience.

- Attachment: The attachment channel taps into how individuals experience and view themselves and key others and how previous relational experiences manifest in their current interpersonal interactions, including with the therapist. The therapist takes notice of pivotal relational experiences that have shaping influence on one's view of self and other, as well as habitual affect regulation strategies. Careful tracking and accurate reflection allow the therapist to discern the themes (e.g., of loss or abandonment and/or violation) that best characterize a client's interpersonal history. As clients' stories unfold, key scenes or poignant interpersonal experiences are identified, and the therapist "gets acquainted with the characters that live in their clients' minds" (Yalom, 1989). The therapist gets to know the individuals who are intrinsically linked with the echoes of trauma and the key attachment figures and aspects of self that are potential allies in resolving those echoes as the therapeutic process unfolds. In addition to attending to possible current relationship resources (e.g., positive intimate relationship), risk/vulnerability (e.g., long-standing and severe family history of depression and/or suicidal ideation or attempts), and resiliency factors (e.g., feeling of competence in specific areas) are noted.
- Relationship: The relationship channel refers directly to the therapeutic alliance. Like other therapies, the therapeutic "relationship," the alliance, is a necessary but not sufficient condition for positive treatment outcome. In EFIT, the alliance is given careful attention at the outset of therapy and is monitored throughout the therapeutic process, with attention paid also, as appropriate, to potential contextual differences between therapist and client. Difficulties with trust are anticipated in clients with histories of trauma, especially at the outset of therapy, and are addressed with careful attunement and sensitivity. Throughout the process, attention is given to the therapeutic relationship or alliance, and any concerns that may emerge are immediately attended to if and as appropriate.

  Issues of trust are commonly at the forefront of the clinical picture, particularly with interpersonal trauma. The EFIT clinician anticipates being challenged and potentially put off balance in the initial phase of therapy, as the client either naturally questions and provokes as a means of assessing the clinician's stability as a "safe, stronger, wiser other" or remains hidden until ready to risk opening up. As always, careful attunement guides the establishing of a therapeutic alliance, giving clients the opportunity to share their experiences of trauma, potentially for the first time, from the vantage point or distance that is currently safe and within their "window of tolerance." The therapist builds a foundation for future work through accurately reflecting and validating a client's earlier experiences, as well as their experience in the "here and now," such that the client feels seen and heard.
- Emotion: The therapist attends to the way emotion is expressed (or not expressed, in the case of numbing or detachment), as well as the manner in which emotion is regulated (e.g., anxious, avoidant, or a combination of both). The therapist attends to what the client says, but also how it is said, that is, the therapist focuses on

> both process and content. Specific process elements might include body language or facial cues and voice tone, as well as related shifts that might occur as a client talks about various topics. For example, a tone of anger might be detected in the context of an event that likely engendered a sense of helplessness. As the therapist engages with the client's experience, the therapist tracks how the client expresses and regulates emotion. Core features of emotional disorders are noted (e.g., heightened anxiety, vigilance, behavioral avoidance, social withdrawal, self-criticism). Attention also is given to "emotional handles," or poignant phrases, images, key words, or metaphors that represent the client's inner felt experience.

In the CARE model, these four channels are mutually informing as the therapist continually attends to these four critical dimensions of a client's experience throughout the course of therapy. The therapist shifts between each of the CARE dimensions to ascertain the most clear complete picture and "felt understanding" of the client's experience, much like an optometrist using a phoroptor (fancy piece of equipment) during an eye exam shifts between various combinations of lenses while collaborating with the patient to discern optimal sight. As the therapeutic process unfolds, the therapist moves fluidly between assessment and intervention and back again, continually assessing the pulse and confluence of these four perspectives all the while gauging therapeutic interventions accordingly. For example, a therapist might focus on their alliance (relationship) during periods of a client's immediate uncertainty when a client's responses are notably overregulated in discussing a childhood memory. As the therapist attends to the client's experience, they may shift to contextual influences shaping this unfolding scene (context). Reflection and validation might then soothe the nervous system of the client and continue to propel the process forward. At times of high racial tension and stress in the workplace, for example, the therapist will shift focus to context and providing support in this arena. When the alliance is strong and solid and external stressors are low and support high, the therapist can then proceed to interventions aimed at joining the client in further discovering and exploring aspects of painful material.

Personal Reflection

Reflect on a client you have worked with that has a traumatic history. Make an observation based on your experience using each of the four dimensions of the CARE approach.

Context: ____

Attachment: ____

Relationship: ____

Emotion: ____

Case Conceptualization and Treatment Planning

Assessment of contraindications is essential in EFIT. In general, clients exhibiting psychotic or antisocial features are not likely to be suitable candidates for EFIT. Further, it is important to assess the capacity of the client to safely engage in the therapeutic process. The therapist gives particular attention to a client's affect regulation capacity and potential vulnerability to resort to either substance abuse or violence or to be at risk for self-harm or self-injurious behaviors. Referral for additional services might be indicated either prior to or while engaging in a course of EFIT (e.g., home supports, substance abuse treatment, psychiatric consultation to consider medication).

Therapist pacing and attunement guide the assessment process. There are times, for example, when a slower pace is necessary with clients who present with signs of dissociation or are highly avoidant or intellectual. In the case of complex or developmental trauma (e.g., early childhood, chronic exposure to trauma in the absence support), particularly in the absence of any systematic treatment to date, a longer and more arduous therapeutic process, especially in Stage 1, should be anticipated. Viewed through the developmental attachment perspective, it would be anticipated that if key aspects of development (i.e., self, social, and emotional development) are thwarted by trauma early on, the reshaping and revision of models of self and other will take time, requiring intermittent periods of intervention followed by consolidation. A thorough assessment guides practical matters, including the scheduling of sessions, with attention to self and social and emotional resources, but also with respect to any current personal and/or social stressors (e.g., illness in the family, work-related stress).

In EFIT, it is helpful to stage the process in a manner that both capitalizes on momentum and attends to clients' windows of tolerance. In some cases, weekly sessions will be too frequent, while in other cases, longer periods between sessions will lead to a feeling of stopping and starting over, with little progression along the way. The initial assessment guides the clinician, and a collaborative conversation with the client regarding resources (e.g., emotional, social, and other resources such as finances or childcare), which sets the stage for a commitment to the therapeutic process in Stage 1. In cases involving complex or developmental trauma, clients may engage in an important piece of work, leave therapy for a period to consolidate these gains, and then return again to build on and continue the therapeutic work they started. Also common are situations in which clients re-initiate treatment at key developmental transitions (e.g., marriage, birth of a baby, loss of a parent). In cases involving first responder trauma, continued therapy is helpful in addressing previous trauma, as well as allowing for more immediate processing of likely exposure to additional traumatic events, increasing first responders' resilience to work-related stress, and trauma exposure in particular.

Clinical Example: A First Session in EFIT

Sandy presented at the initial session with a tone of skepticism and disillusionment, citing a history of abuse and traumatic experiences ranging from childhood bullying, sexual abuse, and assault, and an adult history of unstable intimate relationships, including physical and emotional abuse. She has "never been able to let it go," she asserted, referring to her history, and indicating that it has "never been addressed." Now in her early 40s with two young children and an adult stepson, she described her current relationship of about 13 years as positive and stable and her partner as reliable and trustworthy. "He is perfect," she said, but she does not want to "burden him."

Much as she did as a child, rather than reaching to her parents, her tendency is to retreat and withdraw. Similarly, she does not tend to rely on her friends and family for support. Work and school have always been a refuge and a place of success, but she currently is unhappy in her work environment and struggling with the competing demands of work and family impacting her mental health. During periods of overwhelm, she becomes more difficult to reach and finds herself lecturing her partner and their children and then retreating into a "dark place" of depression, shame, and guilt. At such times, she seriously contemplates suicide "for the benefit of [her] family; they would be better off without [her]."

Throughout the session, she sat with a strong posture, forthright and articulate, illustrating this same reliance on her intellect and verbal ability as a means of coping, though at times tearful. Drug and/or alcohol use were not contributing factors nor did she report a personal or family history of substance abuse. Sandy stated that she has been in counselling since her early 20s. She has "tried everything . . . books, hypnosis, tapping, talk therapy . . . and shared this story a lot of times to no avail . . . this feels like a last-ditch effort." She also has "taken every medicine under the sun" and continues to take medication, saying "[she] wouldn't do well without it."

Exercise 10. 4. Type of Trauma

The clinical example above best illustrates an example of

a. Simple trauma.
b. Complex trauma.
c. A case in which EFT is contraindicated.

Exercise 10.5. Resiliency Factors

The clinical example of Sandy highlights a number of resiliency factors. Identity the resiliency factors you observe. Circle all that apply.

a. A currently positive work environment and work satisfaction
b. A strong and broad support network that she relies on regularly
c. Relational resources, including her relationship with her intimate partner, as well as friends and family
d. A history of success educationally and vocationally

Exercise 10.6. EFIT Session Goals

Key goals for this session for the EFT clinician will be one or more of the following. Circle all that apply.

a. To instill a sense of hope in the (therapeutic) process
b. To establish safety, with respect to suicide risk in particular
c. To work toward establishing a strong therapeutic alliance
d. To provide the client with a sense of the therapeutic roadmap, allowing for some sense of transparency and predictability in the process

In the initial session. the EFT clinician explored indications of suicidal ideation and inquired about her partner's awareness of these thoughts. Sandy had informed him about six months prior to the session, but when asked to promise her safety to him (imaginally, in the session), she indicated that "it [felt] out of [her] control" and that she "didn't want to break a promise to him." As the session progressed toward a conclusion, as an alternative means of establishing safety, the EFT therapist used Move 3 of the EFT Tango to bring Sandy in contact with her younger self, the part of her that was alone during a very difficult time of bullying in her mid-childhood. After numerous other attempts to have Sandy commit to a suicide contract, it was the encounter with her younger self that shifted Sandy's inflexible stance and opened a space that allowed her to express a commitment more fully to the therapeutic process and to her own safety throughout it.

Sandy's negative model of self was notably visible as she shared her perception that maybe she "did have that coming," referring to years of poor and cruel treatment from others, including incidents of bullying in childhood. The therapist first asked Sandy about a visual image representative of herself at that time as a means of evoking contact with that younger self. Promoting immediacy and deeper experiencing, the therapist asked about her appearance, her facial expression, and, in particular, her eyes. As the encounter with this younger self became more vivid and alive in the room, the therapist was then able to experientially bring Sandy in touch with the depth of her isolation. This provided a frame for her means of coping currently that, though adaptive at that earlier time, was now a barrier to self-compassion and her ability to embrace the love of precious others in her life who wish to give it to her. The therapist was able to use this experience or encounter to conclude the session with a summary of the experiential process, weaving in elements of psychoeducation through validation and reflection and then describing the therapeutic roadmap.

Exercise 10.7. Instilling Hope and Trust in the EFIT Process

Given strong indications of skepticism and suicide risk, the therapist endeavored in the initial session to instill a sense of hope and trust in the process. As illustrated, in EFT, an effective means of instilling a sense of hope and trust in the process (and the therapist) is to

a. Refer clients to the literature in the area of trauma.
b. Provide them with a series of homework assignments.
c. Cite examples of previous successes with clients.
d. Provide them with a new experience in the session, in the "here and now" and then use that experience as an anchor to celebrate success and explain the therapeutic process.

Exercise 10.8. Summarizing the Session

As an EFT therapist, write out what you would say to Sandy at the end of this session in summarizing the initial session, and providing a roadmap for the EFT therapeutic process. Elements to consider include

- Help Sandy understand how her previously adaptive ways of coping now entrap her.
- Provide her with a "roadmap" or understanding of how the EFT process will liberate her not by taking these coping strategies away or addressing each and every traumatic event but by diminishing the automaticity of her coping responses/ attachment strategies and providing increased flexibility and agency during times of stress and threat.

- Help Sandy see where she is headed, with the support of the clinician and the EFT process, with the goal of increasing transparency (and further solidifying the therapeutic alliance) and providing Sandy with a greater sense of predictability and agency.

Now in your words, what would you say to Sandy in summarizing these key points?

____

____

____

____

____

____

____

Reflections/summary statements serve a number of purposes in EFT. They are often used to

- Capture essential emergent themes within a session.
- Anchor the therapeutic process providing the client with increased awareness,
- Increase awareness by bringing the client toward deeper emotional experiencing.
- Consolidate any therapeutic gains within the session (Move 5 of the Tango).
- Stabilize a moment of therapist uncertainty or when the therapist has been "put off balance" by a challenging comment or expression of emotion (e.g., anger) from the client.
- Reflect a moment for the client to increase their awareness of how their actions/reactions impact relationships.
- Provide guidance for the client between sessions.

EFIT Stage 1: Forming an Alliance, Pacing the Process, and Dancing the Tango

The previous case highlights the importance of assessment as a guide to case formulation, clinical decision making, and therapeutic pacing (e.g., with attention to the "therapeutic window/window of tolerance" such that interventions are paced with the aim of challenging but not overwhelming personal resources). In Sandy's case, in addition to noting a significant history of trauma (including childhood trauma), the EFT therapist attended to various cues suggestive of significant self, other, and affect regulation capacity. Sandy was able to access feelings of sadness and vulnerability in the first session. She identified key support figures, including her intimate partner; she described a history of success educationally and vocationally, suggestive of likely positive regard in these arenas. In light of these resources, the therapist made the decision to introduce the Tango early in the therapeutic process. Sandy's skepticism, disillusionment, and suicide risk were considered best addressed with a new felt experience that would instill a sense of hope and thereby facilitate a commitment to safety and to the established therapeutic process. Sandy committed to six scheduled sessions to be followed by a review to determine whether additional sessions were needed or whether therapy might be suspended for a period.

The EFIT therapist paces the focus on the use of the EFT Tango in cases of significant developmental trauma or clinical presentations characterized by significant numbing and detachment or significant developmental trauma, particularly in the absence of a reliable relational resource outside the therapeutic relationship. When a significant trauma history is being shared for the first time, the therapist can expect to spend considerable time allowing clients to break the silence and isolation that has characterized their trauma history and to help them to make sense of and begin to order their experience (Tango Moves 1 and 2). A comprehensive understanding of the client's attachment history and a strong therapeutic alliance, along with carefully attuned reflections and interventions will provide the client with a sense of being "heard and seen," as well as increased personal awareness and emotional capacity. This work provides a requisite foundation for staging "encounters" (Tango Move 3) and subsequent Tango Moves and ultimately advances progression through the therapeutic process. Initial accounts of a client's personal history might appear disorganized and incoherent and require a number of sessions to share, particularly with complex trauma.

Further, it can be anticipated that the establishment of a solid therapeutic alliance is likely to be more difficult and that the therapist will be confronted in various ways. Given experiences of violation and/or abandonment in key relationships, the issue of trust—a central feature of the therapeutic alliance in any effective psychotherapy—is likely to be challenging, particularly at the outset of therapy. Maintaining a sense of empathy and understanding that current attachment strategies were once survival mechanisms under conditions of isolation and intolerable threat helps the clinician maintain therapeutic clarity and emotional balance within the session.

Early sessions with Sandy often included a tone of anger, frustration, and skepticism as she shared her doubts that her ability to deal with overwhelm would ever improve. She considered the therapist's optimism unfounded given that the therapist did not really know her or know what she was like outside the sessions (and the depth and breadth of her "character flaws"). The therapist viewed Sandy's response through an attachment lens, though the initial experience of her negative tone was unnerving. This allowed her to maintain emotional balance and to hear Sandy's protest as an expression of her high expectations for herself (and others), her deeply entrenched negative model of self, and her significant fears associated with trusting and believing in another and in the therapeutic process.

Exercise 10.9. Maintaining Balance in the Face of Protest

As an EFT therapist, how might you handle this type of protest from Sandy (e.g., expressions of anger and/or mistrust in the therapist and/or the therapeutic process)? Some tips for regaining balance and providing a supportive response that do not derail the process but instead continue to propel the therapeutic process forward are as follows:

- Tune into her felt experience and use it as a guide to imagine how others in Sandy's life might experience such protests and/or angry tones.
- Focus on the protest using an attachment understanding and de-personalize and normalize the reactivity in view of Sandy's history and her prototypical interactions with others.

- Use reflection or a summary statement to ground yourself and slow the process.
- Speak directly to the underlying fears and concerns Sandy is expressing from a place of empathy and compassion and from the position of a "stronger, wiser other" or temporary attachment figure and ally in the process.

With these tips in mind, list two key elements that you would include in your response to Sandy. As possible, practice with a colleague how you would respond to Sandy. Building on the two key elements you identified, what would you say? Together, notice how these responses impact Sandy's protest and felt experience.

Response 1.

____

____

____

____

Response 2.

____

____

____

____

Additional exercises: For additional personal reflection exercises, see the online resource page.

Managing Intrusive Symptoms, Numbing, and Shame

Other considerations regarding therapeutic pacing and "titrating" interventions in Stage 1 include managing flashbacks and/or dissociative experiences in the session, as well as indications of strong affect (e.g., intense hyperarousal) and/or numbing/detachment (i.e., hypoarousal). At times, the therapist will need to "contain" strong surface/secondary emotion to make room for deeper more primary emotion through interventions such as validation, reflection, and slowing the process, and at other times, the therapist will seek to "heighten" emotion (e.g., through evocative questioning aimed at assisting clients in attending to their bodily sensations and associated emotional experiences). In the case of Sandy, once "in the room with her younger self," the therapist might ask, "What is happening in your body as you see her little face, her eyes . . . what happens inside of you as . . . ?" Such inquiry focuses clients and assists them in attending to their felt experience, experiences that are normally outside their awareness or that were unsafe to encounter at earlier times, experiences that might be "frightening, alien, and unacceptable."

Recurring shame and self-blame responses also are acknowledged in Stage 1. Micro-interventions such as empathic attunement, empathic reflection, and validation can be used in Stage 1 to "tame" shame (and dampen the barrier to self and connection) by acknowledging indications of shame and providing a context for such experiences in reference to the client's attachment history. The therapist may use process explanations to help clients make sense of and/or order their experience. The therapist might, for instance, in Stage 1, say some version of the following, "For children who grow up in homes where their caregivers are unreliable or inconsistently reliable, their best choice is to shut down or numb out or to become caregivers rather than rely on care from another and be deeply disappointed; for children who grow up in difficult or abusive homes, to believe that those they should count on most are not there for them or are unreliable is too terrifying; it is better for children to believe they must be bad, to believe it is them, that it is something they did or did not do (to believe it is about "self" provides individuals with a greater sense of "control" or "agency" and helps them to deal with the profound sense of abandonment). Such interventions quiet the impacts of shame and self-loathing but do not fully address them.

The therapist recognizes that shame can be acknowledged in Stage 1 but can only be worked through in Stage 2 (upon a platform of safety and stability, at the end of the Stage 1 therapeutic process). That is, though models of self and other become more flexible and open in Stage 1, deep and sustainable shifts, including shame resolution, occur in Stage 2, through deeper levels of processing and against the backdrop of a strong therapeutic alliance and the markers of stabilization. Various markers of stabilization include, for example, increased compassion for self, as well as an increased understanding that current coping methods were effective survival strategies in earlier times and in other contexts but are now thwarting growth and self-cohesion. Other markers of stabilization include an increased capacity to encounter emotion in new ways, a "greater window of tolerance."

Exercise 10.10. Managing a Disruptive Emotional Moment

How does the EFT therapist contain a disruptive emotional moment in-session (e.g., flashback, intrusive thought)? Mark all strategies the therapist might use to support a client in this moment.

a. As in regular EFT, the therapist slowly tracks, reflects, and organizes the strong emotions/images as they occur.
b. The therapist validates, normalizes, and explicates strong emotional responses. ______
c. The therapist coaches the client in affect regulation skills. ______
d. The therapist can use grounding techniques, talking a client through a flashback and reflecting present realities, as in, "Can you feel your back against the chair, feet on the floor? Can you breathe slowly? This is what happened. . . . " ______

Exercise 10.11. Strategies for Recurring Shame and Self-Blame

Which of the following strategies would the EFT therapist *not* employ in working with a client's recurring shame and self-blame responses?

a. The therapist normalizes self-blame as often being the only coping mechanism open to the survivor and as preferable to complete helplessness. ______
b. The therapist frames self-blame as an alternative to the loss of an abusing or abandoning attachment figure and complete isolation. ______

c. The therapist tracks the impact of self-blame and the hiding stance that goes with shame on the present relationship. ______
d. The therapist actively uses his/her acceptance and empathy to counter self-blame. ______
e. The therapist mainly works on extensive insight into the survivor's past and the creation of his or her model of self. ______

Propelling the Process Forward With the EFT Tango

As described here and in other contexts (Johnson, 2019), the EFT Tango is central in guiding the clinician's interventions within session. The following example highlights the moves of the Tango in session 4 with Sandy.

Mirror and Reflect Present Process

In Tango Move 1, the EFT therapist looks for themes that reflect clients' sense of themselves and others and their prototypical patterns of managing difficult affect. The therapist gives attention to process and content and from the vantage point of careful attunement and a secure base exploring the following:

- How does the client tell her story? How does she put her inner world together?
- How does she relate to others? Do these interactions feel good or bad?
- How does the client interact with the therapist in the session? Does she seem to feel safe with the therapist?
- How does the client speak about her feelings? How well can she contain and regulate emotion?
- How does she deal with vulnerability? Do these ways of coping keep her stuck and constrained and ultimately end up contributing to anxiety, depression, or trauma-related symptoms, or to feelings of helplessness or hopelessness and associated thoughts of self-harm?

In mirroring/reflecting, the EFT therapist helps to give clients a more coherent story of their "inner" and "between" worlds, of their emotional ("within") and social/relational ("between") functioning. Woven into such reflections, the EFT therapist uses validation to help make sense of current behaviors in the present context based on historical experiences, thereby guiding the client toward greater understanding and, eventually, self-compassion. With trauma clients in particular, pacing is critical, and efforts are made to repeat their narratives to help them feel heard and understood but to also help their narratives become more coherent—with the overarching goal of providing clients with a clear anchor from which to move forward therapeutically.

Clinical Example. Sandy came into session 4 wondering aloud to the therapist, "How can I be wrecking the best relationships in my life?" Expressing a sense of hopelessness, she said that it all felt "so deeply seated." As session 4 progresses, Sandy explores these dark feelings, and the therapist captures Sandy's present experience through mirroring, validating, and reflecting Sandy's pain, distress, and echoes from her trauma history, which all make it challenging for her to take it in.

Sandy: In the days between our sessions, I had a feeling of progress. I had hope, and then I spiraled down in such a harmful way. I felt like all the work before was lost; my behavior reverted. It's my anger, it's like a light switch—suddenly angry, volatile—I'm aware of it, but I can't stop it. It feels like everyone around me is intentionally pushing my buttons. I just feel so out of control; I get so hurtful. What am I doing to my children? What am I doing to my husband, to the safest, most precious relationship I've ever had? It's just not fair to send them through this spin cycle, so that's when I think about just leaving [committing suicide] for them because it doesn't feel like there will ever be a time that I could manage it.

Therapist: Yeah, so, Sandy, I actually think we could work on that. For me, it doesn't feel like a setback because I appreciate that the process can be bumpy. What I hear you saying is that you have some automatic responses in situations that trigger you because of legitimate and valid scars associated with your childhood. This is the picture I have; in the first session, you came in, and we talked quite a bit about your history and about significant events that impacted you and the way that you feel about yourself. You also talked about your husband and your home, your current family as a safe haven. You talked about ways that you didn't feel treated well in your school, your mom was a teacher at that time, and she couldn't or didn't protect you. So, the way you learned to cope, I think, was to get quiet and retreat and to maybe get small and less visible. Is that right?

Sandy: Yeah, I make a lot of rules of self-governance. I try to predict what other people are going to do. I have a plan for each sort of circumstance, I rehearse a lot of things in my mind . . . if someone called on me and I was unprepared, then I would be blindsided, and that would give them an opportunity to hit the soft spots. . . .

Therapist: Yeah, Sandy, I hear you, and I think you've spoken with me about this before; you described it as being super prepared and perfectionistic almost, right? And if we keep speaking about the process to date, I think in the next session in particular, that younger part of you was a bit more present in the room and visible and easy to connect with, and we talked about ways that we might be able to give her a voice around this. (Sandy nods.) And now, to come back to today, what I heard you say earlier was that, before you were taken to this angry place, there was a feeling of being dismissed, that your words, your guidance didn't matter—you didn't matter—and then internally you get taken to this other angry place; does that feel right? (Sandy nods.) So, Sandy, I think today, if you could again connect with and embrace and give voice to that part of yourself that has been dismissed, the more that you can openly share your vulnerability, the more I think that we can undo the automaticity of that coping response—the more you can have flexibility with it. I also hear you speak about that next very dark place that you go, after you get angry, and that you feel like your family would be better off without you. Of course, there would be nothing more devastating than that for your family; of course, they're hurt by your anger, but there would be nothing more difficult to recover from than that. . . .

Sandy: I feel like my children's love for me is by default. They don't know what they're doing, they don't know what they're feeling, they don't love me because of who I am or the things that I do; they love me because they don't know any better, and if I was gone, they might have an opportunity to learn about real love, not just default love. . . .

Exercise 10.12. Therapist In-Session and Process Focus

Identify three ways the therapist in the example just presented focused on process rather than content:

1. ____

____

2. ____

____

3. ____

____

Move 2: Affect Assembly and Deepening

As the therapist carefully tracks and remains attuned with the client, the key aim of Move 2 is to help the client become more deeply absorbed in her experience. The most effective means of deepening experience is to "stay still" with it by staying present with the client. The therapist helps the client crystallize her experience by using her images or emotional handles (e.g., key emotionally loaded words or phrases). As the elements of emotion are put together piece by piece, the inner organization of the emotion—the structure—is changed. The affective picture becomes more complete, ordered, and whole, and the client's capacity to regulate affect is expanded. In reflecting on the elements of assembling emotion in an EFIT session, the therapist considers the following:

- *Trigger:* What is the *scene*, *cue*, or *situation* that gives rise to the strong feeling?
- *Basic Perception:* What is the client's basic immediate and initial reaction (e.g., "I react, and then I realize I reacted")? It is typically associated with an undercurrent of threat and danger that is often unclear or at an implicit level of awareness.
- *Body Response.* In exploring body response, the EFT therapist maintains a stance of "soft, slow, and specific" and a position of curiosity (e.g., What's in your body right now? What is happening for you now as you share this?).
- *Meaning:* The EFT therapist seeks to provide clients with a more cogent sense of their experience (e.g., What do you say to yourself? What does this mean? The therapist is seeking to gain an understanding of the attachment significance).
- *Action Tendency.* The EFT therapist helps clients to become more aware of their reflexive, automatic, and inflexible responses under conditions of perceived threat or danger (e.g., Do you run? shut down? numb out? lash out? cling? Some combination of these?).

Clinical Example. Notice how the therapist assembles and deepens moments of Sandy's emotional experience and how this leads to new experience and understanding. As the session continues, Sandy begins to focus on times from earlier in childhood. She is in her childhood bedroom. Mistrustful and fearful others are going to attack and reject her, Sandy is crippled with worry. Focusing initially at a bodily level, the therapist works to get more specific and precise about what Sandy's emotion is, what it means, and what she is drawn to do.

Therapist: Sandy, where does worry sit in your body? What's the physical sensation?

Sandy: Right here . . . tight . . . (Sandy points to her chest.)

Therapist: Tight in your chest . . . right . . . okay. . . .

Sandy: Hard to swallow. . . .

Therapist: Yeah, so if we stay really still on the bed and focus on the tightness, and I heard you, it's hard to swallow, but if you let that grow and really feel into the tightness, what is that like? What happens?

Sandy: It just feels like there's no way out. There's no way around it; there are no options.

Therapist: Trapped . . . and alone? That's good, Sandy; keep breathing. What's happening with the tightness as you breathe?

Sandy: It's moving up. . . .

Therapist: It's moving up . . . yeah . . . yeah . . . you're doing a good job, Sandy. Again, if you stay focused on it, if the tightness could speak, in this moment, just here, now, what would the tightness say?

Sandy: I don't know.

Therapist: As you sit on the bed and feel yourself against the wall . . . and you see the door . . . and you hear the sounds . . . and you're shut in your room . . . alone. . . . (soft, slow voice)

Sandy: Everything feels pointless. I feel angry.

Therapist: What does the anger say in that moment?

Sandy: Just leave me alone. Get lost! Just violent, frustrated anger. . . .

Exercise 10.13. Assembling Emotion

Identify the elements of emotion in Sandy's experience found in the transcript just presented.

Trigger: ______________________________

Basic Perception: ______________________________

Bodily Response: ______________________________

Meaning Making: ______________________________

Action Tendency: ______________________________

Move 3: Engaged Encounters

In EFIT, as the EFT therapist comes to know the client's inner life and the key figures that have impacted definitions of self and other, an engaged experiential encounter becomes possible. Encounters might be with the therapist, a younger part of self, or another attachment figure (e.g., parent or other relative, spiritual figure, partner). In some cases involving trauma, it might be appropriate to set up an enactment with an "offending other," but again, the therapist does so with a clear goal in mind (e.g., to provide the client with a "voice" to express what was not possible to express in earlier times) and with attention to ensuring that the client maintains a safe distance from the other, feels held by the therapist, and is not put in a position that might be experienced as "re-traumatizing." More generally, the choice of "other" is guided by the therapist's goal or intended outcome. Goals for the encounter might include evoking more vulnerable, deeper emotion; challenging strategies that "protect but imprison" the client; making contact with a younger part of self that was shut off, shut down, or "frozen in time" as a means of survival and is now in distant contact with the older self; facilitating self-compassion through contact with a younger part of self; and resourcing the client by setting up an encounter with a key and reliable other.

Clinical Example. As Move 3 unfolds, the therapist walks alongside Sandy and symbolically holds her hand as she more directly encounters her younger, wounded self and continues to intervene in a manner that heightens the immediacy and poignancy of the scene through highlighting visual imagery with specificity, with sound and with "full color." This allows both client and therapist to enter the scene more fully with all their senses. Young Sandy feels misunderstood and alone. Consistent with what is often seen in cases of trauma, the encounter isn't clean and easy. Distressed and dark as she is in her own life now, Sandy struggles to comfort young Sandy. Still, the therapist facilitates the beginnings of a poignant shift as Sandy more and more fully enters the scene and meets directly and authentically with young Sandy.

Therapist: If I stay alongside you, Sandy, what do I see in your room?

Sandy: It's an old house, and it has a solid wooden door that's "orangey brown" and makes a really loud sound when it closes and, gosh, I don't remember what's on the walls, but there's a big poster on the back of the door with all the dog breeds on it and a double bed and a little tape player. . . .

Therapist: What is the bedspread like? (Additional detail is solicited with the aim of deepening the experience.)

Sandy: I don't know. I don't think the blankets are on the bed. I think they're pushed off in a mess. We're sitting on the bed with our feet up and our knees up, leaning against the wall. . . .

Therapist: Sandy, how might you impact young Sandy? In your body, what are you drawn to do as you see her?

Sandy: Just sit there with her. . . .

Therapist: Yeah, just sit beside her. . . .

Sandy: Don't try to convince her of anything. . . .

Therapist: Yeah, that's good, Sandy, and as you glance at her and feel her, even from a distance, what's happening inside your body?

Sandy: I don't like being ignored. (Therapist nods.) She's ignoring me; she's very spiteful. She's just turned her back on me, literally.

Therapist: And as you stay really still with her . . . I get it . . . there's a part of you that feels frustrated and rejected, but there's some other part of you that has compassion and empathy, at least in the sense that you actually know what's going on inside of her, which is why she wants you to stay, but she, for her own reasons, can't and won't say that. . . . I guess maybe it would hurt too much if you then left, she would be so vulnerable. So, you are staying really still with her, right there beside her, even though she can't communicate that to you directly, you can feel it because you can feel her little body and now as you sit super still. . . .

Sandy: Just feels unbelievable that someone so young would have to feel things so heavy. It's not fair. (starts to sob)

Therapist: That's right, Sandy; it's good to let yourself cry, let her sob, that's the best thing to do, you're absolutely right, let yourself sob, from your chest and the tension and that feeling in your throat, let yourself cry and release it. Are you okay to keep staying here? (Sandy nods.) What happens now as you breathe?

Sandy: It's easier, not so tight. . . .

Therapist: So, now what's happening for her? What do you see and feel?

Sandy: I don't know how to describe it; she's so hesitant to soften.

Therapist: To be impacted by your presence. It's okay; we're going to need to be patient, so if we keep breathing, Sandy, what's going on now?

Sandy: We're just sitting, and it feels to both of us like I'm not permanently there; when I get up and leave, she'll be alone again.

Therapist: If your gut could speak to her, right here, right now, in that bedroom, what would your gut want to say to her? I think we understand it; young Sandy's not going to talk. It's too scary to talk; it would hurt way too much to speak and then to be alone again, right? I think that's what's going on for her, so if your gut could speak to her, what would it say?

Sandy: Everything seems so flimsy. . . .

Therapist: Well, we won't expect her to give us anything back because that's just not how it's going to work with kids and especially with somebody like her who's been so hurt and felt so alone and feels so trapped, so we won't . . . but I hear what you're saying as well, that it's hard to find the right words to land on her in any way that might have an impact. So, if we stay out of our brains and just be in our guts with her, on the bed, in the room with the wood door, if your gut could speak to her, what would it say?

Sandy: I would want her to know that I've been there, and I understand. I want to tell her that it gets better, but I'm not going to lie to her.

Therapist: What would your gut say to her about your commitment to her? If your gut could speak, because that's the only part you really have control of, you can't control the kids at school, or what's happening on the other side of the door. (Sandy nods in agreement.)

Exercise 10.14. Deepening Emotions and Shaping Encounters

In the transcript just provided, which of the following responses would be *least effective* in deepening emotion and shaping an encounter between older, wiser Sandy and her younger self with sensitivity to the current distance between younger and older Sandy?

a. Therapist joins with Sandy and enters what experiential therapists call "the phenomenological world of the client" (see, for e.g., Rogers, 1961) by entering a scene with as much detail and with as many of the senses as possible, thus fostering immediacy and heightening emotion.
b. Therapist titrates the intensity of the encounter by following the lead of the client, carefully tracking, and introducing interventions that draw on Sandy's felt experience rather than reflecting her experience (e.g., "What are you drawn to do . . . ?" vs. "I notice you. . . . ").
c. Therapist continually and consistently asks Sandy to draw her attention to her body/her felt sense and to be guided by that aspect of her experience (vs. her thoughts/cognitions) to keep Sandy in her felt experience.
d. Therapist focuses exclusively on the meaning and content generated through the encounter to explore further and use to inform personal insight and future goals.

Processing the Encounter

Following the encounter, it is important to process the individual's experience of the encounter (Tango Move 4). The therapist may use a series of evocative questions to process her experience. These might include "What shifted? What was the bodily/felt sense? What was it like for you to say that? What was it like for that younger part of you to hear that? What do you feel now as you share?"

Clinical Example. As we can readily see, this is a complicated encounter. Young Sandy has a lot of painful events still to come in her life, and older Sandy is unwilling to deceptively reassure her, in some sugar-coated way, that everything is going to be fine. In processing this moving interaction between older and young Sandy, though, the therapist focuses on the potentially soothing impact (on young Sandy, who remains withdrawn and apprehensive) that may come from her older self's compassion, honesty, empathy, and adult Sandy's sincere wish to join and accompany and stay present with her on this painful journey.

Therapist: Sandy, do you have a sense of what [young Sandy] felt as you sat beside her quietly, and . . .

Sandy: She didn't want me there . . . "get lost" . . .

Therapist: Did she feel your presence and comfort? . . . (Sandy nods.) So, there was a part of her that was taking it in and another part of her that wanted to push you away. . . . So, with that understanding, Sandy, what feels right to say to her, from your gut? . . . I guess you could share that understanding, maybe, or just be still with it, I'm not sure. . . .

Sandy: I feel like everything I say will just go into thin air . . . like, why bother? She's not going to believe it anyway. She's fluctuating between a loneliness—her normal feeling—and now something else, but she's not used to this new feeling, so she doesn't feel like she's supposed to want me to be there or enjoy it at all. . . .

Therapist: Yeah, so tell me if I get this right, Sandy; the thing I hear you saying, or reflecting, to [young Sandy] would be some version of, "I hear you and see you and feel you. It's been a lonely journey, and even when you thought and believed that things might be different, they weren't different, and your only recourse has been to be alone, to curl your little self up in this room, on the other side of the door, and listen to what's happening outside it but really struggle hard not to be affected by it and not to let anybody in and, well, not to hope or believe." But as you sat beside her, this older, wiser part of her, of me, when you sat alongside me (therapist now speaks for younger Sandy), there was a part of me that's impacted by your compassion and empathy and wants to be warmed by that, but it's been a long road, a long journey alone, so there's another big part of me that feels angry and frustrated and wants to just push you, like I push everybody else, but I actually didn't do that. I turned away, but I didn't push you, and I'm not going to push you, but I'm also not going to let you in fully; that's way too scary because then, if I am alone again, that will be devastating, that will hurt more than anything. So, what would reassure her, Sandy? I think the only reassurance would be to know that maybe you'll come and go, and maybe there'll be times when you have your attention on her and bring her into the room but you're not going to leave her. Do you feel like you could assure her of that . . . that you are going to come in and out of her life and bring her into the room, in small and big ways, but it won't be an ever-presence because you're not going to be able to promise that, does that all feel right? Sandy, what does that feel like for you?

Sandy: It feels honest . . . and manageable . . .

Exercise 10.15. Processing the Encounter

In reviewing this interaction, which themes/key aspects (e.g., level of impact on emotion, felt bodily sense, model of self and other) of the interaction did you notice the therapist processing with Sandy and with her younger self? List three themes/aspects of the interaction the EFT therapist would want to highlight in processing the encounter. (Hint: The goal of Move 4 is to help the client begin to process, through the lens of attachment, what just occurred; what happened? What was the impact of the encounter?)

1. ____

   ____

2. ____

   ____

3. ____

   ____

Integrating and Validating

Move 5 is an important means of consolidating the gains that have been made, making them explicit, and helping the client own what happened (e.g., "Did you see what just happened? Look what you did"—the therapist explicates and replays the sequence of events, reflecting the process of change to make it more real, concrete, and specific). As appropriate, the therapist also highlights the contrast between what happens when the client risks remaining still in vulnerability, moving outside the "protection that has become her prison." Move 5 also can be a time of celebration. At times, emotional processing will deepen further at this point as the therapist helps the client organize and process this new experience and thereby reorganize the client's internal system.

Clinical Example. As session 4 moves toward a close and adult Sandy continues to sit in contact with young Sandy, the therapist validates and integrates what has just occurred in a way that engenders hope and facilitates more coherence and further orders Sandy's experience.

Sandy: She's (referencing young Sandy) is not near the end of it; there's no light at the end of the tunnel for her; she still has some horrible things to go through. (Therapist nods.) And I can't reassure her that she's any better on the other side of it.

Therapist: That's right, we are not going to be able to change . . . her . . . your history . . . but she doesn't have to be alone in it this time . . . and in so doing, we don't change history, but we change the impact, not completely, and not in a way that we never get triggered or never get impacted, but the more that you can embrace young Sandy and help her to know that she doesn't have to be, not anymore, alone in the world . . . the more that you connect with her, the more that she develops trust and belief and hope, and the more that she has a representation of you in her little tiny body, the more that you don't actually have to be there . . . she can call upon that representation of you . . . she can call upon that experience of you sitting still beside her on the bed. (Sandy nods in acknowledgment.) Yeah, because that's how it is for us, right? You don't always have your husband beside you, but in a real time of need, do you feel like you could call upon a representation of him to support you? (Sandy nods). And your kids, could they do that with each of you? (Sandy nods.) That's our goal, that's what we wish for and strive for, not to be ever-present physically but emotionally. . . . (Sandy nods.) And she's not trusting yet, but your honesty will help her to build trust.

Exercise 10.16: Integration and Summary Statements

Write a reflection/summary statement that captures the process to date based on the information and transcripts of Sandy's engagement in therapy to date. What would you say to her? Write out your response and, as possible, share your response with a colleague.

____

____

____

____

In Stage 1 of EFIT, as clients move toward stabilization (the end of stage 1 and into the stage 2 process), clients gain increased awareness of their triggers and coping responses and the ways their automatic (previously adaptive) coping responses have left them stuck in their current circumstances and have been barriers to growth and new more positive relational experiences. With this newfound awareness, clients can begin to more fully enter into engaged encounters with key others who have either been instrumental in shaping their models of self and other or who can be allies in the Stage 2 therapy process (e.g., the therapist, an imaginal other, a key attachment figure). At this point, clients demonstrate improved emotional balance (are more able to manage stress with less numbing/avoidance or reactivity) and are more able to engage in exploration with self and others. That is, they are moving toward increased accessibility, responsiveness, and engagement—the central defining feature of a secure attachment. Their models of self and other are more accessible, there is increased flexibility, and there is movement toward increased self-acceptance and compassion.

Exercise 10.17. Markers of Stage 1

The markers of stabilization/Stage 1 markers include all *but* which of the following? Identify the incorrect marker.

a. Increased awareness (e.g., of fears, vulnerabilities and longings)
b. Increased awareness of patterns in key encounters with significant others, as well as increased capacity to enter into engaged encounters with others
c. Greater emotional balance (less numb or reactive)
d. Improved exploration (accessibility/openness, responsiveness, and engagement) with self and key others
e. Movement toward greater self-acceptance and compassion
f. More access to, increased flexibility, models of self and other
g. Improved capacity to challenge maladaptive thinking patterns through cognitive restructuring

Exercise 10.18. Client Outcomes in Stage 1

As the therapeutic process in Stage 1 unfolds, we can expect Sandy to demonstrate all of the following *except* (Select the answer that goes beyond stabilization.)

a. A better understanding of circumstances that trigger her.
b. A better understanding of the underlying meaning including her typical response.
c. Greater emotional balance.

d. Resolution of personal blocks and shame responses.
e. Increased empathy and self-compassion.
f. Greater understanding of the way echoes of trauma and prototypical responses/action tendencies impact current relationships.

Stage 2: Working Through Trauma and Restructuring Self and System

Throughout Stage 2, the EFT therapist actively and directly moves toward accessing and modifying Sandy's model of self and other by choreographing additional encounters, at deeper levels of experiencing, with her younger, more vulnerable self. As the therapist continues to join older, wiser Sandy in her childhood bedroom, encounters are choreographed with the goal of facilitating more compassion from older Sandy and gradually opening younger Sandy up to taking that in and accepting and internalizing that compassion from her older self (and, by extension, from the witnessing and supportive therapist). The therapist's focus in Stage 2 is to support the client in moving into deeper levels of experiencing, that is, Level 4 or above on the Experiencing Scale (Klein et al., 1969), for longer periods, leading to productive experiencing (i.e., shifts in models of self and other). For further discussion of the EFT process and the Experiencing Scale, see Johnson (2019, p. 50).

Clinical Example. At one point in the Stage 2 EFIT process, Sandy recalled an incident of childhood sexual abuse. She reported that it had been bothering her and had been a recurring theme over the past two weeks. She described it as being unattached to any emotion and as connected to many other related images and memories. For the most part, however, she explained, she was unwilling to engage with any of the memories, including the most frequently recurring memory.

With attention to principles outlined (e.g., therapeutic pacing, Sandy's current window of tolerance with respect to any family or other stressors), the therapist helped Sandy to first describe the memory, then enter the related "scene" as a means of allowing her to feel and move through the emotion that she could not have possibly felt and experienced during that actual childhood time of intolerable threat, when she was alone and defenseless in the face of trauma. Instead, at that time, her best recourse was to freeze, go numb, shut down. The therapist takes Sandy back in the scene with her "older, wiser self" at her side with the therapist in close proximity, tracking and attuned, and holding space and safety, with high doses of RISSSC. Sandy was able to allow herself to fully feel and work through this traumatic incident, which was representative of other traumatic experiences involving violation. This "corrective emotional experience" allowed Sandy to liberate herself from the weight of the unprocessed emotion/trauma that she had been carrying, all alone, for so many years. Sandy's discovery and deep emotional processing were indications of her increased capacity to protect (and be protected by) and to give (and take in) the love of another as "older, wiser Sandy" led her "younger self" away from this toxic, damaging scene, and the two innocently and tranquilly walked down a rural secluded road toward home, her arm draped over her "younger self," with the dust of the road kicking up behind them.

Sandy's window of tolerance had expanded, her models of self and other were now open to revision, and various signs of greater self-cohesion, coherence, and confidence emerged in the sessions that followed. In session and at home, she had indications of increased emotional balance and capacity to love and be loved. Sandy spoke of increased closeness with her partner, of increased capacity to manage everyday stressors without resorting to uncontrollable anger and rage, and, although she still experienced those "dark spaces" at times, she described them as less frequent and more short-lived. As the therapist continued to choreograph various encounters (Move 3 of the Tango) within session, and as Sandy continued to gain greater flexibility with her previously automatic responses and began to respond to triggers with increased vulnerability (rather than reactive anger), key others in her life similarly responded to her differently. Rather than shrinking and retreating from her earlier angry responses to feeling dismissed, for instance, her husband reached back with compassion when she described feeling hurt and alone during times of threat or stress. Similarly, as she responded to her children from a softer place, with the same clear rationale and moral compass she had always upheld, they more easily and readily responded to what she was saying and began to internalize the values she was imparting.

In summary, as the reshaping of self and other continued to evolve both within and between sessions, various elements of change became apparent. These key elements of change have been identified based on numerous studies with distressed couples (see also Johnson, 2019). The microelements associated with EFT change events are as follows:

- Active engagement with vulnerabilities and needs
- Asserts personal needs coherently and directly
- Able to receive comfort and affirmation from a supportive other
- Able to give attuned support to another

Exercise 10.19. Micro Elements of Change in EFT Stage 2

In what ways does the Stage 2 clinical example illustrate the microelements highlighted here? Identify each of the elements evident in Sandy's experience.

a. There are indications of greater attunement both within and between sessions (with her younger self and with her family).
b. There are indications of increased capacity to take in the care and love of others (again, both within the session, with her younger self, and outside sessions, with her family).
c. Sandy is more able to actively engage with her vulnerability and needs, express them directly, and inhabit a "softer self" with her family.
d. All of the above

EFIT Stage 3: Consolidation

The Stage 3 process across all modalities is focused on consolidating and integrating the therapeutic gains that have been made over the course of EFT treatment. In EFIT, individual clients gain greater access to and awareness of the strategies that have "protected" but "imprisoned" them and are able to unlatch from what were reflexive and automatic strategies under conditions of stress or perceived threat or danger. They are able to gain a greater sense of agency/choice. What were rigid responses now become more flexible. What was a scattered narrative, filled with gaps and uncertainties, now has more structure and coherence. The echoes of trauma that once trapped them are now better understood in the context of their life history and framed as a means of survival, when they had no other choice rather than a source of shame or self-loathing.

At the stage of consolidation, clients are better able to see themselves and others differently, from a position of greater self-coherence, awareness, and competence. During times of stress or when faced with threat or danger, though initially put off balance, they become more able to regain emotional balance, problem solve, and seek and accept the support of others. With revised working models and an expanded capacity to use emotion as a compass, by this stage of therapy, moreover, clients are better able to use this compass to guide everyday problem solving, as well as face more significant decisions and/or existential dilemmas surrounding loss and love. By this stage, clients have moved beyond symptom reduction and improved coping; they are now able to engage with themselves and their emotional worlds and with those who matter most in ways that allow them to live fully and to continue to grow from their experiences.

Consolidation with a trauma focus includes focusing on the clients' vulnerabilities and traumatic histories in cases of developmental trauma and/or the cumulative impact of multiple exposures such as in the case of first responders or military personnel. Triggers that impacted them at the outset of therapy, such as the anniversary of specific traumatic events (e.g., witnessing the traumatic loss of a loved one in a motor vehicle collision or a friend in combat), will often still persist. At the conclusion of therapy, however, now with a felt sense of security in self and others, clients will tend to be more able to manage and "get in front of" the triggers (e.g., anniversaries) that previously immobilized them or crippled them with heightened anxiety and hyperarousal. Such individuals also are more likely to return for additional sessions at other key developmental transitions or during periods of stress or new trauma exposure against this backdrop of a positive therapeutic outcome and with increased attachment security. In summary, with clients' capacity to grow now unleashed and their belief in humanity now renewed, individuals with trauma histories become able to face the challenges of life with more resilience. Their histories and associated vulnerabilities still present, future possibilities nevertheless appear brighter, as their capacity to risk, explore, and thrive increases and as the grip of past traumatic experiences loosens, and associated impacts fade further into the background.

SUMMARY

In this chapter, we have focused on how to address the echoes of trauma in the context of individual therapy. In addition to focusing specifically on understanding the impacts of trauma from an attachment perspective, the chapter included an overview of some of the key considerations that bear upon clinical assessment and case conceptualization, as well as treatment planning. Readers are encouraged to not only review this workbook chapter but also engage in further study through readings (such as those suggested later), online and other specialized trainings and conferences, and the review and study of various training tapes and related educational materials.

The clinical example (Sandy) used in this chapter includes excerpts from a related training resource/DVD set featuring Drs. Susan M. Johnson and T. Leanne Campbell. The resource is titled *EFIT—Creating Core Change in Emotionally Focused Individual Therapy* and is available through the International Centre for Excellence in EFT. Other related resources are available through www.eftvancouverisland.com.

ANSWERS AND SUGGESTED RESPONSES

Exercise 10.1 Trauma Through an Attachment Lens

Answer: Model of self, model of other, affect regulation strategies

Exercise 10.2. Affect Regulation

Answer: Anxiety and avoidance

Exercise 10.3. Attachment Resource

Answer: Secure base

Exercise 10.4. Type of Trauma

Answer: B. Complex trauma

Exercise 10.5. Resiliency Factors

Answer: Both **C** and **D**.

Exercise 10.6. EFIT Session Goals

Answer: All answers are correct.

Exercise 10.7. Instilling Hope and Trust in the EFIT Process

Answer: D. Providing clients with a "felt experience" and then providing a "more cognitive" frame for that experience, including congratulating them and helping them to see how they arrived at that "felt experience" (Move 5 of the Tango) provides them with an opportunity to consolidate such gains in session and, over time, creates such "felt experiences" outside of session.

Exercise 10.8. Summarizing the Session

Suggested Therapist Summary: "So Sandy, the thing I hear you saying . . . is that . . . those childhood experiences shaped your future in various ways . . . in terms of the way that you felt about yourself . . . and the way that you've related with others . . . and the way that you've felt able to assert yourself with others . . . not always, but at various times . . . but your resilience has been your work ethic . . . and your intellect . . . your great ability to articulate yourself . . . and sometimes it works, and sometimes it doesn't . . . but in any case . . . nothing has fully allowed you to move on . . . from some of those poignant experiences . . . and I recognize that today . . . we focused on one of those incidents, and the way that it works is we don't have to necessarily address every one of those incidents . . . but enough that you have control of them rather than them of you . . . and enough that . . . that beautiful younger Sandy is not just an image from the past that you can connect with . . . but eventually, she becomes more and more a part of you . . . and things feel more whole and coherent and complete . . . and slowly . . . she's able to appreciate and enjoy . . . and find refuge . . . in the arms of [your husband] and others . . . that surround you . . . as much as parts of you do now . . . I get . . . that some of you does, at times . . . and that it's not always sustainable . . . is that it? Am getting it right?"

Exercise 10.9. Maintaining Balance in the Face of Protest

Suggested Therapist Responses

1. Validate Sandy's experience given her history of being unable to rely on others and her lack of progress in spite of working hard in other therapies at other times over the years.
2. Stay close to the therapeutic process and highlight any gains that have been made, contrasting her typical means of coping (with stoicism and her verbal capacity) with times that she has allowed herself to be vulnerable and make contact with that younger part of herself, whose only recourse was to retreat and hide.

Exercise 10.10. Managing a Disruptive Emotional Moment

Answer: A, B, and D

Exercise 10.11. Strategies for Recurring Shame and Self-Blame

Answer: E

Exercise 10.12. Therapist In-Session and Process Focus

Suggested responses to focus on the process/present moment:

1. In response to Sandy suggestion that she suffered a setback due to her angry response, the therapist does not try to talk Sandy out of her thoughts or encourage her to challenge them but instead again provides her with a historical/childhood context for understanding the automaticity of her responses.
2. The therapist conveys the expectation that the process is not likely to be linear but rather bumpy.
3. Even when Sandy shows some resistance in responding to the therapist's interventions, the therapist remains focused, and attempts to turn Sandy's attention to her younger more vulnerable self as a means of containing self-contempt and facilitating access to deeper more vulnerable emotions and compassion for self.

Exercise 10.13. Assembling Emotion

Answer: Possible Responses to assembling Sandy's experience

Trigger: feeling dismissed or unimportant
Basic Perception: helplessness and lack of control
Bodily Response: tightness

Meaning Making: "I am alone"; "I don't matter"; "I have no impact/no respect"; "I can't count on anyone."

Action Tendency: shut down/retreat and/or argue and lecture/get angry

Exercise 10.14. Deepening Emotions and Shaping Encounters

Answer: D. The cognitive and content focus would be less effective in helping Sandy gain a deeper experience of the encounter.

Exercise 10.15. Processing the Encounter

Answer: Some possible themes to highlight include:

1. The therapist now moves Sandy away from her body/felt sense by posing questions that allow her to begin to cognitively process what has happened, e.g., "What that was it like when . . . ? What happened in the moment when?" The therapist joins Sandy in reflecting upon and making sense of the therapeutic process.
2. Level of impact, i.e., how much was younger Sandy able to take in older Sandy's bid for contact and connection?
3. The therapist uses "parts language" to highlight that there is a part of younger Sandy that wants to believe/wants to take it in/wants to be liberated from her long-standing prison of isolation, and there is another part (likely larger given the ongoing distance between them) of her that continues to be afraid.
4. In emotionally focused individual therapy (EFIT), at times when clients get stuck or when it is too much to ask Sandy to be the voice of the younger part in this case (again, because the distance between them is still wide), the therapist then speaks for the younger self in an effort to show older Sandy that her efforts were not futile, but instead only partially impactful and that the process is still unfolding.

Exercise 10.16. Integration and Summary Statements

Some of the key elements to include in your summary statement are as follows. Check to see if your summary statement includes

1. Summarize and validate Sandy's stoicism, skepticism, and self-reliance as well as her main attachment strategy for dealing with stress or threat (e.g., to be prone to anger and lecturing vs. directly expressing fear or vulnerability) as adaptive in the context of her childhood and earlier adult history.
2. Contrast Sandy's presentation in the initial session with her presentation at other times in the process (e.g., when she taps into her vulnerability as she engages in an encounter with her younger self).
3. Outline, with specificity and with careful attunement (using Sandy's words and her account of her experience), signs of progress to date (e.g., return to the moment of hope she felt, and what provided that hope early in the therapeutic process).

Exercise 10.17. Markers of Stage 1

Answer: G. Improved capacity to challenge maladaptive thinking patterns through cognitive restructuring

Exercise 10.18. Client Outcomes in Stage 1

Answer: D. The process of working through shame and revising view of self and view of other is the focus of Stage 2.

Exercise 10.19. Micro Elements of Change in EFT Stage 2

Answer: D. All of the above

11

FACING TRAUMA TOGETHER THROUGH EFT

In this chapter, we focus on healing the echoes of trauma, including relationship trauma (i.e., "attachment injuries") in the context of couple therapy. Building on previous chapters, we begin with a brief overview of the potential impacts of trauma and their adverse effects on relationship functioning. Emotionally focused couple therapy (EFCT) practices are explored when working with couples in which trauma is a factor in treatment, and a clinical example is used to illustrate how the emotionally focused therapy (EFT) therapist weaves the impacts of trauma into the couple's interactional cycle in Stage 1. Next, the trauma implications for Stage 2 work are considered following the same clinical example through withdrawer re-engagement. A final section focuses on the impact of attachment injuries on the EFT process and the process for resolving these injuries and final comments pertain to the EFT consolidation stage (Stage 3).

THE IMPACTS OF TRAUMA ON RELATIONSHIP FUNCTIONING

In the previous chapter, we reviewed the shaping impact of trauma on attachment strategies and mental health outcomes and the potential buffering resource of secure attachment to trauma's impact. Here we review the relational impacts of trauma from an attachment perspective, noting specifically how a client's capacities to interact and authentically connect with others can become severely restricted. Specifically, in the wake of trauma, individuals' self-perceptions and trust in others risk being colored by self-blame and self-criticism, social mistrust, and in some cases deep disillusionment surrounding humanity in general. The presence of "protective" strategies, which may have previously served the adaptive purpose of helping to shield them from the full onslaught of trauma-related distress, now become a "prison" of loneliness and isolation within a couple relationship. Trapped in the rigidity of negative models of self and other, and crippled by a narrowed capacity to order and make sense of their emotional experiences individuals with trauma histories frequently struggle to reach to and rely on their partner and struggle to hear and take in their partner's acceptance and care.

Guided by this sort of pervasively negative internal compass, the repetitive blocks to connection often amplify earlier experiences of being essentially alone in the world. In cases involving complex or developmental trauma, the sense of self is often damaged and infused with shame and self-denigration. Clients frequently say they do not know themselves and that their internal experiences seem distant and foreign. There is an inability to organize or regulate their own bodies or their emotional lives. They are blocked—from

DOI: 10.4324/9781003039457-14

themselves and from connection. In some of these cases, a long-standing reliance on more primitive coping strategies (e.g., numbing, dissociation, and other even more overtly destructive means of coping, such as substance abuse and infidelity) lead to disappointments, scars, and attachment injuries in their key relationships, the very relationships that also hold the capacity to attenuate the long-term impacts of trauma. In short, the absence of a secure base of attachment tends to perpetuate the impacts of trauma and prevents healing, both personally and interpersonally. A secure attachment relationship, on the other hand, is the natural healing arena for the wounds of trauma.

Exercise 11.1. Consequences of Trauma in a Couple's Relationship

Identify the possible relational impacts of trauma on a couple's relationship.

a. Self-protective strategies lead to isolation and loneliness _______
b. Difficulty in knowing personal experience and expressing needs _______
c. Pervasive negative view of self and enduring shame _______
d. Struggles to regulate emotional experience with partner _______
e. Increased likelihood of attachment injuries _______
f. Absence of relationship resources for trust and support _______

Working With Trauma and Couples in Stage 1

If secure attachment represents the natural antidote for the wounds of trauma, then it follows that, whenever possible, inclusion of a potentially reliable and trustworthy significant other in the therapeutic process is desirable. How best to do this? First, against the backdrop of previous chapters, we recognize the essential role of assessment in couple therapy, including special considerations with couples in which one or both partners have a trauma history. Next, a case example will be used to illustrate the effective use of EFT in using the relationship as a resource in healing trauma while also strengthening the relationship bond, allowing for greater resilience both personally and relationally and a wider window of tolerance as therapy progress.

Many of the same principles and challenges described in working with individuals are relevant with couple treatment. For instance, the EFT therapist can expect the therapeutic alliance to be more sensitive to rupture. Similarly, although assessment is always important in EFT, once again, it becomes critical when echoes of trauma shape either (or both) partner's personal history and/or if the relationship is characterized by a history of one or more attachment injuries. Therapeutic pacing and various clinical decisions are guided by initial and ongoing assessment of a partner's capacity for affect regulation and possible contraindications, including vulnerability to substance use disorders and domestic violence, as well as the capacity of the relationship to manage challenging what might be a well-established and long-standing cycle of distress. At minimum, the EFT therapist needs to provide emotional and physical safety in the session and work with couples to generate curiosity and some level of increased openness and engagement without heightening the risk of additional trauma and/or the exacerbation of trauma between sessions.

Given that the echoes of trauma tend to prime and exacerbate the negative cycle between partners, regulating and transforming emotion and shaping corrective interactions with significant others in EFT is likely to be more difficult when one or both partner(s) have trauma histories. As such, therapists can expect the course of therapy to be longer (e.g., 30 sessions) and can anticipate more setbacks along the way. It also is likely that there will be greater need for affect containment through therapist validation, accurate reflection, and slowing pacing, particularly important at the outset of treatment and in cases involving developmental or complex trauma. Education about traumatic stress and how it impacts relationships can be helpful for clients, and consultation with other therapists who may be providing individual psychotherapy provides useful guidance in the EFT couple therapy process.

The impacts of trauma can be considered on a continuum, and issues of flexibility and capacity are paramount concerns. Secure attachment is associated with greater capacity for flexibility and adaptation, allowing the individual to live fully and to grow from new experiences. Attachment strategies characterized by anxiety, avoidance, or a mixed combination, on the other hand, might be restrictive depending on the client's capacity to adapt. As viewed on a continuum, clients' reactions might range from being highly automatic, rigid, and reflexive (akin to a "narrow window of tolerance") to more flexible and adaptive. In cases in which healthy development was thwarted by trauma early on (e.g., chronic childhood abuse in the absence of any secure connection or support), more rigid and negative models of self and other would be anticipated, as well as more automatic and reflexive affect regulation strategies. Also relevant in couple therapy is the rigidity of the relationship cycle of distress, which can be seen continuously from very rigid and automatic in highly escalated couples to more flexible and adaptive in more securely attached partnerships. To summarize, in EFCT, the therapist assesses each partner's personal resources (e.g., self and coping resources, affect regulation capacity/window of tolerance), as well as the relationship resources (e.g., Is the couple isolated, or do they have significant social support? How rigid is the negative interactional cycle? Do one or both partners have a trauma history, and, if yes, what are the impacts relationally? Can either partner be a resource to the other at this time? Is the relationship history also marked by trauma (i.e., attachment injury) and, if yes, has the trauma been resolved?).

Exercise 11.2. Trauma and Couple Therapy Assessment

Identify three questions or topics you would give attention to in the assessment of a couple facing the impact of trauma in their relationship.

Focus or Question 1.

____

____

Focus or Question 2.

____

____

Focus or Question 3.

____

____

As in EFIT, the therapist's pacing is crucial in working emotionally with couples dealing with the echoes of trauma. Along with the CARE model (**c**ontext, **a**ttachment, **r**elationship, **e**motion; see Chapter 10), assessment variables such as those highlighted earlier guide case conceptualization, clinical decision making (e.g., is individual psychotherapy concurrent to couple therapy recommended?), and therapeutic pacing. Inevitably, for those who have endured interpersonal trauma, especially chronic childhood abuse at the hands of a parent or caregiver, attachment strategies will come alive in the therapy room and need to be addressed with attention to pacing, that is, with attention to the "therapeutic window/window of tolerance" such that interventions are paced with the aim of challenging but not overwhelming the resources of either the partners or the relationship. Throughout the therapeutic process, interventions will be titrated with attention to the partners' and the couple's window of tolerance. At times, the focus will be on heightening emotion, and at other times containment will be needed (especially with highly escalated couples, particularly in Stage 1) with the goal of stabilization/de-escalation and with the byproduct being a stronger therapeutic alliance and increased safety in the session and within the relationship.

Reflection/summary statements provide an effective and purposeful means of slowing negative down interactions, empathically holding and containing emotion or deepening underlying feelings, and seizing therapeutic opportunities for education and/or consolidation. In the initial phase of Stage 1, for example, as the therapist summarizes the therapeutic process, educational components can be woven into summary statements, allowing for increased understanding of the impact of trauma both personally and relationally and the means by which EFCT will continue to address such echoes. The following clinical example illustrates how the EFT therapist contextualizes the impact of trauma in the couple's negative cycle.

Exercise 11.3. Summary Statements and Psychoeducation

Use the following clinical example to identify examples of the therapist validating and providing educational support. Underline the key educational components in this example of a therapist's summary statement.

Clinical Example. After a number of years of individual and group psychotherapy, as well as successful treatment of various addictions (i.e., alcohol, drugs, pornography), Randy invited his wife Karen to engage in a course of couple therapy with an EFT therapist. Guided by attachment theory and by the EFT roadmap, following the assessment phase and with a solid alliance established (Step 1), the EFT therapist identified the classic pursue/withdraw cycle of distress (Step 2), as well as the personal and relational contexts in which it evolved. Here, the EFT therapist summarizes the cycle while also weaving in key elements of Randy's trauma history and its impact on the couple's relationship.

Therapist: It makes sense, Randy. What I hear you say, and what we commonly see with others who have come from difficult home environments, is that when you were a little boy, there was no choice but to shut down and hide during times of danger. There was no safety to speak up and no space for your feelings. It was adaptive to shut down and to build a wall to "shield" yourself . . . and what also happens, over time, and especially when there is no refuge, is that the wall that protected you as a little boy becomes an automatic response during difficult times. So when you get any hint of disapproval or criticism or when people that matter to you show any signs of frustration, your "natural" reaction, your "visceral" response, is to pull away or hide or shut down . . . but the problem with that in this relationship, in the relationship that matters most, is that the strategy that protected you as a little boy is the one that also keeps you from getting close to Karen, to your beautiful wife . . . and Karen's experience of your wall, though she understands why it was so important when you were little is to feel shut out and alone. When she reaches to you (and although she also understands that she hasn't always reached in the best ways) and you turn away, she feels rejected. Not being allowed to be close to you is painful for her. She feels like she is not important and that there is no space for her.

Working With Trauma With Couples in Stage 2

As Karen and Randy moved through the first stage of EFT (de-escalation/stabilization), they were able to acknowledge their pursue and withdraw positions and the underlying feelings associated with those positions in their negative cycle. As a couple, they were increasingly able to understand how the echoes of Randy's traumatic history had impacted their relationship over the years. Specifically, Randy's childhood experience of physical and emotional abuse, abandonment, and peer rejection and bullying in adolescence impacted his limited capacity to believe in himself and trust others, including Karen. The gridlock of their marriage's negative cycle often left Karen feeling frustrated and alone, and Randy felt defeated in his ability to give Karen what she needed, which compounded his feelings of shame and unworthiness. Through their work in Stage 1, the couple had a foundation to begin the process of withdrawer engagement and pursuer softening. Provided next is an example of the initial stages of withdrawer engagement with Randy and the ways in which the EFT therapist integrates traumatic experience.

As is commonly the case in working with couples, with trauma in particular, the process of withdrawer engagement happens incrementally, session by session. The EFT therapist observes the moment-to-moment experiencing in the session as the couple is triggered by and reacts to the nuances of their interpersonal cues and missteps that maintain both the relational negative cycle and personal difficulties (e.g., Randy's propensity to rely on numbing and dissociation as a coping strategy). Reflecting such interactional sequences and validating defensive strategies provides increased awareness and helps build trust in the therapeutic process (Tango Move 1). As the therapist observes and accurately and empathically reflects, the opportunity becomes greater for deeper, more primary emotions to emerge.

Once identified and assembled, the goal of Move 2 of the Tango is to further develop, deepen, and distill the primary/deeper emotion. As a curious and empathically attuned observer, the therapist asks questions to illicit greater clarity. When the felt sense has changed, when one partner (in this case, Randy, with his propensity to withdraw) has slowed down, explored, discovered, and shared the deeper emotional experience with the therapist (temporary attachment figure), and the emotion can be felt as distilled and tangible, an enactment/encounter is choreographed (Tango Move 3). The encounter provides a rich opportunity for the couple to connect in a powerfully new and different way ("in the here-and-now") that deviates from the stuck rigidity of the negative cycle (e.g., conflict or withdrawal) and that also challenges and curatively departs from the sorts of automatic, self-protective responses (i.e., shutting down, distancing, avoiding) that tend to emanate from the unresolved reverberations of trauma. Once the new bonding event or "corrective emotional experience" has occurred, it is processed with each of the partners. An illustration of processing the encounter might include the therapist saying:

Therapist: A few moments ago, Randy, when you took the risk of sharing what goes on behind that wall, the way you feel, empty and alone, and in what you describe as your "inner hell, and when you looked into Karen's eyes, what did you feel in your body? In your chest? In your throat? What happened in that moment? What did you feel from her eyes? What did you hear her eyes saying?

Personal Reflection: Imagining Randy's Response

Reflect on your own response. Imagine a moment where you felt empty and alone. How would you respond to each of these questions?

- What did you feel in your body?
- What happened in that moment?

Now imagine you are sharing this with the attention and caring of a loving other. How might you respond to these questions?

- What did you feel from their eyes?
- What did you hear their eyes saying to you?

Finally, imagine if you, like Randy, found sharing vulnerably a significant threat and often did not feel entitled to share these feelings. What would you need most from your therapist in exploring and sharing your experience?

The goal in this moment is to draw Randy's attention specifically and intentionally to his body and to his partner's nonverbal/bodily cues and away from any cognitive appraisals that are likely to be colored by his trauma history and associated expectations based on his negative model of self and other. It is here, in the moment-to-moment processing, that he can begin to both attend to and be guided by his own inner experience and be impacted by the responsiveness of his partner. As the EFT couple therapist takes partners away from their typical ways of interacting and from defensive and automatic coping strategies, new possibilities for relating emerge, and existing, and often long-standing, models of self and other begin to be challenged.

In processing the "enactment/encounter," both Randy and Karen said that they felt closer, and both conveyed a better understanding of the impact that they can have on one another, both positive and negative. As he described his bodily feeling, rather than speaking from a more cognitive and distanced vantage point, Randy told Karen that he experienced a powerful sense of warmth and connection. No longer feeling alone, he could take in and appreciate her welcoming presence. Similarly, Karen felt in that powerful moment that she could experience and deeply sense more of the husband that she had been married to for over 30 years. She could feel him. She could see him. Rather than being let in only "a crack," as had been more common in their previous interactions, Karen felt like Randy had taken the risk of opening the door widely to reveal a fullness that she had rarely if ever seen before. She felt soothed. She felt grateful.

In Tango Move 5, the goal is to integrate and summarize what happened. This is always a key aspect of the therapeutic process and all the more important in working with trauma. Entering, engaging in, and sharing new emotional experiences can be disorienting and destabilizing. As alluded to earlier and similar to what was described in the context of EFIT, reflections/summary statements associated with Tango Move 5 can serve to anchor the couple, as well as the therapist. More important, they can provide a valuable opportunity for consolidation, a sense of predictability and control and ownership of a new and powerful healing experience. When provided toward the end of a session, reflections can include not only a summary of the moment-to-moment processing and interactional sequences in the session (punctuating the final phase, Move 5) but also a summary that again highlights the impacts of trauma on personal and interpersonal functioning and the manner in which the relationship can be used as a resource in both challenging the echoes of trauma (e.g., avoidance and withdrawal) and strengthening the bond between the couple, leading to further trauma resolution and increased resilience.

After making experiential contact with the vulnerability, he felt during a difficult event in his childhood, an event that represented that of many, involving themes of loss, abandonment, and a sense of aloneness during periods of threat or danger, Randy was able to share his vulnerability with wife Karen, and she was able to respond from a place of compassion, authenticity, and accessibility. This time, he was not alone. Initially destabilized by the felt experience within session, by this new encounter, access to a secure base, a safe haven, Randy was bewildered. He wondered aloud, "Is this how it was for you in your childhood? Is this how it could be?" As Karen honestly responded affirmatively, then later followed her response with a reminder that this is what Randy gives to their grandchildren, with ease and sincerity, access to his emotions continued to flood forward as he vacillated between grieving all that "was not" and "has not been" in his childhood and at other times in his life, and cherishing the love he now had access to, in the "here-and-now" in the session. The therapist then moved into Move 5 as a means of both summarizing and closing the session. This transcript excerpt illustrates the final moments of a session representing the initial stage of withdrawer engagement with Randy.

Therapist: I want to give you as much space as you need, but I'm also aware that it's exhausting? Are you okay? You tell me when you're ready.

Randy: I'm fine. I'm okay. I feel comfort, and I feel—I just feel some strength, warmth, love. I feel safe and loved, and I need it. I need it. (still crying)

Therapist: And you deserve it. Absolutely, you deserve it. Yes. And you're taking it in, which is so good. And in so doing, it puts you right back in touch with the sense of loss that of course you would feel, in terms of what you didn't have as a little kid. And you vacillate between cherishing this moment and wanting to hold onto it but then knowing also what's been missing, right? That's the back and forth you're doing, which is perfect. (Randy nods as Karen looks on with compassion as she holds Randy's hand.)

Randy: I feel so good, Karen. It feels good. It really feels good.

Karen: It's okay. Let it out. Do you need a Kleenex?

Randy: No, no. (Karen acknowledges Randy and stays alongside him, looking on with compassion and continuing to hold his hand.)

Randy: I feel so good. I've never experienced this before. It makes me so sad. Why did it have to be that way? I'm just holding on to you. (Randy now clenches Karen's hand more tightly.) Everything you're giving me right now, no one has loved me like that before.

Therapist: Let her hold you. What are you feeling, Karen?

Karen: I feel his pain, but there's also a sensation of being needed. (Therapist nods.) And so that gives me strength.

Therapist: That he'll let you hold him. (Karen nods. Randy also acknowledges permission to continue to bask in this new experience of secure connection.)

Randy: I love that. I love this.

Therapist: Yeah, that's good. You know what, Randy? It's back to what I said earlier, that when you find your way there, then you have more flexibility. It's not going to be perfect, but do you see what happened? Do you see what you did? How you got there? Karen, earlier, do you remember? (Karen nods.) The thing that happened is that Karen said, "Occasionally, that wall, that hole, that whatever it is, can be a teeny bit porous at times, and I can get glimpses of you—I can get glimpses of him." And what you did today, Randy, is you took the risk, of not just taking a glimpse and then going back; you actually took a real leap of faith and allowed yourself to be seen, and felt, and heard. And in so doing, you felt a kind of love, and security, and support, that you said you'd never felt before, right? (Randy nods.) And while that's beautiful and amazing, it also brings you right back in touch with what wasn't and what hasn't been. And there's lots of grieving to do around that. And that's where you guys are now, right? Vacillating between these two things. And it'll be okay. You'll come up for air, over the next week or two, for sure over the weekend. As much as you can live in this space, it'll help you through it. It's going to be profound. I think it already is, and it'll be sustainable. Does that make sense? (They both nod.) And what Karen says is that in those times, not only does she feel needed, I think, but in those moments, Karen, do you feel like you have more than a little glimpse of him?

Karen: Oh, absolutely.

Therapist: Yeah. All of you, right? (Therapist turns to Randy.)

Karen: Yeah, he's all there. Yeah.

Therapist: And that's part of what she's been fighting for and struggling for. She's been patiently, patiently there, waiting for you. And the more that you risked revealing yourself and sharing with her, the more special and important she felt—what a gift you just gave her. You said, I've never, ever, ever, ever, ever felt this way in my life. (Therapist uses soft slow voice to further deepen and hold the experience.) You risked with her, and she was there. That's a beautiful treasure that you have, and share, and have worked toward.

Randy: Yeah. You just break me up when you said, "Never experienced before." Whenever you say that, it just evokes so many emotions.

Therapist: You both did amazing. Beautiful. A gift.

Karen: Is that right? A gift? (Randy nods in agreement.)

SUMMARY COMMENTS

As highlighted, the powerful impact of Karen's care and compassion left Randy vacillating between two contrasting emotional planes—i.e., profoundly cherishing the wonderful connective feelings with Karen on the one hand but also simultaneously being faced with intense grief and loss over how unsafe and alone he felt so often as a child. As Randy flipped back and forth between this joy versus grief, it prominently emerged that he was profoundly drawn toward, and beautifully astonished by, the relational safety and connectivity that he experienced with Karen in the here-and-now in the session. As Randy allowed himself to sit in this elated feeling, he was able to begin to steep himself in, for the first time ever, what it could be like to feel truly safe, comforted, and loved by another.

Building on this momentum, as Randy continues to grieve what he did not have as a young boy and continues to embrace what he has with Karen, models of self and other are transformed, and the impacts of trauma are similarly offset. Additionally, as the couple continues to progress through Stage 2 of the EFCT process, and Randy feels increasingly empowered and competent, more space for Karen and her needs is created. It is at this juncture that relationship traumas/attachment injuries can be addressed. At times, as was the case with this couple, the Attachment Injury Resolution Model (AIRM) represents both a key change event (e.g., withdrawer engagement or pursuer softening) and a means of moving couples toward forgiveness and reconciliation. Provided next is a brief review of the definition of attachment injuries followed by an overview of the AIRM approach. For ease of reference, we refer to this same couple for illustrative purposes.

Addressing Attachment Injuries in Emotionally Focused Couple Therapy

Attachment theory has been called a theory of trauma because it emphasizes the extreme emotional adversity of isolation and separation at moments of vulnerability. Attachment injuries are defined as relationship traumas or wounds that result when one fails to experience the expected availability and support from their partner, especially during a time of vulnerability or crisis. These specific events result in a change in the couple's felt sense of security. Relationship incidents that involved betrayal, deceit, or otherwise breach trust in the relationship may result in an attachment injury. Attachment injuries may appear in therapy in the wake of infidelity or an affair (either recent or remote). They may also commonly appear surrounding other perceived abandonment or betrayal at key moments of prior vulnerability, transition, and/or crisis when the need for support and comfort from the partner was high and perceived to not be forthcoming. Such situations might include miscarriage, life-threatening medical diagnoses, the death of a parent, or immigration to a foreign country.

The impact of these events can be difficult to fully understand without appreciation for the attachment implications of these injuries. Wounded partners use phrases like, "My hurt just didn't matter to him," "You let me down," or "I promised myself, never again—never again—would I let myself need you." These injuries can disorganize attempts to seek comfort and care from a partner who is now both a source of comfort and a source of pain or threat. Couples struggle as defensive relationship patterns are organized by attachment-related fears that have no clear path to resolution. At times, injured partners have trauma-like experiences, including intrusive memories and flashbacks of these events, often alternating between numbing associated feelings and becoming hyper-aroused and accusatory. Subtle echoes of the original wound or any emotional risk can evoke extreme fight or flight responses. These events often shatter assumptions about the safety of their shared emotional world, including their view of their partner, their relationship, and even their own worth and importance.

Couples often have struggled to address the injury and forge some kind of resolution. Attempts may have failed in the past and compounded mistrust and heightened global relationship distress. The offending partner might have attempted to discount, deny, or dismiss the injury, further reinforcing the injured partner's cynicism surrounding token repair attempts or efforts to gloss over a breach of trust. These events are not general hurts; they are compelling wounds that shatter attachment assumptions about the dependability of the other.

Frequently, the attachment injury is disclosed at the outset of therapy (e.g., in the case of a recently disclosed affair). The impact of the injury must be addressed and understood in the context of the relationship history and negative interactional cycle in this initial phase of therapy. Attachment injuries arise very compellingly at moments of potential risk, especially in the second stage of EFT, when partners are asked to reach for the other, confide needs and fears, and put themselves in the hands of the other. In Stage 2, the couple has a platform of increased safety, awareness, and accountability such that the injury can be fully worked through, and healing and reconciliation are attainable. The EFT therapist's role is to foster forgiveness and reconciliation around these wounds so that trust can be re-established and the emotional reconnection that occurs in change events in Stage 2 of EFT can be propelled forward and/or completed through the resolution of an injury. Preliminary research tells us that if the EFT therapist works with and resolves these injuries, then the couple is able to create a powerful forgiveness event and go on to create a more secure bond (Makinen, & Johnson, 2006; Halchuk, Makinen, & Johnson, 2010).

Exercise 11.4. Defining an Attachment Injury

Which of the following statements are descriptive of attachment injuries? (Check all that apply.)

a. They are potential bonding moments, when attachment needs are tangible, yet turn into a nightmare of finding oneself alone, helpless, and desperate. ____
b. They are instances of general hurt and a reflection of a general lack of trust. ____
c. They are disappointments and are the primary cause of marital distress. ____
d. They are specific events that shatter attachment assumptions and plunge a vulnerable spouse into isolation and helplessness. ____
e. They are moments of abandonment, when a spouse fails to respond at a moment of urgent need. ____
f. They are not defined by a set of content features but by their attachment significance. ____
g. These injuries shatter a basic sense of trust and block relationship repair. ____

Exercise 11.5. Trauma-Related Symptoms

When these events arise in the therapy process, they remind the therapist of the symptoms of post-traumatic stress in the following way: (Check all that apply.)

a. The injured spouse reports flashbacks or intrusive memories and ruminates on the injurious event. They cannot "let it go." ____
b. The injured spouse appears disorganized. She or he flips between clinging to and distancing the other, since the other is paradoxically both the potential solution to and source of fear. ____
c. The injured spouse, especially when there is a potentially risky engagement with the other, numbs out and avoids the risk. ____
d. The injured spouse avoids any situation when he or she is "in the hands" of the other. ____
e. The injured spouse shows exaggerated sensitivity and hypervigilance for any further signs of abandonment and betrayal. ____

Exercise 11.6. Attachment Injury Statements

Identify the attachment injury statements.

a. "You are always saying hurtful things. You just brush me off. I feel hopeless." ____
b. "And then, as I told you the diagnosis—the 'sentence'—you got all cold. You just stepped away and said, 'Oh don't panic. It will be okay.' And then you ignored me, focused on all the details of the tests and how to arrange them. I was alone." ____
c. "You drove me to the hospital. I was in labor. And you left me there. I asked you to hold me, but you didn't. You asked how long it would be, and then you left, to finalize that so-important deal. And I had the baby by myself. Something shut down in me that night. And we have never been able to talk about it. Something is still bitter—hopeless. I gave up on us." ____
d. "'Never again,' I said. Not after that time when our little one was so ill—never again would I count on you. And I never have." (Becomes very still, quiet, and distant.) "I thought he was dying." (Voice becomes hard and fast.) "But we have worked together. We made it—sort of." ____

Attachment Injury Resolution Model

The process of resolving an attachment injury in EFT has been delineated and empirically supported through the study of successful resolution events (see Makinen & Johnson, 2006; Zuccarini, Johnson, Dalgleish, & Makinen, 2013). In brief, the AIRM process follows a set of steps that directs the focus of the EFT therapist in working through the relational impact of the injury and guiding couples toward repair and re-engagement of a trusting bond. These steps begin with a focus on the impact of the injury and proceed to processing the attachment significance of the injury and related losses. This enables a more complete expression of remorse and apology. The process concludes with new risk of vulnerability from the injured partner met with an effective and available response from the offending partner.

Steps in the Attachment Injury Resolution Model (AIRM)
(*Zuccarini, Johnson, Dalgleish, & Makinen, 2013*)

Impact of the Injury

1. Injured partner (IP) describes the incident in which he or she experienced a violation of trust that damaged his or her belief in the relationship.
2. Offending partner (OP) discounts, denies, or minimizes the incident and his or her partner's pain and moves into a defensive stance.

Differentiation of Affect: Attachment Significance of the Injury

3. IP stays in touch with the injury and begins to articulate its impact and attachment significance.
4. OP begins to hear and understand the significance of the injurious event.

Re-engagement: Vulnerably Sharing Impact and Owning Responsibility

5. IP tentatively moves toward a more integrated articulation of the injury and allows the other to witness his or her vulnerability by expressing grief at the broken trust and fear concerning the specific loss of the attachment bond.
6. OP becomes more emotionally engaged and acknowledges responsibility for his or her part and expresses empathy, regret, and remorse.

Forgiveness and Reconciliation

7. IP then risks asking for comfort and caring that was unavailable at the time of the injury.
8. OP responds in a caring manner that acts as an antidote to the traumatic experience.

Clinical Example. Returning to the example of Randy and Karen, through a focus on withdrawer re-engagement, Randy was better able to face his shame and find new ways to be more responsive to Karen. As Randy moved through the withdrawer re-engagement process and showed signs of accessibility, Karen was able to come forward and open up about her own enduring attachment injury surrounding infidelity within the marital relationship. Over the years, she had disavowed her needs in the relationship (as she had at other times in her life in other relationships) and had struggled with feeling alone and undesirable.

Next we follow the AIRM process as the therapist guides Karen through expressing the impact of Randy's breach of trust while also acknowledging the impact on their relationship at a fundamental attachment level. In turn, we see Randy's struggle to respond to the impact of his actions, honor and own the pain he caused, and offer remorse and a heartfelt apology for his actions. This example concludes with Karen's reach for support and Randy's accepting response.

Exploring the Impact of the Injury

Initially, the therapist must balance a focus on processing the account of the injury and its impact for the injured and offending partner. These sessions may be challenging for the therapist as the intensity and emotional impact of the injury may heighten reactivity between partners, and volatile emotions may be difficult for partners and therapist alike to manage. The therapist will work with these reactive moments by tracking and reflecting the partner's surface emotions and actions, while validating the different emotional realities each partner is responding to in the present moment. In the following transcript, the therapist guides each partner to face the impact of the injury as Karen recalls a moment that brings the impact of the injury to light.

Karen: I just get this sick feeling in my stomach that something is wrong. He comes through the door and "Where have you been? . . . "Oh, I was buying you a Christmas present" . . . "Well, the stores closed several hours ago, so then what did you do?" and then I become the interrogator . . . I'm looking for something I don't want to find. . . .

Therapist: Karen, as you talk about this, do you have that sick feeling now, in this room, in your body?

Karen: Oh, it comes back . . . yeah. . . .

Therapist: I know it's hard, but if you could focus on it, could you focus on it, let it grow, stay with it, stay still with that feeling in your stomach?

Karen: I'm so used to pushing it down.

Therapist: It is helpful to be back in the moment.

Karen: It was a long time ago, but I still get that feeling every once in a while when I don't know where he is. . . . I can hardly even breathe. . . .

Therapist: Karen, are you able to share with Randy now, in his eyes, that sick feeling, that feeling in your body, and if you can just let it speak—uncensored.

Karen: I don't know how to speak uncensored about it, actually, but I'll try.

Therapist: Well, you could just speak from your body, try to just let your body speak, let your body say what it hasn't been able to fully say.

Karen: In that moment, I can hardly breathe. I feel like I'm going to throw up. I'm overcome with fear, fear that something horrible is about to happen and I'm powerless, absolutely powerless, and it's going to hurt, not just me but my whole family, my children.

Therapist: It's good to breathe (turning to Karen). Randy, are you able to share, from your eyes, what you feel from her body? What happens inside of you, if your body could speak back to her, what would your body say? . . . as you take in her tears? (soft, slow voice)

Randy: I'm feeling your pain. I did to you . . . I became the monster that my father was. I did this to you.

Karen: (Now sobbing and her voice intense, here the impact of the injury is felt and coherently expressed at a deep level of experiencing.) How could you do that?! How could you do that to me?! And to us?!

As the session continues, the therapist supports both Karen and Randy as they walk through this painfully difficult moment when the injury is given voice. Commonly, the intensity and direct expression of pain trigger the offending partner's withdrawal or minimization. In this moment, Randy initially responds with empathy but then moves to shame and ultimately freezes. He goes "blank." The therapist supports Randy in staying present and grounded in this specific moment.

Randy: Karen, the thing that I want to say here is . . . oh man . . . I've gone blank here . . . how could I do that? I've just . . . I've gone blank here. . . .

Therapist: That's okay. Karen, in the moment when you shared so beautifully and Randy turned to you and touched you, did you feel seen and heard and felt in that moment . . . in your body, not in your brain because, of course, your history and your experience is going to tell you not to trust, but I trust your body, we trust your body, what did your body feel in that moment?

Karen: I don't know.

Therapist: Did you feel held? When he hugged you, did you feel held?

Karen: I felt held, but I also felt "make it stop," but that might be in my own head.

Karen's mistrust is normalized and validated even as Randy struggles to be present to her pain. The therapist highlights Randy's responsiveness and attempts to respond as he struggles to send a clear and coherent supportive response. The AIRM guides the therapist to lean into Karen's uncertainty as a manifestation of the injury's impact on the couple's attachment bond and support Randy in remaining present to the injury.

Exercise 11.7. Exploring the Injury Impact

Which of the following therapist actions focus on exploring the impact of the injury event? Mark the two therapist actions focusing on the injury.

a. The therapist reflects the negative cycle and its attachment significance. ____
b. The therapist creates an enactment in which the injured person tells the other how hurt he/she is. ____
c. The therapist helps a partner stay in touch with a compelling emotional reaction that captures a relationship trauma and begin to articulate its impact and its attachment significance. ____
d. The therapist confronts the partner about their betrayal of the injured spouse. ____
e. The therapist helps the other partner hear and acknowledge the injured partner's pain and see it in attachment terms—as a reflection of the injured partner's need for caring. ____

Differentiating Affect and Attachment Significance

As the couple is better able to organize their experience of the injury, partners are more able to explore the attachment significance of the injury. Deeper themes of hurt, loss, and fear enable the couple to more fully face the loss of trust and form a common understanding of not only what happened but also how this happened to them. This shared story provides a platform for the couple to face the injury together, fully acknowledging and making sense of the impact of the injury on the injured partner and the bond they share. Through this process, the therapist uses more evocative interventions (e.g., heightening, empathic conjecture, and evocative questions) to access and expand attachment related-affect associated with each partner's view of self and other. The therapist helps the couple face the shattered assumptions and confidence about the trust and security in the relationship, also developing a shared narrative for the injury and its relationship to the couple's relationship history.

Clinical Example. The session continues as Karen makes sense of the attachment significance of the injury including her ability to receive genuine reassurance and comfort from Randy. The therapist supports Randy's ability to focus on the relationship impact and demonstrate his understanding of the impact of the injury on the relationship and Karen. Specifically, earlier in this session, Karen described various ways that Randy's infidelity and lack of affection and interest only added to her sense of insecurity as a romantic partner and maintained her long-standing view of herself as a "caregiver" (messages she had received in childhood and that were reinforced in her vocation as a care provider). At the time of this attachment injury, she resolved to stay in the relationship for the sake of her family and was resigned to self-sufficiency and to never fully trust again. The following years of marriage provided additional evidence of her fate as Randy continued to struggle with various addictions and betrayals of trust accumulated.

Karen: Make this history, this pain stop. . . . I don't know if I can trust. I feel like his hug was genuine, but I've been fooled—I've been fooled so many times. I am so embarrassed to tell you how many times I've been fooled.

Randy: I know, without you, I wouldn't be here today. What I want to say is that it seems like there were two people. I fell in love with you because you were—you are—a wonderful, beautiful lady. When I first saw you, I fell in love with you. I was always remorseful after (various incidents of betrayal), but I could never escape what was in me. I was always fighting good and bad all my life, but I was living with some terrible feelings, very, very bad feelings, and I hate them, I hate them (voice intense and crying)—they're a curse, and no matter how I tried, I always lived with them, and I created you the same way, I created the fear in you, the "can't depend on anybody," "can't trust anybody." I'm so sorry for what I did to you. I can hardly live with myself for doing that to you (sobbing) . . . it is awful. . . .

Therapist: Karen, you can let yourself cry . . . it'd be good.

Together the couple and therapist walk through Karen's uncertainty and Randy's attempts to reassure, show remorse, and stay present to Karen's struggle to trust. As Randy shares his deep pain and remorse powerfully and authentically and how profoundly sorry he is for the hurt and damage that he has caused Karen, Karen tearfully listens. As the therapist holds and supports both partners, Karen's fear and wariness are validated while the therapist introduces the notion of allowing her body, in this moment, "in the here-and-now" to be the relied-upon barometer of trust. Initially, Karen struggles to respond. As the therapist keeps her focused on her bodily felt experience, tracking, reflecting, and validating, Randy then shares more deeply, powerfully, and authentically how sorry he is for the damage he has caused to Karen. As Randy acknowledges the ways in which he has instilled fear and mistrust in Karen, the same fear and mistrust his father instilled in him, there is opportunity for Karen to feel seen and heard, for her needs to matter—for Karen to matter. Focused on her felt experience in the moment, Karen is able to express that she can feel Randy's genuineness and appreciates it but that she remains frightened.

Exercise 11.8. Attachment Significance of an Injury

Which of the following therapist actions focus on helping a couple process the attachment significance of the injury and its relationship importance? Mark the two actions that promote attention to the attachment impact of the injury.

a. The therapist discusses the rewards of striving for forgiveness to both. ____
b. The therapist helps the injured one move to a complete, clear, and integrated expression of his or her loss and pain. ____
c. The therapist coaches the offending spouse in how to make an apology. ____
d. The therapist supports the other spouse to stay engaged, own responsibility, and express regret, remorse, and grief. ____
e. The therapist relates the injury to deeper childhood wounds. ____

Re-engagement Around the Injury

The process of working through the attachment injury takes a more explicit present focus on the injured partner's experience of the injury, focusing the "broken" attachment bond. The depth of experiencing for the injured partner promotes a greater felt awareness of the injury as this is shared directly with the offending partner. The therapist turns to shaping a vulnerable encounter around the injury as the injured partner risks vulnerably sharing the impact and meaning of the injury to their partner and the offending partner is guided to respond in an emotionally engaged manner, taking responsibility for the impact and effect of the injury, and expressing deep felt remorse and apology.

Randy: I can't escape how I feel as this all unravels, what an awful person I was, to hurt you, it's not right. (Karen is crying as Randy speaks of the magnitude of the injury/injuries and the impact he has had on her, referencing in particular her earlier expressions of nausea and questioning, "How could you do that to me? . . . and to us?")

Therapist: Karen, let yourself cry; it's good if you can breathe and cry; you can cry together.

Randy: I always loved you, I always loved you, I always loved my kids, I hated myself. (sobbing, his voice intense)

Therapist: It's good to breathe, Karen, it's good; let yourself feel it. (Karen is present and engaged.)

Randy: I'm sorry, I was just trying to survive, I was just trying to get by and be good. I have tried my hardest to deal with this stuff. I would not be here if it wasn't for you, believing in me, seeing some love in me when no one else could. (now sobbing) It's true, that's what love is about, and I see what I've done. I see how I've damaged you. If I could change it, I would, in a minute. I'm sorry, you're a beautiful person, you're strong and smart, compassionate, you're all those things. I wish I could make you feel better. (Here Randy speaks directly and explicitly to the "damage" he has done, the ways he has impacted Karen's view of herself. Earlier, he said, "I hated myself," i.e., it wasn't about you, any flaws in you, you were enough, you are enough, it was about me, and my history. The therapist now turns to Karen to see if she can take it in.)

Therapist: Karen, what is happening inside for you? Are you able to share how that lands on you? How that feels for you, from your body, as you're able? You can take your time and breathe.

Karen: Self-preservation . . . getting through . . . not crying too hard or too loud, that's been my way, trying to be as inconspicuous as I can. I do feel that. I felt the genuineness in what you just told me. I appreciate that.

Therapist: Karen, did you take it in?

Karen: I did, but I'm frightened of it. I know he is working as hard as he can but that we can't change what happened or even how I responded, that none of that can be changed.

Therapist: But you can change the impact, as you're beautifully doing. It's so hard, but you're doing it now. You don't have to be alone in it.

The therapist makes space for Karen to process Randy's apology and to begin to take in his deep remorse. Note the focus of Randy's regret focuses on the hurt and broken trust Karen has expressed. Randy's shame is now in the background while Karen's hurt and injury experience has his foremost attention.

At this point, Karen turns to some recent events in which Randy "had her back," took care of her, and was there for her, and she allowed him to care for her. Randy then recalls, yes, she had mentioned "You seem to really be listening to me." He then replies, "I like those comments because it sometimes feels like I'm not progressing. It's nice to get that type of comment." As the couple continues to process the gains, Karen also notes that they are more able to come back from difficult periods, process, and repair. Here the therapist normalizes and validates the couple, indicating that missteps in relationships are normal and that being able to back up and repair is the desired outcome.

Following this interchange, the therapist processes this new encounter with Karen.

Therapist: As Randy so beautifully shared his feelings about you, and with you, and his "sorries"—I think he said "sorry" a few times—what happened inside of you?

Karen: I felt like I saw the unedited version of that apology and that it was completely genuine. I felt that. I definitely did.

Therapist: Did you feel like he could see you and feel you?

Karen: Yeah, I think he is . . . yeah. . . .

Randy: I do.

Karen: You're getting misty-eyed; what is that?

Randy: I don't know whether it's happiness, sadness . . . I feel very comfortable and connected.

Karen: Do you? (Karen inquisitively looks at Randy.) I've always felt a connection to him, and it's always been so hard to find that it was blank on the other side sometimes.

Therapist: Karen, where are you now, in terms of your protective armor? What do you feel inside, about that part of things, going back to the beginning?

Karen: I still probably just default to self-protection, but it doesn't keep me from being vulnerable.

Forgiveness and Reconciliation

In the final steps of the AIRM process, the injured partner is invited to risk reaching for their partner, often with needs that were neglected or abandoned previously. The therapist supports the injured partner in working through fears and reluctance to trust the repair. These new bids for caring and comfort are deepened and shared with the offending partner. In processing these encounters, the therapist promotes the accessible and emotionally engaged response of the offending partner who is now in a position to reassure and comfort. Throughout these AIRM steps, the therapist remains focused on facilitating a deeper emotional engagement and shaping engaged encounters between each partner, thereby providing an antidote to the injury and promoting greater confidence in the security and significance of the repair.

Clinical Example. The therapist invites Karen to reach to Randy from a new place of trust and vulnerability. As Karen risks expressing her needs to Randy, the therapist helps Karen clarify her attachment-related need and highlight the vulnerability she often protects.

Karen: Even when I do tell you what I need, I probably don't do it from a place of vulnerability. I probably do it from a place of guardedness, right?

Therapist: Karen, this is the perfect opportunity, if you can allow yourself. . . .

Karen: I do need you to sometimes just listen to me and hear, oh, she's asking me to do this because she loves and trusts me. When I ask you for something that I need, I want you to feel like I love and trust you, and that's why I'm asking for it. I'm not asking you for it because I don't love you or don't trust you to make the right decisions. Does that make sense at all? (Here Karen is referencing the many occasions that Randy would get caught in his shame/negative self-view and hear her bids for connection/expression of needs as criticism rather than a direct and open request.)

Therapist: I hear you saying I need you to see me. I need you to put aside your shame, which, actually, Randy, I feel like you beautifully did . . . and your guilt about the past . . .

and when I make a request or when I reach to you, I need you to see me and feel me and hear me, is that right, Karen? (Karen nods in agreement.) Did that happen today for you? Or is it happening now?

Karen: Yeah, I think it did . . . yeah . . . I feel more connected than when we came in, so I think it is.

Randy: Could you say that once again? . . . 'cause I just want to hear those words again about . . . when you ask me . . . it's because you trust me. . . (Randy shares this with a tone of disbelief, dismay, and uncertainty.)

Karen: and I love you. . . .

Therapist: Yeah . . . it's not about what you haven't done . . . it's about what you could do . . . that's what she's saying . . . and today . . . she risked trusting, from a deep place of vulnerability, which is huge for her, and in her brain, she still goes to this place of, maybe I shouldn't, or maybe I'm not worthy, or maybe I'm not supposed to be cared for. You're supposed to care for others. There's all these voices in her head, but when she took the risk of quieting those voices and struggling, from a deep pit in her stomach and a deep place in her body, the thing that happened, the thing that you did, is you, Randy, you beautifully put aside your shame and guilt, and you were there for her, in a time of great need, and you told her that you love her, and you told her about the way you see her . . . with compassion . . . and caring . . . she's smart . . . and beautiful . . . and you told her that you have always loved her.

In the AIRM process, the therapist turns to the offending partner to promote a caring response to the injured partner's need. Here Randy expresses the impact of Karen's vulnerability and need for him. In this the couple finds a more authentic experience of their love and a resource for growth into the future.

Randy: It's hard for me . . . it was hard for me . . . to feel that anyone needed me . . . would want me.

Therapist: Are you feeling it now?

Randy: Yeah . . . it's like . . . there's some light in there . . . but . . . wow . . . it just seems like there was a wall there . . . it wasn't getting through . . . I think I'm feeling that . . . I'm learning that . . . I'm seeing that . . . yeah . . . yeah . . . I've been searching to feel good . . . to feel wanted and needed . . . for so long . . . it just never penetrated like it should.

Therapist: Do you feel like you guys can stay in this space?

Randy: I'm feeling a comfort in it. I'm feeling more connected. I'm feeling like a part of me . . . that was kind of blocked . . . has opened up. . . . I feel differently than I ever have . . . ever . . . for so long, I was blocked . . . this is so different.

Therapist: That's good, Karen; you can feel him?

Randy: I also understand where you're coming from . . . how could you, with so much history, how can you believe me now?

Karen: But I . . . I do believe you actually. . .

Randy: We have to live it.

Karen: Yeah . . . I not only believe you . . . I actually . . . I think I feel . . . your authenticity.

Exercise 11.9. Healing an Attachment Injury

The final two steps of the process of forgiveness and reconciliation and healing the attachment injury require.

a. The creation of a contract to make sure similar injuries do not occur ____
b. An enactment in which the injured spouse can ask for comfort and caring—often related to one's need at the time of the injury ____
c. The offending partner's receptive, loving, available response to the injured partner's reach of vulnerability
d. An agreement that the couple forgive each other and to make amends ____
e. The consolidation of the injured partner's post-traumatic growth

Exercise 11.10. AIRM Relationship Outcomes

The successful completion of the AIRM process results in the following relationship outcomes: (Mark all that apply.)

a. That the relationship is defined as a potential safe haven. ____
b. That basic trust is restored between the spouses. ____
c. That the injury is better understood and forgiven. ____
d. That the impasse is overcome and partners can complete the EFT process. ____
e. That positive cycle of bonding and connection can then occur. ____
f. That a clear coherent narrative of the injury is integrated into the relationship context and is owned and accepted by both partners. ____

Exercise 11.11. AIRM Summary

Now use the following therapist summary to identify the key themes of attachment injury resolution. Note how the therapist highlights key shifts that the couple has taken in this injury conversation.

Therapist: Randy, you had done a lot of work already, both of you together, around your relationship, yourselves, each other. But when I met you, Randy, I think there was still so much trauma, nonetheless; you took huge risk, to open yourself up in a way that allowed you also to be seen and heard and felt, in different ways. And Karen, like she's always been, in all the beautiful ways that you articulated today, was caring, compassionate, and present for you, and patient with you, and as she made that space for you, you became, more of you, and she had more of you, which made more space for her, and that's what was happening on your holidays, in lots of different ways that may feel or sound small, but they're huge, right? It is what gave Karen the confidence today, I think, and me, too, to know that you could be there for her and make space for her, and when she risked undoing some of her own voices and experience from the past, not just between the two of you but also in her childhood . . . like you're not supposed to need and want and ask—you're supposed to give to others. When she shared her pain about the past and you beautifully said sorry, that made more space for her as well. And I think there's more—and that's going to be her challenge, to not guard herself off but to risk being open and vulnerable. Truly, in the moments before you said, "Will you marry me?" that is what it felt like to me, like a renewal. It's like there's two different people in the room and a different future together. And Randy, you also did a beautiful job of saying, I don't want to be that person, I want to get rid of the past, and then you reassured Karen . . . or this is how it sounded to me . . . I'm not wanting to erase the past and pretend it didn't happen; it did happen, and I know I hurt you, but I want to be different. I want to be a new guy for you, the guy I've always wanted to be, and I feel capable of that. And then, beautifully and spontaneously, Randy said, "Will you marry ME?" . . . "ME" . . . and I think that "ME" . . . that's a really important word.

Now in your own words, summarize the new experiences that the therapist highlights for each partner in working through this injury.

1. Karen's New Experience:

   ____

   ____

   ____

   ____

2. Randy's New Experience:

   ____

   ____

   ____

   ____

Exercise 11.12. Identifying Key AIRM Themes

With respect to the clinical scenario involving Randy and Karen described, identify key themes related to attachment injury repair. List two key themes below.

Theme 1.

____

____

Theme 2.

____

____

AIRM AND STAGE 2 CHANGE EVENTS

In considering the AIRM process, it is relevant to note that, at times, as highlighted earlier, the process might take more than one session, particularly when shame is a significant barrier for the offending partner, making it difficult for that partner to fully engage with the injured partner's pain. In such cases, one or more sessions might need to focus on resolving some of that shame (and particularly when layered, with roots in childhood for example, and with links to previous partially and/or unresolved trauma). It also is relevant to note that as the AIRM process unfolds, Stage 2 change events (e.g., withdrawer engagement or pursuer softening) might be initiated and/or completed. That is, for example, and now moving away from the earlier case example, as the injured partner shares her pain surrounding the loss of a parent and the associated sense of grief associated with feeling that she was alone in this loss—that her partner let her down—she might reach a level of experiencing that is deep enough and sustained long enough to connect with the needs and longings characteristic of withdrawer engagement. This would both propel the AIRM process forward, as well as the larger and more encompassing Stage 2 process. As the AIRM process unfolds, the pursuing partner is similarly commonly challenged in various ways (e.g., to take in the love of another, to believe it, to reach openly and directly for needs to be important/special to be met), and the pursuer softening key change event might either be initiated or completed in the AIRM process.

With the blocks to connection caused by relationship injuries repaired, as sessions progress through the Stage 2 process and beyond, the EFT therapist can anticipate that the processes of withdrawer engagement and pursuer softening and associated shifts in models of self and other and affect regulation capacity will be ongoing, with gradual and sustainable change along the way. Once again, as the EFT therapist moves fluidly between assessment and intervention, the way is paved for ongoing growth, both within and between sessions. Now firmly embedded in the EFT process, with attachment theory as its compass, a clear roadmap and an enduring beacon of light are provided for therapist and couple alike. By Stage 2, the healing journey is well underway, and the impetus for ongoing growth and connection is momentous.

Exercise 11.13. AIRM and Forgiveness

The attachment-injury concept clarifies how forgiveness can be understood in a couple's relationship. Identify the important ways AIRM informs forgiveness for couples.

a. Helps us understand the nature of the negative events that call for forgiveness ____
b. Integrates forgiveness and injury into a broader theory of marriage and love ____
c. Helps us outline the critical elements in the forgiveness process ____
d. Helps us understand how to translate forgiveness into reconciliation ____
e. Allows for the outlining of the key interventions in the interpersonal process of forgiveness ____

STAGE 3. CONSOLIDATION

The consolidation stage of EFCT focuses on helping the couple consolidate and integrate the significant gains that have been made. New solutions to old problems are highlighted. A spotlight is shone on new ways of being and engaging as the positive cycle is contrasted with the cycle of distress that brought them to therapy. In the case of trauma, it is important to again validate previously adaptive strategies in the context of the couple's personal and relationship histories as a contrast to increased flexibility, both personally and relationally. It also is important to draw attention to any potential ongoing vulnerabilities (e.g., anniversaries that might trigger either personal or relationship distress) with the aim of preventing any significant setbacks and with the overarching goal of promoting resilience. More generally, in this final stage of therapy, the therapist helps the couple construct a coherent narrative that captures their understanding of their histories, the therapy process, and their new understanding of the relationship. This narrative can then be used as a positive reference point and a beacon for the future.

SUMMARY

In this chapter, we have focused on how to address the echoes of trauma in the context of couple therapy. Also addressed in this chapter was the special case of relationship wounds—attachment injuries that occur within a couple relationship—and how best to address them in a manner that facilitates forgiveness and healing and provides for the potential of leaving couples with a stronger foundation than ever in spite of such relationship scars.

The clinical example used in this chapter featuring Randy and Karen (EFCT case) are excerpts from a related training resources/DVD set titled *Escaping the Trauma Trap—Transforming Life-Long Trauma in EFT Couple Sessions* (see www.iceeft.com). For more information about this case and related resources, please visit www.eftvancouverisland.com.

ANSWERS AND SUGGESTED RESPONSES

Exercise 11.1. Consequences of Trauma in a Couple's Relationship

Answer: All answers but F. Although a pervasive traumatic history may have limited a partner's resources of trust in EFT, we assess and explore sources of resilience found in relationships of support and care that also might offset the potential impact of trauma.

Exercise 11.2. Trauma and Couple Therapy Assessment

Possible responses:

1. A partner's relationship history, including resources of resilience
2. A partner's window of tolerance/affect regulation capacity
3. Each partner's level of traumatic exposure or trauma history
4. Rigidity in the couple's negative interaction pattern
5. Negative models of self and other
6. Role of trauma in the couple's relationship (e.g., attachment injury)

Exercise 11.3. Summary Statements and Psychoeducation

Underlining Educational Components

Therapist: It makes sense, Randy. What I hear you say, and what we commonly see with others who have come from difficult home environments, is that when you were a little boy, there was no choice but to shut down and hide during times of danger. There was no safety to speak up and no space for your feelings. It was adaptive to shut down and to build a wall to "shield" yourself . . . and what also happens, over time, and especially when there is no refuge, is that the wall that protected you as a little boy becomes an automatic response during difficult times. So when you get any hint of disapproval or criticism or when people that matter to you show any signs of frustration, your "natural" reaction, your "visceral" response, is to pull away or hide or shut down . . . but the problem with that in this relationship, in the relationship that matters most, is that the strategy that protected you as a little boy is the one that also keeps you from getting close to Karen, to your beautiful wife . . . and Karen's experience of your wall, though she understands why it was so important when you were little, is to feel shut out and alone. When she reaches to you (and although she also understands that she hasn't always reached in the best ways) and you turn away, she feels rejected. Not being allowed to be close to you is painful for her. She feels like she is not important and that there is no space for her.

Exercise 11.4. Defining an Attachment Injury

Answer: All answers but B and C. Regarding C: These injuries can be the primary cause of marital distress, or frequently, they exacerbate already existing distress and vulnerabilities and become a symbolic marker for the security of the relationship. Failed attempts to resolve the injury then compound already existing distress levels. Avoidance of vulnerability and numbing by the injured spouse also erode the couple's connection.

Exercise 11.5. Trauma-Related Symptoms

Answer: All responses are correct.

Exercise 11.6. Attachment Injury Statements

Answer: All but A, which is a statement of general hurt and insecurity.

Exercise 11.7. Exploring the Injury Impact

Answer: C and E are the correct answers.

Exercise 11.8. Attachment Significant of an Injury

Answer: B and D are the correct answers.

Exercise 11.9. Healing an Attachment Injury

Answer: B and C are the correct answers.

Exercise 11.10. AIRM Relationship Outcomes

Answer: All responses are important outcomes of AIRM.

Exercise 11.11. AIRM Summary

Possible Themes

1. Randy takes risk to be open and vulnerable. Randy acknowledged and accepted responsibility for his injuring Karen and showed openness and responsiveness to her pain. Randy symbolizes his own commitment to a new relationship.
2. Karen gained confidence in Randy's availability and risked sharing a need. Karen began to take down her own self—protection in the presence of Randy's reassurance and revisit past fears. Karen accepted Randy's responsiveness and deepened their emotional engagement.

Exercise 11.12. Identifying Key AIRM Themes

Answer: Possible Responses

1. Karen was able to share her pain from a place of vulnerability.
2. Randy was able to manage his emerging shame and respond to Karen's pain. He was able to meet her in her experience from a similarly deep level of experiencing.
3. Randy was able to apologize, from a place of authenticity, and with regard to Karen's experience (e.g., recognizing the impact his actions have had on her over the years).

Exercise 11.13. ASRM and Forgiveness

Answer: All responses illustrate how the AIRM informs an understanding of forgiveness.

12

EMOTIONALLY FOCUSED FAMILY THERAPY

Emotionally focused family therapy (EFFT) reflects a key movement in family therapy with a primary emphasis on the importance of nurturance and connection between family members in contrast to past models that focused more on the dimensions of power and control. EFFT frames the emotional experiences between family members within a context of attachment theory and works to create and maintain secure bonds (Furrow et al., 2019; Johnson, 2019). Secure attachment is generally understood as the degree of confidence a family member has that other family members will provide support, comfort, and protection and will remain emotionally responsive and accessible. Typically, more cohesive families have secure attachment bonds, whereas more conflicted and distant families tend to demonstrate more insecure attachments between family members (Cobb, 1996).

EFFT is a useful modality when a child or adolescent presents with symptomatic or problematic behavior, a parent or parents present with parenting problems or when a family presents with interactional difficulties such as constant fighting or bickering. EFFT works to prevent family breakdown or the isolation of a particular family member. This approach can be combined with other treatment models to increase a family's resilience in facing particular child conditions. For example, an autistic child in residential treatment could also be seen with her family in EFFT sessions (Efron, 2004).

KEY EFFT ASSUMPTIONS IN WORKING WITH FAMILIES

The following assumptions guide emotionally focused therapy (EFT) therapists in working with family.

- Secure attachment is a developmental catalyst that promotes growth and development of family members (Mikulincer & Shaver, 2016).
- A family's health is impacted by level of felt security in family relations and their ability to adapt to the changing needs of family members.
- A parent or caregiver's availability to a child is a key attachment resource providing accessibility, responsiveness, and emotional engagement to attachment-related needs.
- EFFT focuses on the interplay between individual and interpersonal functioning addressing both interpersonal and intrapsychic systemic issues driving distress in the family system.

DOI: 10.4324/9781003039457-15

- EFFT allows the family to shift its focus from negative interactions about one individual member to creating strong attachment relationships between family members.
- EFFT mobilizes family resources and allows for a more flexible and open system in which family members are better able to effectively problem solve.

KEY DIFFERENCES BETWEEN EFFT AND EFT WITH COUPLES

An EFT therapist, in both couple and family sessions, employs the same set of interventions, and choreographs repeated sequences of the EFT Tango. The differences that exist in EFFT arise from the shift in structure from couple to family. Familial relationships have different characteristics than romantic relationships. While parents and children are reciprocal in their emotional impact on each other, they are not mutual or equal in the level of responsibility for caregiving. Attachment in family bonds is centered primarily on caregiving as opposed to connection. Parents are motivated to provide care for their young, while children are born to seek and receive care. The overall goal in EFT with families is engaging parental responsiveness and openness to receive and often translate children's bids for care and to meet their attachment needs.

The markers for the change events of Stages 1 and 2 are different in family work. Stabilization of the family distress in Stage 1 is met when the parents are no longer reactive and stuck in negative patterns of interaction with their children and have shifted their perception of the problem away from the child. Their blocks to responsiveness have been processed, and they have moved into a new position of emotional accessibility and engagement. The restructuring of relational blocks in Stage 2 is achieved when the child is able to clearly express emotional vulnerability and is open to their parent's responding with care, comfort, support, and confidence. The attachment needs of the child are visible, the parent is available, and the child is able to receive and take in the parents' care.

Family relationships require a fine tuning of the EFT therapist's skills in tracking negative patterns and emotional processing. Patterns in families are oriented around caregiving, and when parents are stuck in reactive positions, their responsiveness to their child is either elevated or diminished. The overresponse or underresponse is met with an intensification of the child's efforts to have their needs met or alternatively a shutting down or minimization of their attachment needs. Both sides of this pattern can become locked into repetitive, narrow feedback loops that are loaded with negative affect. The reactive pattern blocks the parents' good intentions to provide care and scrambles the attachment messages between family members.

How emotion is processed in families is slightly different in EFFT. Parents' emotional blocks are processed with the intention of increasing self-awareness of their emotional triggers and promoting ownership of their reactive positions. Parents are encouraged to be transparent regarding their own emotional world while the therapist supports their competency as caregivers. Emotional disclosure by parents helps children differentiate their own experience and creates new meaning out of negative interactions. The therapist creates and maintains emotional safety for children, titrating the depth of the work with the emotional maturity of the child. Children's blocks are processed with the intention of helping children send clear emotional cues regarding their attachment needs. Stage 2 is focused on accessing and deepening of the child's attachment-related affect and helping the parent respond accurately to the attachment bids for care. The EFFT therapist structures parental enactment with an attuned response to the child's vulnerable reach to the parent. The marker for the completion of Stage 2 is the child receiving parental care through taking in of the support, reassurance, and/or acceptance the parent provides.

The end of EFFT is characterized by a secure and cohesive family system, and the overall family climate has shifted in a positive direction. Parents are accessible and attuned to the attachment needs of their children and are able to be there for their children when needed. Children are able to feel protected and safe but are also able to go out in the world with a sense of confidence in a developmentally appropriate way.

EFFT PROCESS OF CHANGE

EFFT follows the same three-stage process of change found in EFT with individuals and couples. These stages include

- Stage 1: Stabilization: Therapist identifies the negative interactional cycle and underlying feelings. The problem is framed as being the cycle and its impact on attachment issues rather than the child or the parent. The goal of reframing the problem is de-escalation.
- Stage 2: Restructuring Interaction: The therapist helps family members articulate and express the attachment emotions and needs directly so that they are more central to the family's awareness and emotional engagement. Family members access and reorganize emotional experience to shape new interactions, that foster secure bonding, and provide comfort, support, and protection for each family member.
- Stage 3: Consolidation: The therapist promotes the integration and consolidation of felt security in the family. Working with family members, the focus is given to strengthening intimate exchanges and the development of family rituals of connection.

Therapist Goals in EFFT

The EFT therapist focuses on the following goals in promoting changes in the family's interactions and emotional climate.

- Modify distressing patterns of interaction that create and maintain attachment insecurity between family members.
- Foster positive cycles of accessibility, responsiveness, and emotional engagement between family members.
- Promote the family unit as a secure base for children to grow in and leave from.

Key Moves in the Process

The EFT therapist works with emotion and actions in a particular way to help move the family from a distressed conflicted state to a more cohesive and responsive place. The therapist begins by framing the family problem in attachment terms and normalizes the family's difficulties as arising out of an attachment crisis. A defiant and distant adolescent with critical and controlling parents can be understood as a family struggling with a difficult stage in family development: the emerging independence of the adolescent, the new and uncertain role of the parent, and a family coping with how to change together. Following the five moves of the EFT Tango, the therapist works to create new emotional encounters between parents and children that promote a felt sense of attachment security.

Throughout Stage 1, parental reactivity is reflected in the present moment and is organized and integrated as part of the negative interactional cycle while also validated and normalized in terms of the positive intention to care. Parents are helped to explore their emotional triggers that lead them to either over- or underrespond and share their softer, more vulnerable emotions with their children. Once safety is in place and parents see more clearly their children's needs, the EFFT therapist helps the child to do access and share their more vulnerable attachment emotion. Interventions are designed to promote parental emotional accessibility and responsiveness and increase the child's sense of the stronger, wiser other that is there for them. The therapist tracks the negative interactional patterns that keep family members stuck and clarifies each member's position in the pattern. The family problem is shifted from the child to the relational blocks that inform the distress in family interactions.

In Stage 2, the therapist creates secure, responsive bonding interactions. Interventions are tailored to be sensitive to the developmental needs of the child. For example, an adolescent's attachment needs are different from a child's needs because of a natural move toward autonomy that still requires parental support. The therapist heightens and validates the family's strengths and reinforces family rituals that promote and encourage family connection and emotional support. If the relationship between the parents becomes a primary locus of the family difficulty as EFFT ends, often couple therapy begins as a further step in treatment.

EFT INTERVENTIONS IN WORKING WITH FAMILIES

EFFT practice includes the same micro- and macro-interventions used in EFT with couples and individuals. Three tasks organize the focus of EFFT intervention, and these include

- Building a therapeutic alliance with each family member without invalidating, alienating, or dismissing another family member. Therapist uses validation, normalization, and empathic reflection to promote felt understanding and a safety in the therapy process.
- Creating a secure base through focusing on and processing attachment emotions (e.g., fears) and accompanying needs (e.g., comfort, reassurance). Therapist uses empathic conjecture, exploration, and inference to expand on each client's frame of reference and access more adaptive responses.
- Engaging new interactions through shaping, fostering, and structuring new interactions between family members. Therapist utilizes enactment exercises within session and gives homework tasks that create new rituals or experiences for family members.

In this process, the therapist also focuses upon the relational blocks that interrupt effective caregiving responses and attachment bids or care seeking responses. Working through these blocks uses empathic reflection, validation, empathic conjectures and evocative responses to access and process underlying core emotional responses associated with these relational blocks. Underlying emotions are understood in the context of attachment seeking and caregiver responding providing both motivation and direction for restoring emotional balance and relational connection. Reactive responses are reframed in terms of predictable patterns of family distress and a parent's caregiving intent.

In EFFT, the therapist tracks negative patterns to identify relational blocks the disrupt caregiving responses and the sharing of attachment needs (See Figure 12.1). These blocks are most evident in specific dyadic interactions, say between a parent and a child. Although the impact of the relational block can also create distress and negative interactions among other family members. The EFT therapist typically organizes treatment around the most distressed dyad and begins working through that relational block with relevant family members.

In assessing relational blocks, the therapist identifies rigid patterns of interaction that are most often seen in family interactions. The therapist focuses on present moment experience (Tango Move 1) to explore the relational patterns including triggers and action tendencies. Emotional experience found in these moments. This leads to the processing of these responses, including assembling and deepening of underlying core emotions that inform a caregiver's perceptions, feelings, and actions (Tango Move 2).

RELATIONAL BLOCKS

More secure relational patterns are created as the therapist promotes greater parental availability and increased child vulnerability. These interaction patterns are formed based on these new emotional responses or positive cycles of attachment security. EFFT differs from EFT with couples in recognizing the hierarchical role of a parent and the primacy

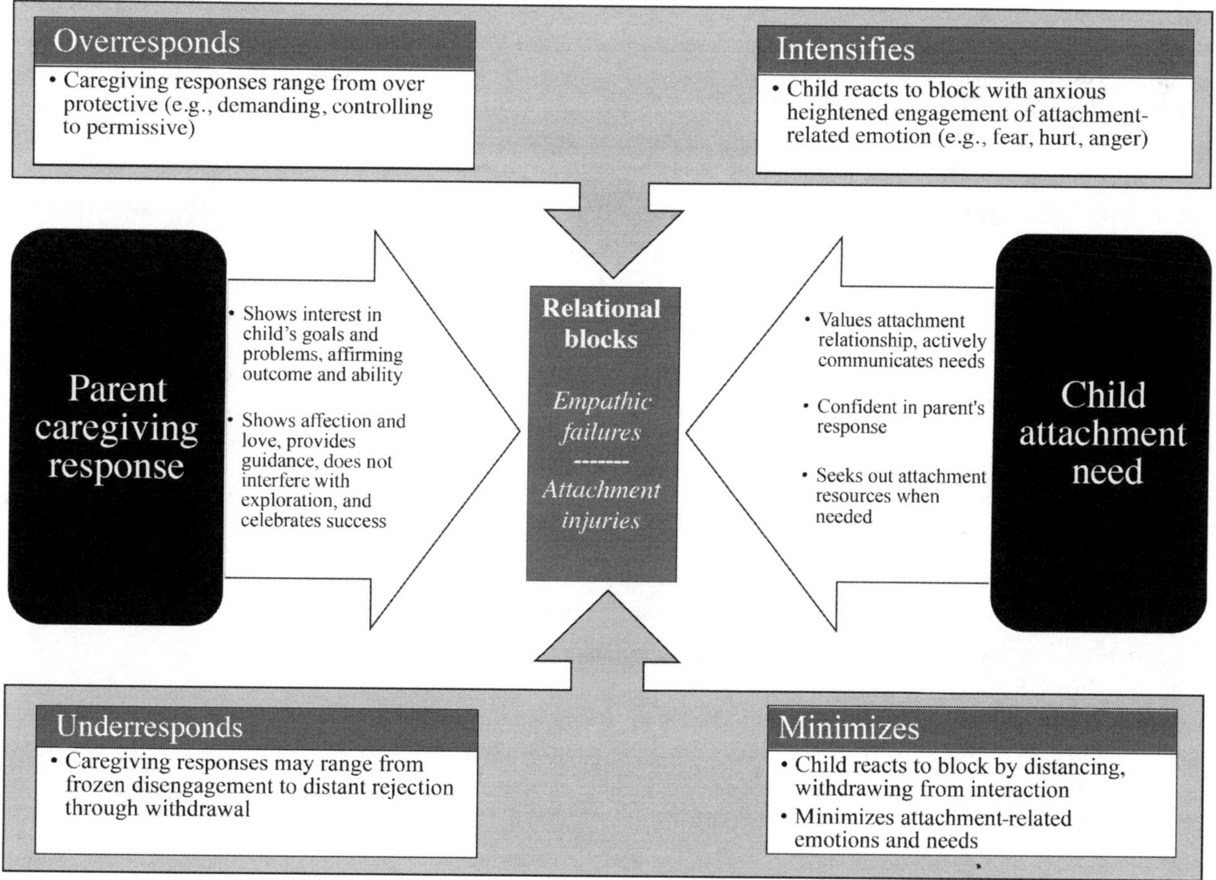

Figure 12.1 Relational blocks in caregiving and attachment responses.
From *Emotionally Focused Family Therapy: Restoring Connection and Promoting Resilience* (p. 121), by J.L. Furrow, G. Palmer, S.M. Johnson, G. Faller, & L. Palmer-Olsen, 2019, New York, NY: Routledge Press.

Source: Copyright 2019 by Routledge Press.

of parental caregiving in response to attachment needs expressed by a child. The EFFT therapist uses heightening interventions, and enactments are used to choreograph change events that promote the child's sharing of attachment related emotions and needs and parental responsiveness and accessibility to a child's vulnerability.

EFT TANGO AND EFFT

A typical EFFT session follows the familiar sequence of EFT related interventions, the EFT Tango. This mental framework orients the therapist to the "here and now" work of emotion work in restructuring family attachment relationships. Each of the five moves works together to engage emotion and transform relationship interactions. Here is a brief example of the EFT Tango from an EFFT session with a mother and son and the relational block they encounter when trying to talk about responsibility and accountability.

Move 1. Mirroring Present Process

The EFT therapist tracks and reflects a family's experience as it unfolds in session. Through attuning to the present moment, the therapist helps the family explore the intrapersonal and interpersonal aspects of their shared experience. The therapist is tuned into the unfolding sequence of action and emotion playing out as family members navigate this moment together. Throughout EFFT, the therapist is focused on moments where relational blocks to caregiving and care seeking organize a family's distress and efforts to manage its impact.

June, Sam's mother, recalls an argument from earlier in the week around household chores and homework. In sharing her experience, June begins:

June: (tense and cautiously) I just asked Sam if he had taken care of the dishes and finished his homework. He was gaming, and I know I was interrupting him. He gave me attitude about that. I tried to stay on point, but the longer the conversation went, the worse it got. I finally pulled the plug on his game and told him this has to change, or his life will go nowhere!

Sam: (rolling his eyes, sarcastically). Yeah, something needs to change. I told you I would get to all that when I was done, but that's not good enough. Never is.

June: (angerly) But that was not our agreement. It's not about being good enough; it's about doing what is expected. Keeping your promises. Following through. I should be able to expect that of you.

Sam: Right, it's just about you. (disengaging and looking away)

June: That's not fair. I am just trying to be a good mom.

Therapist: Yes, that's important, June. I hear the importance even in your voice as you say this. This really matters—Sam matters to you. You want Sam to see you are trying to help, to guide him to help him follow through—that's being a good mom. When you see that Same is not responding or pushing back, you try to help him see the potential consequences—this all feels urgent, so much at stake. But Sam, this all is too familiar. Like another round of how you are not measuring up. It starts with homework and chores and then becomes about your future and failing. You pull back, like there's nothing to say, and this leaves you, June, feeling either more frustrated or defeated, feeling like you are failing too in these moments, not able to be the mom you want.

Acknowledging the familiar dynamic, the therapist validates Sam's escalating frustration at his mom's disappointment and fear. Focusing on the present process, the therapist retraces this typical interpersonal sequence, highlighting the block that emerges when June's efforts to engage Sam led to a well-worn pattern of defensiveness organized by mom's fear for son's future and Sam's own fears and hurt from his mother's lack of confidence in him. The therapist engages the present moment to see the emotional realities that that trigger the mother and son's escalating distress providing an entry point to explore an order these experiences.

Move 2. Affect Assembly and Deepening

As the session unfolds, the EFFT therapist focuses on elements of emotion that begin to emerge, putting pieces of a family member's experience together into a more coherent and explicit whole. Through accessing and processing these experiences, family members often deepen their awareness and understanding of these felt experiences and their links to views self and other. Helping family members to get clearer about their underlying emotional experience is a necessary first step toward the end goal of new, more secure and corrective conversations. The following example the therapist repeats Mom's triggering comment as an access point to explore, assemble, and deepen Sam's felt experience.

Therapist: Sam, what happens when your Mom says, "Your life is going nowhere?"

Sam: (clenching his fist, angry tone) It's ridiculous. I'm taking a break, playing game, and I'm ruining my future! Makes no sense.

Therapist: Right. And you want her to get this. Your anger is a way of pushing back against this. Your anger is trying to stop a message you don't want to hear, that doesn't make sense. Am I getting that right?

Sam: Yeah, it makes me so mad. It's like it's her future, not mine.

Therapist: Sure, of course, it's like her intensity, her fear that things are not going to work out for you, leave you feeling like this is her agenda, her future.

Sam: Like I don't matter anyway, like I don't care, too. It bums me out, then I am left with all this drama. What's the point?

Therapist: It feels futile, and you go away, right? Check out. Get away from the drama. (Sam nods and looks down.) Right, and that's tough because when you go away, it's like you're on your own then. Alone.

Sam: Yeah, and sometimes that's the best thing.

Therapist: Is that what you say to yourself? Like better than I am on my own, alone.

Sam: Better than being told you're a failure.

Therapist: What's it like on the inside when you hear that word—failure? Like you might fail. Like you are not cutting it.

Sam: Hate it. . . . It sucks. . . . makes me sad.

Therapist: Sure, I think anyone would feel that way when they are hearing that they are a failure by someone that matters, like your Mom. So, it sucks to hear that, and you go away—try to distance from that message. She sees you going away.

The therapist links his action tendency (going away) to the trigger (failure message) and helps Sam to begin to assemble his other elements of emotional experience. These include the perception or meaning he makes in these moments, like he is better off alone, and his felt sadness in these moments. After putting these elements together in a summary, the therapist frames this experience in relational terms by highlighting his mother's importance and her lack of awareness to his underlying pain.

Move 3. Choreographing Engaged Encounters

The EFFT therapist uses these newly found experiences to engage family members in structured interactions where these new underlying experiences are made known. More vulnerable expressions of emotion are used to engage new ways of relating between family members who more typically avoid these experiences rather than use them as opportunities for understanding and connection. In this example, the therapist turned to Sam's mother to explore the impact of hearing his hurt and loneliness. June initially saw Sam's escape or avoidance as something to be challenged as irresponsibility, but hearing his hurt, the therapist focused on her growing felt understanding (Tango Move 1). The therapist focused on June's underlying fear of Sam's failure and its tie to her own insecurity of not knowing how to help Sam. Following Move 2, the therapist assembled her fear, focusing on her caregiving intention, making explicit the link between her questioning and her fears that she is not doing enough to help Sam. The therapist asks June: "What would it be like to share some of the fear that takes over when you begin to fear your support is not enough or not what he needs? Can you tell him about your fear?"

June: I'm sorry, Sam. I don't see you as a failure, and I don't think you are going to fail; it's just I get scared sometimes. I worry as your only parent that I am not giving you all you need, and when I get afraid, I get pushy, question you. . . . It's too much, and I don't like it either. I can see why you say it becomes all about me and I don't see what that is like for you. I don't want that.

Move 4. Processing the Encounter

Following this enactment, the EFFT therapist explores the impact of sharing and hearing more about these often, unspoken experiences. The therapist creates space to process these new experiences to begin to make sense of these encounters and what impact sharing these experiences has on how one sees the other or oneself in response. Acknowledging June's initiative, the therapist validates her care and concern for Sam.

Therapist: I can see even as you say this that your care for Sam is so clear; it makes so much sense that when you are not sure your care is enough that you can worry, and this fear leads to lots of questions, not only about yourself but also about Sam. What was it like to share this with him?

June: Good but different. I mean, I want him to know that I believe in him and don't believe he is failing, though I am sure I come across that way. I want him to know sometimes my worry gets the best of me.

Therapist: Even as you say that, I hear a strength in your voice. Like this belief you have is really certain and clear. (June nods emphatically.) And Sam, what was it like for you to have your mom share this, to share about how her fears mix up in her care for you leads to all these questions? Did you hear she cares?

Sam: Yeah. I know she cares. I mean, I know it's not easy for her. It's just the drama, too much too often. Sometimes I just need space.

Move 5. Integrating and Validating

The final move in this process focuses on the experience and the new understandings that resulted from the encounter. New insights and connections between family members are supported, and emphasis is given to the ways in which one's new experience provides new possibilities for further engagement. Through the process of sharing these encounters, one can find new insight and awareness of self and family members.

The therapist summarizes for Sam and his mother what just unfolded in session highlighting the underlying experience shared through the encounter. The process of slowing down their interaction and finding space for Sam's experience of sadness underneath his withdrawal and his mother's heartfelt concern opens new opportunities for the mother to see her son more clearly and to better understand his reactivity but also his need for her confidence. The therapist refocuses on the ways these moments can quickly escalate, when anger and negativity seem inevitable, and how in this moment they can each see a bit more clearly that listening to these emotions and what is going on behind the scenes actually helps them move toward facing these challenges together. Validation of the son's concern, even at an early stage of treatment, creates greater acceptance and understanding of his needs for support in exploration. Acknowledging the mother's intention and care reinforces her awareness and underscore how in this moment her ability to respond in an accessible way opens the door for a different conversation that still takes to heart her concern for her son.

EXPLORING EFFT IN STAGE 1

In this section, we explore key moments in the EFFT process of stabilization. The EFFT approach to assessment and treatment planning are identified. A case example is used to illustrate the EFFT approach including a focus on EFT interventions and the EFT Tango. You will identify interventions, practice formulating responses, and track the unfolding EFFT process.

EFFT Alliance Building and Assessment

Typically, the EFFT assessment process includes a whole-family session, a caregiver session, and child/sibling session. Ideally, the therapist begins treatment with a family session as a common starting point for those involved and an opportunity to see the family in action. Alliance building begins with each member in this conversation, and the session frames the focus of the therapist on the family's experience and the distress associated with the presenting problem. In some situations, EFFT assessment begins with a parent session, particularly when there is a strong child-centered focus and a reluctance to begin with a family-focused session.

The overall goal for this initial family session is for the therapist to gain a felt sense of each member's experience in their family. Attention is given to the presenting problem and a focus is also given to member's description of their family experience. Space is given for each member to speak, and the therapist validates each person's perspective making meaning through the context of attachment experiences and with the family's cultural context. The therapist balances the sharing and blocks attempts to overtalk or minimize another's experience. As the therapist hears from each family member, she begins to organize and knit together these individual experiences and map out a family pattern. By the end of the family session, the therapist offers a summary statement that acknowledges each person's position in the family dynamic and starts to reframe the problem as not solely existing in a problem individual but also in the relationship interactions in the family.

Following the initial family session, the therapist invites the parent or caregiver to a session exploring their experience of the family's struggle. The EFT therapist uses these session(s) to promote parental buy-in, assess the caregiving alliance, gain an attachment history, and honor parental caregiving efforts and intention. Contraindications for conjoint sessions are assessed he therapist, evaluating the parent's goal alliance, the flexibility and capacity to self-reflect, and the degree of negativity directed toward the child. Caregivers may need more time to be heard and for the therapist to have established a strong therapeutic alliance before embarking on conjoint treatment. A sibling or child session may be offered allowing the therapist to hear the child's perspective and to assess for safety. The therapist fosters an alliance with children by inviting them to tell their own story of the family. The therapist is curious about the child's external world and the influence of peers, school, and special interests.

Treatment Planning

In EFFT, the therapist structures treatment plan to fit the unique family situation. Typically, the therapist will prioritize treatment focused on the most distressed dyad in the family unit. The therapist may choose to focus on specific dyads in a family when their reactive patterns make it difficult to access and focus on emotional experience. Dyadic sessions may also be necessary if a child is caught in triangulation between parents or a when siblings are overly aligned with a particular parent. Children who are too young or otherwise vulnerable to family distress may be excused from participating in treatment assuming that their actions are less relevant to the family's distress or presenting problem.

Stepfamily dynamics of the require that family sessions be structured around unique family ties. Often biological or adoptive parents are seen with their children independently from the step couple. This formation allows for healing of ruptures in the caregiving system and strengthening of the new couple bond. Overall, the EFT therapist remains flexible in her treatment and engages with family members who are present and available to work. Sometimes a family member may refuse to participate in a conjoint session, and therapist reaches out to this individual, promoting their value to the family and highlighting the uniqueness of their experience and perspective. However, it is not always possible to work with everyone in the family.

Case Example

Wendy and Jen, both professionals with highly demanding jobs, requested therapy for their family following a series of escalating parental conflicts that resulted in constant fighting over household chores and school responsibilities. The couple has three sons: Jack, Dennis, and Randy ages 18, 15, and 13, respectively. In their initial session, Jen complained about the lack of cooperation and responsibility in the family as a whole. This meant for her that she was constantly reminding the kids to do their chores and to complete their homework. She complained there was constant bickering between the kids. Wendy joined in, stating that there was a lack of enjoyable family time, with the fights at the dinner table and everybody arguing with each other. She said she was "at a loss" and had "no idea" how to change the family environment, especially when conflicts would escalate with Dennis acting out aggressively and angrily toward his younger brother Randy.

Jack was absent from the first session because of work, although his parents added that he was rarely at home, spending most of his spare time with his friends. In session, Dennis was sullen and reluctant to speak, stating he was only present because he was "forced" to attend. He saw very little wrong with the family and stated he was feeling "fine" about his family. Randy was playful, teasing his brother, and did not communicate directly about the family difficulties. He laughed and made distracting comments to the therapist's inquiries. Jen dominated the interview with complaints regarding all three children and chastised Dennis for not contributing to the session. Wendy then expressed empathy for Dennis and stated that maybe everybody was picking on him. Dennis did not respond verbally to Wendy's comment but physically looked like he began to relax.

Exercise 12.1. Alliance Building in EFFT

Imagine as the EFT therapist how you might respond to the parents and children in this session focusing on creating space for each member's experience through empathic reflection and validation. In EFFT, the therapist focuses on validating a parent's caregiving intentions—highlighting the intentions to protect or provide for the child in some way.

1. Identify which of the following therapist responses best promote alliance building with family members. (Mark all the answers that apply)
    a. "I can feel the distress this family is in, and this says to me that when you are not getting along, it matters to each and every one of you. How you show your distress is different for everyone, and what I want to help you do is communicate in a clearer way that actually brings you together, rather than drive you apart." ______
    b. "I want you, Wendy, to have a conversation with Dennis about how to fight more effectively and help him to win his fights." ______
    c. "Jen and Wendy, you are both are trying very hard as parents to try to bring this family together and work as a team, and when you get resistance and

a lack of cooperation from the kids, this upsets you because family life is important to you both; you want the family to work together in a positive way. When this doesn't happen, Jen, you may become louder and more forceful, whereas you, Wendy, find yourself not knowing what to do and being at a loss. The kids react by either fighting back or fleeing; they get into fights with each other, or they leave the house or make lots of funny remarks. Everybody ends up feeling bad and not good about each other." ______

d. "I want the family to go home tonight and make a list of chores and have a family meeting to decide who does what chore and set up a work schedule." ______

e. "I think that this family needs to have some individual work to sort out what is happening and allow you to function better as a family unit. I would suggest that Dennis see our child and adolescent therapist." ______

2. List two reflections you could make that would validate the parents and unearth their positive parental intent.

   a. ______________________________

   ____

   b. ______________________________

   ____

3. List two reflections that would validate the children's experience. As the therapist, practice making sense of their surface or reactive emotions and action tendencies using an attachment perspective.

   a. ______________________________

   ____

   b. ______________________________

   ____

Exercise 12.2. Assessment Sessions

Respond to the following questions about assessment and treatment planning using this case example.

1. List two possible goals you would have in meeting with Jen and Wendy (parent session).

   a. ______________________________

   ____

   b. ______________________________

   ____

2. List two goals you would have in meeting with Dennis and Randy (sibling session).

   a. ____

   ____

   b. ____

   ____

3. In reaching out to Jack, what might you say to him to encourage his involvement in a family assessment session?

   ____

   ____

   ____

Exercise 12.3. Promoting Parental Buy-in

The EFT therapist guides parents who may have a strong focus on the "child as the problem" to expand their concern to include the relationship distress and the family's problematic interactional patterns. This involves promoting parental buy-in to the EFFT frame and process. In responding to a parent's child-focused complaint, the therapist will reflect and validate four themes.

- Reflect the parent's caregiving intention.
- Highlight a parent's unique role, importance, and irreplaceability.
- Empathize with the parent's struggle and need for support.
- Focus on relationship interactions that lead to negative or undesired outcomes.

Now imagine that Jen holds on to the idea that Dennis is the "real problem" in the family and asks you in a parent session to focus your approach on Dennis. Jen urgently interrupts: "My concern is that Dennis is increasingly out of control, and he needs help. I think he needs more attention, and maybe with some sessions with you, he can work out what is truly bothering him. You know he is the middle child."

1. Which two of themes might you use to help Jen "buy-in" to shift toward a family or relationship focus?

   a.

   b.

2. Now form a response to Jen focusing on at least two of these themes.

   ____

   ____

   ____

   ____

Personal Reflection

Take a moment to reflect on a child-focused parent you have worked with when you found it difficult to find their underlying caregiving intent. In what ways did their reactive responses make it more difficult for them to see their role in the negative pattern?

____

____

____

____

Caregiving Blocks

A relational block disrupts caregiving attempts in predictable ways, including over responsive reactions (e.g., Anxious strategies: overcontrolling to overpermissive responding) or underresponsive actions (e.g., avoidance: dismissive attacks to indifference of absence). See Table 12.1 for examples. In working through these blocks, the caregiver is better able to see themselves (e.g., view of self) and their child (e.g., view of other). Accessing and processing caregiver vulnerability improves awareness and attunement toward the child's experience and needs.

Table 12.1
Summarizing Caregiver Blocks

Over Responsive: Anxious Blocks	Underresponsive: Avoidance Blocks
Demanding/critical: anger—negative view of child—overfocus/cares too much/control	Rejecting/cold: uncaring—negative view of child—dismissive/judgmental
Overprotective: anxious—preoccupied with child—lacks self-awareness, emotionally intrusive	Absent/indifferent: preoccupied with own lives
Overly permissive: anxious—enabling: negative view of self	Inadequate/freeze—indecisive, negative view of self, fear of getting it wrong

Exercise 12.4. Identifying Caregiving Blocks

Now reflect on the parent's response in the family. These questions will help you explore the parental blocks in caregiving impacting this family. What would you hypothesize regarding Jen's and Wendy's caregiving response? Note each parent's action tendency when a family conflict erupts with their boys?

1. Which of the following best describes Jen's response (parental block)?
   a. Overresponding: critical and demanding
   b. Overresponding: overly permissive—enabling
   c. Overresponding: overprotective and intrusive
   d. Underresponding: critical and dismissive
   e. Underresponding: distant and distracted
   f. Underresponding: indecisive and disengaged
2. Which of the following best describes Wendy's response (parental block)?
   a. Overresponding: critical and demanding
   b. Overresponding: overpermissive and enabling

c. Overresponding: overprotective and intrusive
d. Underresponding: critical and dismissive
e. Underresponding: distant and distracted
f. Underresponding: indecisive and disengaged

In working through a parent's caregiving block, the EFT therapist will aim to address the following aspects of a caregiving block. These targets include

- Naming and engaging parental reactivity in the present moment.
- Linking triggers to action tendencies: (When . . . then . . .)
- Validating present experience, relationship history, and attachment history.
- Heightening underlying emotions and vulnerability.
- Reframing parental intentions focusing on caregiving intention.
- Enacting parental openness or availability in the moment.

Exercise 12.5. Identifying Parental Intent

How would you intervene to begin to access Jen's core emotion, and how would you frame her experience in attachment terms? Imagine that Jen shares the following in session:

Jen: There is a lot of heaviness in our home. I need to use a harsh response because he asks for it. A simple request, and he doesn't listen; the only way I can get his attention is to come down hard. And come down hard I do. It's the only way I get him to respond.

Review each of the therapist responses below. Underline the parental intent highlighted in the therapist's empathic reflection.

1. "In the face of Dennis not listening, you come down hard. It's like, 'I will do anything to get a response from him.' After all, no response leads you nowhere, and that is pretty hard to take as his parent, yes? You want to have guide him because happens to your son matters. Not being able to reach Dennis is not only frustrating but alarming. You see him behaving in ways that scare you because you want the best for him? Is that right? You help me."
2. "I hear you owning, Jen, that you do come down hard on your son. You know that your response is harsh, and you are also aware there is a lot of heaviness in your home. I am imagining that would be hard for you as Mom, who loves your son. I can see the tears in your eyes as I say this. Can you tell me what's happening?"

Now write your own reflection or conjecture based on Jen's statement. Be sure to highlight her parental intent.

____

____

____

Exercise 12.6. Following the EFT Tango and Micro-Interventions in Stage 1

After each therapist statement, identify the therapist's moves using the EFT Tango. Then identify one or two EFT interventions used by the therapist.

Dennis: It is all my fault. Jen and I do get into arguments, and I get angry. My mom doesn't get angry until I do. I do have an opinion, and that's a problem because it just isn't what she thinks.

Jen: He just doesn't listen. He doesn't want to accept the truth, and whatever I say to him, he just takes the wrong way and immediately starts yelling and swearing. He can't go around like this, intimidating everyone, especially his brother.

Therapist: I can hear as you say this that you very much want to reach your son, and when he doesn't listen and hear what you are trying to say to him, that is really frustrating. And even more so, if he gets angry, you get concerned about the impact on Randy, is that right?

1. Tango Move: ________ Interventions: ________________ ________________

Jen: He is just a big bully. And Wendy says nothing.

Wendy: I don't want any more conflict. (starts to tear)

Therapist: This is a really hard spot here, yes? As parents, you want to be able to shift things in the family. Jen, you do that by offering Dennis the truth, and you, Wendy, stay quiet because you want to avoid conflict. And then what happens for you, Dennis? This has got to be hard for you, too. It/s like you end up feeling that maybe all of this is your fault.

2. Tango Move: _____ Interventions: ________________ ________________

Dennis: I do try to do it her way. I get her intention.

Therapist: You do want to try to please and not disappoint your parents. But right here, right now, your mom she feels like you don't listen. It sounds like you do hear, but there are other times that you have something to say, is that right?

3. Tango Move: _____ Interventions: ________________ ________________

Dennis: (glaring at Jen) And that's when it all goes to shit.

Jen: (scolding) Enough, Dennis. (Dennis swears under his breath and looks away, and Jen looks at the therapist, exasperated.) And THIS is exactly what happens.

Therapist: Right. I see that, and I also hear that you want me to understand what is really going on. All of this happened really quickly, and I would like to be able to slow this all down and figure out together what is happening here. (to Jen) What I am hearing is how much you want to be able to reach Dennis; you want to have influence on him, to be able to help him and focus him in the right direction. And I am guessing that there is a lot going on here that is alarming for you, yes? When Dennis gets angry, which he says he does, and his voice goes up and he acts out, that alarms you?

4. Tango Move _____ Interventions: _______________ _______________

Jen: He can't just be throwing his weight around here. He is six feet tall, and just because he is big and male doesn't mean he can run the show. Someone has to put him in his place.

Therapist: So, this feels out of control to you. When Dennis gets angry, and Dennis, you say that you do, and I get the sense that you don't want to end up getting angry, for you Jen, it feels like you need to do something, to fix it, is that right?

5. Tango Move _____ Interventions: _______________ _______________

Jen: Someone has to teach him. Randy also deserves to be protected.

Therapist: You are trying hard to be the best parent you can be to your son. And when you hear Dennis getting agitated, that is alarming, you say to yourself you need to do something to fix his anger, and it's like you do need to get him to hear you.

6. Tango Move _____ Interventions: _______________ _______________

Jen: I know I come down hard on him. That's the only way he listens.

Therapist: And that's when you get frustrated, yes, you scold Dennis to bring him back in line, and what he doesn't see is that it scares you when you can't reach him, yes? He is your son; you want the best for him, and if he is unreachable, then what's going to happen?

7. Tango Move _____ Interventions: _______________ _______________

Jen: He can't yell and swear and get in people's face.

Therapist: You are right. His anger says to you that he is going to run into trouble with others in his life, so no wonder you jump into action mode.

8. Tango Move _____ Intervention: _______________

Jen: And then everyone will say it is because he has two moms. They expect we can't raise a boy to be a man.

Therapist: There is a lot here. There is fear of what consequences lie ahead for Dennis if you don't reach him. There is fear that the world will judge him and you and Wendy as parents. No wonder you want so desperately to get his behavior under control. (Jen nods in agreement.)

9. *Tango Move* _____ Interventions: _______________ _______________

Therapist: Do you think Dennis knows that under your frustration is fear? Can you share your fear with him now?

10. *Tango Move* _____ Intervention: _______________

Jen: (looking at Dennis) It must look like I am always angry at you. I get that. We have a lot of fights.

Therapist: And this is about being afraid for him?

11. *Tango Move* _____ Intervention: _______________

Jen: I am afraid, buddy. I want the best for you. I don't want you ending up in a jail somewhere.

Therapist: Yeah, that's where your mind goes, to the worst possible outcome for your son? (Jen's faces softens, and she starts to tear.) How is it for you, Dennis, to hear your mom?

12. *Tango Move* _____ Interventions: _______________ _______________

Dennis: (looking down, softly) I don't know.

Therapist: Yeah, this is hard to make sense of; this is new, this isn't anything like you guys have experienced before. This is new to see that your mom is actually afraid for you, that under her anger, she wants the best for you, and she gets afraid that bad things are going to happen to you and your family. This is all about how important you are.

This is so good, Jen, that you were able to share your softer side, your vulnerability, because we are all vulnerable when it comes to our kids. Such a wonderful role model for your son. And this is so different than the fights that usually happen.

13. Tango Move _____ Interventions: _______________ _______________

14. Identify key moments when the therapist is focused on one of the following elements. Using the transcript above identify a therapist statement in the earlier transcript that illustrates each of these six key elements. List the number of the therapist response that best illustrate each of these key elements:

Example: Validating Present Experience: #3

a. Naming and engaging parental reactivity in the present moment (Tango Move 1)

____

b. Linking triggers to action tendencies (When . . . then . . .) (Tango Moves 1 and 2)

____

c. Validating present experience, relationship history, attachment history (Tango Moves 1, 2, 4, and 5)

____

d. Heightening underlying emotions and vulnerability (Tango Move 2)

e. Reframing or conjecturing parental intentions focusing on caregiving intention (Tango Moves 1, 2, and 4)

____

f. Enacting parental openness or availability in the moment (Tango Move 3)

____

15. Practice forming an enactment for this family. What other enactments can you imagine would be helpful in Stage 1 of work with this family? Write an enactment intervention based on the focus you identified.

____

____

____

16. Processing a Child's Response

Dennis then defensively responds to Jen's emerging emotions reflecting her care and concern for him. Dennis: (looking downcast) "It doesn't really matter." (sigh, long pause) "Whatever." How would you join the son's response and begin to access this son's underlying emotions? How would you frame his emotions in attachment terms?

In the next examples, underline the therapist response that reflects his mistrust and therapist prompts that target more core or underlying emotion.

a. "It seems like there is no point. It doesn't matter what you say, right? It's like it won't get heard, so what's the point of saying anything? And if you can't speak or no one will hear you, that has got to feel pretty lonely at times."
b. "It's like whatever. Like you don't really matter here. And that is kind of sad? It's sad for all of us if we don't feel like we really matter, especially to important folks like our family."

EXPLORING EFFT IN STAGE 2

In this section, we explore the focus on restructuring attachment interactions in Stage 2 of EFFT. Key moments are illustrated following a different case example with a similar focus on core EFFT practices, EFT interventions, and the Tango process with a specific focus on child vulnerability.

Case Example

Fatemah sought family treatment to improve her relationship with her daughter Abeer (18 years of age) along with her husband Mohammad. Three years previously, Abeer was hospitalized for a severe eating disorder, having weighed only 80 pounds and almost dying. Abeer continues in individual treatment being of normal weight, although she continued to struggle with her eating. Fatemah felt that Abeer still needed her input, but she was unsure about how to communicate well with her daughter without the conversation becoming defensive. Fatemah recognized that she had made mistakes in the past, including confiding in Abeer about her unhappy marriage with Mohammad. Over the past year, Mohammad and Fatemah were in couple therapy and made good progress in strengthening their marriage. Fatemah also realized through her own therapy that she had been a good mother and had been well-intentioned in her efforts to parent her daughter.

In their initial family session, Fatemah stated that she wanted to be able to advise Abeer without her becoming defensive, particularly around schooling and her boyfriend. Mohammad expressed concern that he often had to "walk on eggshells" around Abeer or face her angry outbursts, which he felt were unprovoked. He choked back tears as he spoke about the sadness he felt over all the family had endured and Abeer's struggles. He stated that he had been terrified he would lose his daughter in the past but could not understand why she was so angry today.

Abeer spoke in exasperated tones, explaining that she never felt good enough for her parents, and no matter whatever she told them, she failed to meet her parents' expectations. For Abeer, this was a long-standing pattern, and in the past she had lived with the constant fear that her parents would divorce. She constantly felt caught in the middle, believing that it was up to her to maintain the peace in the household. As a child, she felt close to her father but lately has found it difficult to engage him without triggering an argument. Abeer did not confide in her mother for fear of her disapproval or judgment, often feeling like a disappointment in her mother's eyes.

Exercise 12.7. Building a Therapeutic Alliance

Based on the information just given, write a therapist response that would empathically reflect or validate each family member's experience.

a. Write a reflection that would make Mohammed's caregiving intention more explicit.

____

____

____

2. Write a response that validates Fatemah concern for her daughter's future and highlights her care and concern for Abeer.

____

____

____

3. Write a response that validates Abeer's surface emotions and anticipates her underlying attachment emotions.

____

____

____

4. Select the therapist statement which would best focus the session on the experiences of family members when they are impacted by family's insecurity or relational distress. (more than one correct answer)

   a. "I would like to set our next meeting at lunchtime, and all of us will bring our lunch, and we will eat together."
   b. "Dad, I would like you to teach Abeer about how to stand up for herself and give her some lessons on assertiveness."
   c. "An eating disorder can take over a family and become the ruler in how family members interact. It seems like the eating disorder has taken siege of your family."
   d. "I wonder what it is like for you, Fatemah, when Abeer doesn't listen to your efforts to mother her? Can you help me understand what happens to you?"
   e. "Are there times in this family when everyone does feel connected and close?"
   f. "What happens to you, Mohammad, when there is an explosion? What is it that you do?"
   g. "Do you know what happens to you, Abeer, when you don't feel that you are measuring up and are disappointing your mother?"

Exercise 12.8. Assessment Sessions

1. Identify two goals you would have in a parent session with Mohammad and Fatemah?

   a. _______________

   ____

   b. _______________

   ____

2. List two goals you would have in meeting with Abeer (the child)?

   a. _______________

   ____

b. ____

____

3. Identify a goal for your family session following these assessment sessions. Where would you place your focus in a session with Fatemah, Mohammad, and Abeer?

____

____

Exercise 12.9. Caregiving Blocks

Review the case description and based on the information provided hypothesize which of the following parental blocks best fit each parent's response.

1. Which of the following blocks best describes Mohammad's response (parental block)?
   a. Overresponding: critical and demanding
   b. Overresponding: overprotective and intrusive
   c. Overresponding: critical and dismissive
   d. Underresponding: distant and distracted
2. Which of the following blocks best describes Fatemah's response (parental block)?
   a. Overresponding: critical and demanding
   b. Overresponding: overpermissive and enabling
   c. Underresponding: critical and dismissive
   d. Underresponding: indecisive and disengaged
3. Which of the following blocks best describes Abeer's response (child block)?
   a. Intensifying: critical and demanding
   b. Intensifying: parentified, caretaker, stabilizer
   c. Minimizing: distant, cold, dismissive
   d. Minimizing: placating, compliant, and invisible

Exercises 12.10. Processing Caregiving Blocks

How would you respond to the following response from Fatemah?

Fatemah: I don't know what to do! The course she is taking I just don't understand. I think she is being influenced by her boyfriend. I mean, she talks and acts like him, using the same language. She just changed her mind at the last minute—I am not sure she thought it through at all, and I am afraid she is making a mistake. It's a lot of money.

Select the response that provides a clear focus on her underlying emotions in attachment related terms.

a. "Fatemah, can we slow down? There is a lot going on for you right now."
b. "I can hear that this is really distressing you when you see your daughter today. It's like she is changing."

c. "It sounds like you feel pretty helpless right now when you say you don't know what to do. That must be so hard, when you want to be there for her, and it feels like you have almost lost her?"

Exercise 12.11. Accessing Child Vulnerability

In accessing and processing a child's underlying emotions in Stage 2, the therapist will focus on assembling and deepening the child's experience including attachment-related core emotions. As the therapist, how might you begin to access this daughter's underlying emotions and frame these core emotions in attachment terms?

Abeer: I can't do anything right! Every time I bring anything to you—my grades, anything—it is never good enough! What did you say the last time I told you my marks? "How come you got a C?" Those marks aren't important, but all I get is criticism. No wonder I don't want to tell you anything!

Select the response below that best focuses on Abeer's underlying emotions in attachment-related terms.

a. "This makes you so frustrated when you hear criticism from your mother, yes? The marks don't matter to you as much as they matter to your Mom."
b. "It's like you can't do anything right. No matter how hard you try, you can't please your mom, yes? So, it makes sense then that you would want to pull away and not share with her."
c. "What's most important to you is how your Mom feels toward you. It's like the marks don't matter. What matters is how your Mom sees you. When you hear she is disappointed, it feels like she is disappointed in you and that really hurts. Of course it does. Down deep, you want your Mom to be proud, yes? "

Stage 2. EFFT Session 5, Mother and Daughter

The focus of Stage 2 in EFFT shifts to child vulnerability after parental openness and accessibility have been established. The EFT therapist intervenes to create new, secure bonding interactions between the parent and child. In this case, Abeer's fears and attachment longings are accessed and expressed, and the therapist provides support for Fatemah's more accessible and responsive engagement of her daughter's attachment emotions and needs. Stage 2 is complete when Abeer is able to reach for and receive her mother's comfort and care.

Exercise 12.12. Transcript Review of Tango and EFT Interventions

As treatment progressed, Fatemah expressed her fear that she was no longer able to reach her daughter. In working through her fear, Fatemah was better able to see that fear led her to focus almost exclusively on Abeer's behavior and performance. In turn, Abeer was able to express the hurt underlying her frustration and anger and let her mother know that her opinion of her truly mattered. In the following transcript, please follow the therapist focus on underlying emotion, attachment-related themes, and new opportunities for engaged encounters. Please identify the Tango Move and intervention the therapist uses with each therapist statement.

Fatemah: I am still worried about how we are doing. I need to be able, as her mother, to express my concern for her. I wouldn't be doing my job as a parent otherwise.

Therapist: It's really hard for a mom not to worry. I think that is the job of moms everywhere.

1. Tango Move: _______ Interventions ________________________________

Fatemah: I can't help but feel she is making a mistake, that she doesn't know what she is giving up.

Abeer: Why can't you just trust me and let me make my own mistake? I can't tell you anything! I know from the look on your face how you feel—you make it abundantly clear!

Fatemah: But I don't know why you don't talk to me. You know I can handle it. I want you to let me know what is going on with you.

Therapist: This is where you get caught in the cycle because you as her mother wants to do a good job parenting and protect your daughter. Abeer, you hear all this protection as disapproval and judgment, so you withdraw. Fatemah, you are left not knowing what is happening with Abeer, which is scarier still because it's like you can't reach her or have any influence. I would expect what you want is to be able to talk to each other.

2 Tango Move: _______ Interventions ________________________________

Fatemah: I want to be able to talk to Abeer, but sometimes I just don't know how. She doesn't want to talk to me.

Abeer: (rising voice) It's not that I don't want to talk to you, but what do you expect? I just hear how I am screwing up. You think I want to hear that?

Fatemah: I am just trying to be your mom.

Therapist: (soft, slow voice) It sounds like it's really painful for you, Abeer, to go to your mom and to see disapproval. It's really important to you how your mom feels about you.

3. Tango Move: _______ Interventions ________________________________

Abeer: Of course, it is important. She must know that.

Fatemah: I don't know that. It seems more like you just want to get away and that you are so angry with me for the past.

Therapist: That's so hard for you to think that Abeer is mad at you, particularly when you think of the past.

4. Tango Move: _______ Interventions ________________________________

Fatemah: (crying) I don't know how I can get over the past. I thought I was such a good mom. I was so involved in Abeer's life—I did everything with her, and with the eating disorder, I didn't see it—I didn't see it at all.

Abeer: I was a good liar. There was no way you could know—I covered it up.

Therapist: This is a really painful part of your relationship for you, Fatemah. It sounds like it's really hard for you to get over what happened, and you feel so guilty as a mom that this happened to your child. That you weren't there to protect her or take care of her. That hurts as her mom, yes?

5. Tango Move: _______ Interventions ______________________________

Fatemah: (crying) I don't think I can ever forgive myself. It should never have happened.

Therapist: And you wonder how Abeer feels about it also—could you talk to her about that now?

6. Tango Move: _______ Interventions ______________________________

Fatemah: (looking at Abeer) I am so sorry that it happened.

Abeer: You've said that before. I know that you feel that way, and I don't blame you—that's not what pisses me off!

Therapist: What happened in the past is not so alive for you now, Abeer, as it might be for your mom. When your mom feels bad about the past, you feel bad also and feel maybe a little guilty for your mom's feelings?

7. Tango Move: _______ Interventions ______________________________

Abeer: I want to get over the past. I feel like a big screw-up when you talk about it. I want you to see what I have done and how I have got better. You don't give me any credit! You know how hard I have worked and the number of therapists I have seen—does any of that sink in!?

Fatemah: I know you have worked hard, and I am not worried about your eating. I just don't know what to do.

Abeer: You could start with not being so critical and cutting of me. I am not the little kid who was stuck in hospital and not able to eat. I have changed a lot since then.

Therapist: I get the sense that it is more about what is happening today with your mom and the disapproval that is so hard to bear.

8. Tango Move: _______ Interventions ______________________________

Abeer: (looking at her mom) I have been working really hard to get out of this. All my life I have been trying to please people. I would do anything for someone else, and that was something that you taught me to have compassion for others—you know, even the sick squirrel on the street.

Fatemah: Yes, but that is what I am afraid of—that you will get stuck there, just pleasing others and not looking after yourself.

Abeer: I am trying to take care of myself. I need to feel good about me (starts to cry), and I don't.

Therapist: (soft, slow) This is the hard part, yes Abeer? It is so hard to feel good about you. Your tears are saying how hard this is. It is so great that you can let your mom see some of this pain. This pain that you have been carrying for so long, all by yourself.

9. Tango Move: _______ Interventions ________________________________

Abeer: (Fatemah moves closer to Abeer and puts her arm around her.) I am working on it.

Therapist: (slowly, softly) Yes, but that gets so tiring when you are working on it all alone. You have been all alone for a long, long time. You have been trying to get your mom to see, and she has been trying to fix it for you, but the hard part is that you don't feel good about you, and that hurts. It's kind of like (proxy voice) "I am hurting, Mom; can you see me? Can you see my pain?"

10. Tango Move: _______ Interventions ________________________________

Fatemah: (Abeer crying) You know, I think that is when I am feeling bad about me—it's hard for me to feel good inside.

Therapist: You can understand this pain, Fatemah, the pain of feeling bad inside. What's it like to see Abeer's pain right now?

11. Tango Move: _______ Interventions ________________________________

Fatemah: (looking at Abeer) I feel sad for you, baby. And I feel like I have caused some of that pain.

Therapist: You have tried very hard to mother Abeer without really knowing how. Like most of us and when things have gone wrong, it is so scary, that you lose control and try to make things better by fixing things. But right here, right now, Abeer is letting you see her pain. She is saying (proxy voice), "Can you see me? Umm can you see my pain?"

Fatemah: I want to be there for her.

Therapist: Can you tell her?

12. Tango Move: _______ Interventions ________________________________

Fatemah (looking at Abeer) I am right here, hon. I don't want you to feel alone.

Therapist: (leaning toward Abeer, using a soft, slow voice) Can you feel your Mom beside you? What's that like? She is right here, saying she sees your pain and that she doesn't want you to be alone.

13. Tango Move: _______ Interventions ________________________________

Therapist: (soft, slow voice as Abeer nods) And you need your Mom. You have said that in many different ways, and now you are letting her see how vulnerable you feel. It takes so much strength and courage just to say "I hurt. I am in pain."

14. Tango Move: _______ Interventions ________________________________

Fatemah: (stroking Abeer's arm) Yes, I see your strength. You are amazing.

Therapist: Do you feel your mother sees how much you hurt and maybe how scary it is to not feel good about yourself and to feel so alone?

15. Tango Move: _______ Interventions ________________________________

Abeer: I hate my life. I sometimes wonder if I am going to make it.

Fatemah: (looking at Abeer) Ohh, but I want so much for you to be happy.

Therapist: (to mother) Yes, of course, you do, but right here, right now Abeer is sharing her pain, how hard and dark it gets for her sometimes. Can you be with her there?

16. Tango Move: _______ Interventions ________________________________

Fatemah: (to Abeer, in a strong and steady voice) I want you to know you are not alone. You can count on me. Please tell me what you need.

Therapist: What you are saying is really important, Fatemah. This is a really good question. You want Abeer to know that you are there for her and that you want to listen. Can you tell her?

17. Tango Move: _______ Interventions ________________________________

Fatemah: (looking at Abeer) You know that your grandmother and I are not close, and what I want for us is to be close. I want you to know that I will be there for you, that you can come and talk to me anytime, and you know I will try to remember just how grown up you are, and I will try to listen and not tell you how to be. I do trust you, and I want you to trust me. I am there for you.

Abeer: I know. I do want to come to you. What do you think matters to me most? You know, I do want to talk to you.

Therapist: You hear that your mother wants to be there. But what is that you need from her? What is it that Abeer needs for Abeer?

18. Tango Move: _______ Interventions ______________________________

Abeer: (pause, looking down)

Therapist: This is so hard. You're asking for you. You have been so busy looking after everyone else. But you are saying it's hard, you get down and discouraged sometimes, and you have been saying how much how your mother sees you affects you. To have her confidence in you, to have her see you. Can you imagine what that would be like?

19. Tango Move: _______ Interventions ______________________________

Abeer: (raising her head, softly) I want you to believe in me.

Therapist: Yes, you want Mom to believe in you, especially at times when it's hard to believe in yourself. None of us can do this alone, and right now you are letting your Mom in, in a way that she can be there for you. (pause) What do you see when you look at her face?

20. Tango Move: _______ Interventions ______________________________

Abeer: (crying) I know that she loves me. (Mother and daughter embrace.)

Therapist: And that feels good. This is so moving to see the two of you together right now. Fatemah, I see your tears. Abeer, I see your tears. This is so beautiful that you can talk to each other in this way. So different than how it has gone in the past. This is all about how much you matter, Abeer, and how much your love as mother matters.

21. Tango Move: _______ Interventions ______________________________

Exercise 12.13. Assembling Emotions in Stage 2

Identify the different elements of emotion you see in each response. Then write a reflection that would begin to assemble her experience.

1. Fatemah: "When I see her going to her boyfriend, it makes me so sad. I worry about the kind of influence he has, and I worry about what is going to happen to her."
   a. Trigger: ______________.
   b. Bodily Response: ______________.
   c. Meaning: ______________.
   d. Action: ______________.

Response:

____

____

____

2. Abeer: "You can be so cutting. I know I can give it right back, but you have no idea. I just go to my room and stay there. It rips me up inside. I stay there until it goes away."
   a. Trigger: _______________.
   b. Bodily Response: _______________.
   c. Meaning: _______________.
   d. Action: _______________.

Response:

____

____

____

Exercise 12.14. Deepening Emotions in Stage 2

Select the therapist response that would most likely heighten Abeer's pain when she says:

Abeer: You can be so cutting. I know I can give it right back but you have no idea. I just go to my room and stay there. It rips me up inside. I stay there until it goes away.

1. Select the therapist response that would most likely heighten Abeer's pain in response to her mother's critical attacks.
   a. "Your mother doesn't really see your pain, just your anger."
   b. "It rips me up. Her words can cut so deep. Deep down this is so very painful."
   c. "What would you want your mother to know about this pain?"
   d. "It makes sense that you defend yourself in these moments. It's the only way to stay safe."
   e. "Your pain is deep, and you go away till the pain also goes away."
2. What metaphor would you use to heighten Abeer's experience?

   ____

3. Now write your own response using this metaphor to help Abeer begin to speak from her attachment-related emotions. What would you say to deepen her felt awareness of this pain?

Response:

____

____

____

Exercise 12.15. Enacting Encounters in Stage 2

Practice forming an enactment following Abeer's comment. In your enactment focus on enacting Abeer's attachment-related needs.

Abeer: I want you to respect my opinions and decisions. There are things I can figure out, and I do take things seriously. I can see that I have made mistakes in the past, and maybe it's hard for you to trust me, but I have a good head on my shoulders, and I can look after myself properly.

1. Now write an enactment response to help Abeer begin to speak from her attachment-related needs. What would you have her to share with her mother?

   Response:

   ____

   ____

   ____

2. Following Abeer's enactment of this need, how would you respond to Abeer to support the reach she made with her attachment need?

   Response:

   ____

   ____

   ____

3. Write a similar response to Fatemah focusing on promoting her accessible and responsive reply to her daughter's clear and compelling attachment need?

   Response:

   ____

   ____

   ____

This family continued to work in therapy. The next step was to include Mohammad and Abeer. Dyadic sessions were held with the father to open up the communication between Abeer and her father and restructure their interaction. Mohammad was withdrawing from conflict, and Abeer was being angry and explosive with her father to get a reaction. In session, Abeer was relieved that she could talk openly with her father and he did not run away. Mohammad was reassured that he could have an open conversation with Abeer that did not escalate into conflict but brought them closer. Mohammad stated, "I feel like I have my daughter back." Abeer was able to let him know that she really did need him, and when he withdrew from her, it sent her a message that "I am not worth it." Mohammad reassured his daughter and let her know how proud he was of her, which Abeer received with a big smile.

In Stage 3, the family group was reunited, and a session was held to reinforce the new positive patterns of accessible and responsive interactions and create a new family narrative of strength, connection, and confidence. Abeer was registered in a college program in a nearby city and was making plans to leave home. She now felt ready to leave home as she had "a home to come home to." Rules of engagement were established in this family with the agreement made that issues would not be fought about or ignored. The family now shared a new confidence in the availability of the other. Fatemah and Mohammad had revitalized their romantic relationship and functioned well as a parenting team. Abeer continued to struggle with occasional bouts of depression, but she was able to reach for help when she needed it and felt the security of her parent's emotional presence. Overall, the family climate had shifted from tension and hostility to warmth and relaxation.

SUMMARY

EFFT is an effective and powerful modality to address fractured and conflictual relationships among family members. Attachment theory guides the therapist in identifying the relational blocks in the caregiving system. The goal is to restructure the family dance in the direction of accessible and responsive interactional patterns so that parents are emotionally available to their children. The therapist utilizes the interventions of the EFT Tango to process both parental blocks to caregiving and child blocks to reaching and receiving care. Secure attachment is established when children can send a clear emotional cue to available and responsive caregivers and children's attachment needs are met. The processes of EFFT differ in the hierarchical or generational elements and how emotion is processed with parents and children. The multiple members and overlapping cycles in families are managed through the use of the decision tree to determine how to structure the assessment and treatment sessions. The EFFT therapist titrates the intensity and level of emotional engagement to fit the developmental needs of the child. EFFT is a therapeutic intervention that restores and rebuilds secure attachment bonds with the goal of resourcing the family unit to face problems and life challenges together.

ANSWERS AND SUGGESTED RESPONSES

Exercise 12.1. Alliance Building in EFFT

1. **Answer: A, C, E.** Responses b and d are incorrect. b is a directive focused on positive connotation of fighting behavior, and d is a behavioral focused problem-solving task.

2. **Possible Responses:** Four possible responses are listed next. Reference to parental intent is underlined in each response.
    - "Jen I can see that you want your family to work together in a positive way, and when that doesn't happen, as a mom, it is frustrating as you want the best for your family."
    - "Jen, it looks like it is really important to you that Dennis have a voice and express himself directly because if you don't know what is happening for him, how do you fix it?"
    - "Wendy, I see that you want happy times for you and your boys, and when it is only fighting, that must be very discouraging, yes?"
    - 'Wendy you are very attuned to how Dennis is feeling. I see you coming to his defense right now, like you want to protect him, or help make sense of what it might be like for him. Does that fit?"
3. **Possible Responses:** Three possible responses that validate the children's experience using the attachment frame.
    - "Dennis, I guess I wouldn't want to say much if I felt like I didn't have a choice to attend, or I don't know, but maybe what's going to happen if I do speak up?"
    - "Randy, I can see that maybe you are trying to create some fun times right here, right now, with your jokes and teasing; maybe then there won't be fights?"
    - "I am happy that the two of you did come to meet me today. I hear that this is not your favorite thing to do, but I am imaging your family is important."

Exercise 12.2. Assessment Sessions

1. **Parent Session Possible Goals:** Strengthen the alliance, empathize with parent's struggles, assess caregiving alliance, assess attachment histories
2. **Sibling Session Possible Goals:** Strengthen the alliance, provide space for children's perspective, assess for safety, assess sibling dynamic, and foster sibling support
3. **Possible Response:** "Jack, I appreciate that you are in a different place in the family than your brothers, and I would appreciate getting your perspective, hearing your take on this family situation. You no doubt see things in some ways different from others, and I would really appreciate hearing from you and what you see that might help me better understand how I can help your brother and moms.'

Exercise 12.3. Promoting Parental Buy-in

1. Any of these four themes will be useful in promoting greater parental buy-in from Jen. These themes include reflecting care giving intention, highlighting parental uniqueness, validating impact on parents; and focusing on relationship patterns.
2. **Possible Responses:**
    - "Jen, I hear the urgency and your concern. This matters so much, and you are really concerned for Dennis. I appreciate how difficult this is sometimes, especially when he gets really angry and then pulls away. You see his need

for support, and I also see how important you are to him. In these moments, you can lose that connection, and you both end up on opposite sides. I think our work together can make a difference there."

- "It's hard as parents to balance these different needs and demands from each of your sons. I know that you as his mom fear that you are losing touch with Dennis, and that is something I can help you talk about in a new way. I see how much you care and how important you are as his mother, someone he has counted on and while it is very hard to see, he still needs you as his mom."

Exercise 12.4. Identifying Caregiving Blocks

1. **Answer: A**. Jen's behavior is often critical and demanding and her approach to moments of uncertainty is more often to take charge or take control even if her anger is driving family members away from her.
2. **Answer: B**. Wendy also seems to over respond to situations, especially as she is more likely to keep the peace by responding to others. In moments of conflict, she is more likely to freeze and seek to please either Jen or Dennis.

Exercise 12.5. Identifying Parental Intent

1. "In the face of Dennis not listening, you come down hard. It's like, 'I will do anything to get a response from him.' After all, no response leads you nowhere, and that is pretty hard to take as his parent, yes? You want to have guide him because what happens to your son matters. Not being able to reach Dennis is not only frustrating but alarming. You see him behaving in ways that scare you because you want the best for him? Is that right? You help me."
2. "I hear you owning Jen that you do come down hard on your son. You know that your response is harsh, and you are also aware there is a lot of heaviness in your home. I am imagining that would be hard for you as Mom, who loves her son. I can see the tears in your eyes as I say this. Can you tell me what's happening?"

Exercise 12.6. Following the EFT Tango and Micro-Interventions in Stage 1

1. Tango Move 1 Interventions: validation, empathic reflection
2. Tango Move 1 Interventions: empathic reflection, tracking interaction
3. Tango Move 1 Interventions: validation, empathic conjecture, evocative question
4. Tango Moves 1, 2 Interventions: validation, empathic reflection, and empathic conjecture
5. Tango Move 2 Interventions: empathic reflection, tracking interaction, empathic conjecture
6. Tango Move 2 Interventions: empathic reflection, validation, empathic conjecture
7. Tango move 2 Interventions: empathic reflection, evocative question
8. Tango Move 2 Interventions: validation, empathic reflection, empathic conjecture
9. Tango Move 2 Interventions: empathic reflection, heightening (RISSSC)

10. Tango Move 3 Interventions: enactment
11. Tango Move 3 Interventions: evocative response
12. Tango Move 4 Interventions: validation, evocative response, evocative question
13. Tango Moves 4, 5 Interventions: validation, empathic reflection
14. Key Elements in Working through a Parental Block

    The therapist responses may include more than one of these elements in a given talk-turn. Listed below are examples of different talk-turns that illustrate this focus.

    a. Naming/engaging reactivity: See therapist response # 2, 3, 4.
    b. Linking triggers: See therapist response # 4, 6, 7.
    c. Validating: See therapist response # 1, 3, 6, 8, 12.
    d. Heightening: See therapist response # 9.
    e. Reframing/conjectures: See therapist responses # 5, 6, 8, 13.
    f. Enactment: See therapist response #10.
15. **Possible Stage 1 Enactments**
    - Jen, can you tell Dennis right now that when you get alarmed and yell, that you are actually scared that you can't reach him?
    - Wendy, when you go quiet and don't say anything, it's not because you don't care; it's because you are trying to calm things down. Can you let Dennis know that right now?
    - Dennis, can you tell your mom right now that when you get frustrated and shut down, it's because you are feeling pretty bad about yourself?
16. **Processing a Child's Response**
    a. It seems like there is no point. It doesn't matter what you say, right? It's like it won't get heard, so what's the point of saying anything? And if you can't speak or no one will hear you, that has got to feel pretty lonely at times.
    b. It's like whatever. Like you don't really matter here. And that is kind of sad? It's sad for all of us if we don't feel like we really matter, especially to important folks like our family.

Exercise 12.7. Building a Therapeutic Alliance

1. **Possible Responses for Mohammed**
   - "Mohammad it is really sad for you that your contact with your daughter today is filled with negativity. It seems like you miss being close to her?"
   - "It is hard for you as Dad to not know how to reach your daughter. You feel unsure and uncertain and as her father, and you want to be able to talk to Abeer."
   - "It sounds like it is hard to understand your daughter today. As her father, you want to be able to understand her, to know how she is feeling, and when you don't, that feels very unpredictable."

2. **Possible Responses to Fatemah**
    - "Fatemah, it sounds like you feel disappointed in yourself as Abeer's mother in the past, and that impacts how you are with her today? I hear you do want to be there for her, as her mother, but you are unsure of how to do that?"
    - "I am guessing that when Abeer is defensive with you, that impacts you and throws you off balance? You want to be able to reach your daughter, and when that doesn't happen, that is hard?"
    - "It sounds like you care deeply about what happens to Abeer. When you see her making decisions that may impact her in a negative way, you are really concerned, yes? You want to be able to take care of her and protect her."
3. **Possible Responses to Abeer**
    - "This is really hard, Abeer, to feel like you are a disappointment to your parents? I would imagine you want them to be proud of you, and it hurts to feel that you are not good enough in their eyes?"
    - "It's been hard and scary for you in the past, and you have worried a lot about your parent's marriage. You took on the responsibility to try and keep them together. That is a lot for a young girl."
    - "It is really good that you can let your parents know today how you are feeling. You have been very open, and that says to me that you do want them to understand."
4. **Answers: D, E, F, G.** D. invites Fatemah to explore her experience when triggered by Abeer's avoidance. e invites the family to reflect on their experience of closeness and connection. F. focuses on Mohammed's action tendency in response to family conflict. G. is an evocative response that engages Abeer's experience in the face of her mother's disappointment and disapproval.

Exercise 12.8. Assessment Sessions

1. **Parent Session Possible Goals:** Strengthen the alliance, empathize with parental struggles, assess attachment histories. Assess caregiving alliance and how the relationship has changed with the marital therapy.
2. **Individual Child Session Possible Goals**: Provide more space for Abeer's perspective. Assess for safety and potential benefit of individual therapeutic support.
3. Sessions would begin with a focus on the most distressed dyad, which is Fatemah and Abeer. Possible Goal: Strengthening the alliance, tracking relationship pattern between Abeer and Fatemah, reflecting and validating surface and core emotions around relational blocks.

Exercise 12.9. Caregiving Blocks

1. **Answer: D**. Underresponding: distant and distracted. Mohammad is avoidant, underresponsive caregiver. He avoids contact with his daughter and has a negative view of his daughter.

2. **Answer: A**. Overresponding: critical and demanding. Fatemah is an anxious, overresponsive caregiver using criticism and control as a means to reach her daughter. Fatemah has a negative view of child and a negative view of self.
3. **Answer: C**. Minimizing: distant, cold, dismissing. Abeer is avoidant and moves away from her emotional experience and her mother's critical attacks. She has a negative view of others and their availability to her needs.

Exercise 12.10. Processing Caregiving Blocks

Answer: C. Therapist response focuses on her fear and the impact of the loss of influence she fears in her daughter's life.

Exercise 12.11. Accessing Child Vulnerability

Answer: C. Therapist focus on the underlying hurt and the attachment needs to be seen, accepted and loved.

Exercise 12.12. Transcript Review of Tango and EFT interventions

1. Tango Move 1 Interventions: validation, normalization
2. Tango Move 1 Interventions: Empathic Reflection, Tracking Interaction
3. Tango Move 1 Interventions: Empathic Reflection, Empathic Conjecture, Present Focus
4. Tango Move 1 Interventions: Empathic Reflection, and Empathic Conjecture, Present Focus
5. Tango Move 2 Interventions: Empathic Reflection, Attachment Reframe
6. Tango Move 3 Interventions: Enactment
7. Tango Move 4 Interventions: Validation, Empathic Conjecture
8. Tango Move 4 Interventions: Empathic Conjecture
9. Tango Move 2 Interventions: Validation, Empathic Conjecture, Heightening (RISSSC)
10. Tango Move 2 Interventions: Heightening
11. Tango Move 1 Interventions: Empathic reflection, Evocative Question
12. Tango Move 3 Interventions: Restructuring Enactment
13. Tango Move 4 Interventions: Evocative Question, Heightening
14. Tango Move 4 Interventions: Heightening, Validation, Empathic Reflection
15. Tango Move 4 Interventions: Evocative Question
16. Tango Move 3 Interventions: Validation, Refocusing on Attachment Affect, Enactment
17. Tango Move 3 Interventions: Validation, Restructuring Enactment
18. Tango Move 4 Interventions: Empathic Reflection, Validation
19. Tango Move 4 Interventions: Heightening, Empathic Reflection, Evocative Question

20. Tango Move 4 Interventions: Validation, Evocative Question
21. Tango Move 5 Interventions: Empathic Reflection, Reflecting Interactions, Heightening,

Exercise 12.13. Assembling Emotions in Stage 2

1. Fatemah: "When I see her going to her boyfriend, it makes me so sad. I worry about the kind of influence he has, and I worry about what is going to happen to her."_____
   a. Trigger: Abeer turning to her boyfriend
   b. Bodily Response: None given in her response, and the therapist may ask an evocative question about her bodily felt sense in these moments.
   c. Meaning: She is at risk, in danger. I can't protect her. I have lost some influence.
   d. Action: Worries

   Possible Response: You see Abeer turning toward others, her boyfriend, and the worries start. "What's going to happen to her? Is she going to be okay. And there's sadness, too. It brings tears to your eyes not knowing if you can keep her safe, and even if you could, would she want that help?
2. Abeer: "You can be so cutting. I know I can give it right back, but you have no idea. I just go to my room and stay there until it goes away. It rips me up inside. I'm never going to be good enough for you."
3. Trigger: Mother's critical comments
   a. Bodily Response: Rips me up inside
   b. Meaning: Not good enough for you
   c. Action: Goes away

   Possible Response: "Her words cut deep, and you can either fight back or go away, but either way these words cut deep, leaving you ripped up inside and feeling like you will never be the daughter she wants."

Exercise 12.14. Deepening Emotions in Stage 2

1. **Answer: B.** This response focuses on Abeer's pain using her words and repeating phrases emphasizing Abeer's underlying pain.
2. **Possible Metaphor**. Open wound, brokenhearted, stabbing pain, cutting to pieces.
3. **Possible Response:** You can go away, but the pain is like an open wound that doesn't fully heal. The words stop but the pain continues. It all hurts so much.

Exercise 12.15. Enacting Encounters in Stage 2

1. **Possible Response:** Abeer, even as you say this, I can hear the strength in your voice. In one way you understand how your parents might find it hard to trust you, but you want them to have confidence in you and know you are taking this seriously and will take care of yourself. Can you them right now how important

this feels that as your mom and dad that they respect your decisions and your way of thinking?

2. **Possible Response:** What was that like to look in your mother's face and to say, "I need you to respect me to have confidence in me"? You said that so clearly; you are really hoping they can take this in. What was this like for you?
3. **Possible Response:** Fatemah, can you hear your daughter's strength in this moment? Do you hear her need for your support and belief in her? What it's like to hear her heartfelt request and to know she sees both her errors and her confidence in her future?

APPENDIX A

EFT SEXUALITY ASSESSMENT QUESTIONS

Compiled by Susan Johnson & Michael Moran

VERSION 1: LONGFORM (LEFTSA)

This version is for use in individual sessions when sexual problems are explicitly referenced in the couple's concern or goals. The goal is to structure an exploration of each client's sexuality and how it plays out in the EFT "within and between" focus. All questions are to be asked respectfully, staying within the client's window of tolerance and in the context of the creating a safe haven alliance.

A) Sexuality in Present Relationship (12 items)

1. In your own words, tell me how you've come to understand the sexual challenges with your partner.
2. Has this always been the case, and if not, when do you remember it becoming an issue?
3. What have you tried in the past to try to rectify the problem?
4. Describe to me the typical sexual interaction with your partner (the dance); give me a play by play. How do you both communicate what you want and need?
5. Do you experience sexual desire at present in your relationship? Does this translate into satisfaction for you?
6. How often do you have sex with your partner? Is this frequency okay for you? Do you have similar sex drives? If not, how do you handle this?
7. Please rate your initial level of sexual satisfaction in your present relationship on a scale from 1 to 10. How would you rate your satisfaction now? If there is a difference, when did you notice this change? What has changed?
8. What is most important for your partner to know about you sexually? Do they know this?
9. When do you feel most turned on and erotic with your partner?
10. What are your three most important expectations in bed? Have you shared them with your partner?
11. What would you like to change about sex with your partner? Can you discuss this with him/her?
12. How important is it for you to orgasm during sex? How often does this occur?

B) Initial Messages and History of Sexuality (7 items)

1. What is your first memory of sexuality?
2. What messages/myths about sex did you receive growing up? How do you think your family of origin experience impacts your sex life now?
3. When you think of sex, what two words come to mind? What image comes to mind or what associations arise?
4. When did you begin puberty? How did you feel about it? How did your family respond to your development?
5. When and how did you first experience sexual arousal, and how did you feel about it?
6. Tell me about your first sexual experiences.
7. Did you experience any sexual trauma or disturbing or unwanted experiences?
   a. If yes—How were these experiences handled? Did you ever talk about them or get support with them or help with any emotional/psychological distress that may have resulted from the trauma?
   b. If yes, how do these experiences impact your sex life now?

C) Present Sexuality (8 items)

1. Do you feel secure in your sexuality, or are there things you struggle with? (What elements contribute to feeling more/less secure in your sexuality?)
2. How important is sex in your present life? Has this changed over the course of your adulthood?
3. Do you allow yourself to fantasize about sex? What makes fantasies exciting for you?
4. How would you rate your sense of sexual self-esteem—attractiveness? If you can, rate it on a scale from 1 to 10.
5. Are there things you would like to change about your sexuality? Are you clear about your turn-ons and turn-offs?
6. Do you worry about your performance in sex? Is it difficult to remain present and engaged in sexual interactions?
7. How do you address your sexual desire/needs on your own? For example, do you ever turn to things like porn?
8. Are there medications, physical/emotional (e.g., depression, high levels of stress etc.) problems, or even habits that get in the way of you expressing your sexuality?

D) Attachment Style Motives and Strategies (3 items)

1. Do you feel close and emotionally connected when you make love with your partner? Does this translate into hugging, cuddling, and affection after sex?
2. Do you feel anxious during sex and want to check that your partner is feeling desire for you and feels that you are their special partner? How important is this reassurance for you as a reason for making love and during lovemaking?
3. Do you get caught up in looking at things from the outside and thinking about your performance and how attractive you are and find yourself looking for more and more intense sensations in bed with your partner?

SHORTFORM EFT SEXUALITY ASSESSMENT (SEFTSA)

This short form can be used in a couple or individual session where sexual problems are not the identified focus or source of relationship distress but sex is still less gratifying than the couple would prefer.

Ask permission: Can we talk for a moment about your sex life?

1) How generally satisfied are you with the sex you have with your partner? Is there a time when this satisfaction changed for either of you?
2) Describe to me the typical sexual interaction with your partner (the dance); give me a play by play. Is this dance the same as happens in the rest of your relationship, or is it different? Who initiates, and who is less forward? Can you both communicate what you want and need in the bedroom?
3) How often do you have sex with your partner? Is this frequency okay for you? Do you have similar sex drives? If not, how do you handle this?
4) If there are things you would like to change in your sex life with your partner, can you discuss this together?
5) Are there medications, physical/emotional (i.e., depression, high levels of stress etc.) problems, or even habits that get in the way of you expressing your sexuality together?
6) What is the most important part of sex for you both? For some people, orgasm matters more than anything; for others, it matters very little if at all. For some couples, they can't seem to find their desire for each other, or they long to feel closer or more connected in bed. Do you know what matters most to you and your partner?

Additional Questions for LGBTQ Couples

1) When did you first become aware that you were attracted to someone of the same sex?
2) What were the messages that you received from your family/community about being attracted to someone of the same sex?
3) Was there any person you could talk to about these feelings?
4) What did you do with these feelings if there wasn't a safe person to talk with about it?
5) What was your coming-out process like?
6) Did you ever feel like your life was in danger or under threat as a result of your sexual or gender identity?
7) How did you learn about how to have sex with someone of the same sex if this wasn't modeled in your environment (family, culture, etc.)?
8) How do you feel about your sexual orientation/gender identity now?

PLEASE NOTE: There may be times, especially in cases when prolonged sexual dysfunction is present, that obtaining a consult or providing a referral to a sex therapist may be the most responsible decision to make.

Adapted from and informed by:

Althof, S.E., Rosen, R.C., Perelman, M.A., Rubio-Aurioles, E. (2012). Standard Operating Procedures for Taking a Sexual History. *Journal of Sexual Medicine*, 12. DOI: 10.1111/j.1743–6109.2012.02823.x

Iasenza, S. (2020). *Transforming Sexual Narratives: A Relational Approach to Sex Therapy.* New York, NY: Routledge

Johnson, S. (2008) Hold Me Tight. New York, NY: Little Brown & Company.

Johnson, S., Simakhodskaya, Z., Moran, M. Addressing Issues of Sexuality in Couples Therapy: Emotionally Focused Therapy Meets Sex Therapy. *Current Sexual Health Reports, 6 April 2018.* Doi.org/10.1007/s11930-018-0146-5

Morin, J. (1995). *The Erotic Mind.* New York, NY: Harper Collins.

Perel, E. (2015). *Sexuality Conversation Starters.* www.estherperel.com

Weeks, G. R., Gambescia, N., Hertlein, K. M. (2015) *A Clinician's Guide to Systemic Sex Therapy.* New York, NY: Routledge.

APPENDIX B

ATTACHMENT HISTORY

An attachment history involves exploring the history of each person's experiences in attachment relationships. It is particularly important to focus on what people learned about comfort and connection in relationships, past traumas and how people adapted, and how people may have found healing in relationships. The following is a list of possible attachment history questions.

Childhood Attachment Relationships

1. Who did you go to for comfort when you were young?
2. Could you always count on this person/these people for comfort?
3. When were you most likely to be comforted by this person/these people?
4. How did you let this person/these people know that you needed connection and comfort?
5. Did this person/these people every betray you or were they unavailable at critical times?
6. What did you learn about comfort and connection from this person/these people?
7. If no one was safe, how did you comfort yourself? How did you learn that people were unsafe?
8. Did you ever turn to alcohol, drugs, sex, or material things for comfort?
9. At times of crises, what did your family do? For example, did they connect and comfort, or did they fight or distance from each other?

Romantic Attachment Relationships

1. Have there been times when you have been able to be vulnerable and find comfort with your partner?
2. Have there been any particularly traumatic incidences in your previous romantic relationships?
3. How have you tried to find comfort in romantic relationships? Could you be honest and open? Could you ask for comfort?

APPENDIX C

EFT TRAINING NOTE FORM

Date: ___________ Session #________ Length:________ Clients: ________________________________

Therapy Stage: ☐ Stabilization ☐ Restructuring ☐ Consolidation

Aspect of cycle highlighted in session:

Negative cycle

Partner **Partner**

Behavior (pursue or withdraw) | Behavior (pursue or withdraw)

Perceptions and attributions (view of self and other) | Perceptions and attributions (view of self and other)

Reactive emotions | Reactive emotions

Core soft emotions | Core soft emotions

Attachment needs | Attachment needs

Session Content Issues:

Key Emotions, Metaphors, Images, Client Phrases, and Positive Shifts in Session:

Interventions used:

- ☐ Empathic reflection
- ☐ Validation of client realities and emotional responses
- ☐ Evocative questions
- ☐ Heighten/RISSSC
- ☐ Empathic conjecture/interpretation and inferences

How many TANGOs? __________

Steps Covered:

- ☐ 1. Alliance and assessment
- ☐ 2. Identify negative interaction cycle and partner positions
- ☐ 3. Access emotions underlying interactional positions
- ☐ 4. Reframe the problem in terms of emotions, attachment needs, and the cycles
- ☐ 5. Access disowned needs and aspects of self and integrating into interactions
- ☐ 6. Promote acceptance of partner's experiences and new patterns
- ☐ 7. Restructure the interaction and create emotional engagement
- ☐ 8. New solutions to old issues
- ☐ 9. Consolidating new cycles of attachment

Plan for Next Session

REFERENCES

Arnold, M. B. (1960). *Emotion and personality.* New York: Columbia Press.

Barlow, D. H., Farchione, T. J., Fairholme, C. P., Ellard, K. K., Boisseau, C. L., Allen, L. B., & May, J. T. E. (2011). *Unified protocol for transdiagnostic treatment of emotional disorders: Therapist guide.* New York: Oxford University Press.

Bartholomew, K., & Horowitz, L. M. (1991). Attachment styles among young adults: A test of a four-category model. *Journal of Personality and Social Psychology, 61*(2), 226–244.

Bertalanffy, L. (1956). *General system theory.* New York: George Braziller.

Birnbaum, G. E. (2007). Attachment orientations, sexual functioning, and relationship satisfaction in a community sample of women. *Journal of Social and Personal Relationships, 24*(1), 21–35.

Bograd, M., & Mederos, F. (1999). Battering and couples therapy: Universal screening and selection of treatment modality. *Journal of Marital & Family Therapy, 25*, 291–312.

Bowlby, J. (1969). *Attachment and loss. Vol 1: Attachment.* New York: Basic Books.

Bowlby, J. (1973). *Attachment and loss. Vol 2: Separation.* New York: Basic Books.

Bowlby, J. (1979). *The making and breaking of affectional bonds.* London: Tavistock.

Bowlby, J. (1988). *A secure base.* New York: Basic Books.

Bowlby, J. (1980). *Attachment and loss: Vol. 3. Loss.* New York: Penguin Books.

Bradley, B., & Furrow, J. (2004). Towards a mini-theory of the blamer softening event: "Tracking the moment by moment process". *Journal of Marital & Family Therapy, 30*, 233–246.

Bradley, B., & Furrow, J. (2007). Inside blamer softening: Maps and missteps. *Journal of Systemic Therapies, 26*, 25–43.

Brennan, K. A., Clark, C. L., & Shaver, P. R. (1998). Self-report measurement of adult attachment: An integrative overview. In J. A. Simpson & W. S. Rhodes (Eds.), *Attachment theory and close relationships* (pp. 46–76). New York: Guilford.

Brubacher, L. (2017). Emotionally focused individual therapy: An attachment-based experiential/systemic perspective. *Person-Centered and Experiential Psychotherapies, 16*(1), 50–67. doi.org/10.1080/14779757.2017.1297250

Brubacher, L. L. (2018). *Stepping into emotionally focused couple therapy: Key ingredients of change.* London: Routledge.

Brubacher, L. L., & Wiebe, S. A. (2019). Process-research to practice in emotionally focused couple therapy: A map for reflective practice. *Journal of Family Psychotherapy, 30*, 292–313.

Cassidy, J., & Shaver, P. (2016). *Handbook of attachment* (3rd ed.). New York: Guilford.

Cobb, C. L. (1996). Adolescent-parent attachments family problem-solving styles. *Family Process, 35*, 57–82.

Collins, N. L., & Read, S. J. (1994). Cognitive representations of attachment: The structure and function of working models. In K. Bartholomew & D. Perlman (Eds.), *Advances in personal relationships, Vol. 5. Attachment processes in adulthood* (pp. 53–90). London: Jessica Kingsley Publishers.

Crespo, C., Davide, I. N., Costa, M. E., & Fletcher, G. J. (2008). Family rituals in married couples: Links with attachment, relationship quality, and closeness. *Personal Relationships, 15*, 191–203.

Denton, W. H., Burelson, B. R., Clark, T. E., Rodriguez, C. P., & Hobbs, B. V. (2000). A randomized trial of emotionally focused therapy for couples in a training clinic. *Journal of Marital & Family Therapy, 26*, 65–78.

Denton, W. H., Wittenborn, A. K., & Golden, R. N. (2012). Augmenting antidepressant medication treatment of depressed women with emotionally focused therapy for couples: A randomized pilot study. *Journal of Marital and Family Therapy, 38*(s1), 23–38.

Dickstein, S. (2004). Marital attachment and family functioning: Use of narrative methodology. In M. W. Pratt & B. H. Fiese (Eds.), *Family stories and the life course: Across time and generations* (pp. 213–232). Mahwah, NJ: Erlbaum.

Doherty, W. J. (2001). *Take back your marriage: Sticking together in a world that pulls us apart.* New York: Guilford.

Efron, D. (2004). The use of emotionally focused family therapy in a children's mental health center. *Journal of Systemic Therapies, 23*(3),78–90.

Eisenberger, N. I., & Lieberman, M. D. (2004). Why rejection hurts: A common neural alarm system for physical and social pain. *Trends in cognitive sciences, 8*, 294–300.

Ekman, P. (1992). Facial expressions of emotion: An old controversy and new findings. *Philosophical Transactions of the Royal Society of London. Series B: Biological Sciences, 335*(1273), 63–69.

Fraley, R. C., & Waller, N. G. (1998). Adult attachment patterns: A test of the typological model. In J. A. Simpson & W. S. Rhodes (Eds.), *Attachment theory and close relationships* (pp. 77–114). New York: Guilford.

Frijda, N. J. (1986). *The emotions.* Cambridge: Cambridge University Press.

Funk, J. L., & Rogge, R. D. (2007). Testing the ruler with item response theory: Increasing precision of measurement for relationship satisfaction with the Couples Satisfaction Index. *Journal of Family Psychology, 21*(4), 572.

Furrow, J. L., Edwards, S. A., Choi, Y., & Bradley, B. (2012). Therapist presence in emotionally focused couple therapy blamer softening events: Promoting change through emotional experience. *Journal of Marital and Family Therapy, 38*, 39–49.

Furrow, J. L., Palmer, G., Johnson, S. M., Faller, G., & Palmer-Olsen, L. (2019). *Emotionally focused therapy with families: Creating connection and restoring resilience.* New York: Routledge.

Gottman, J. M. (1994). *What predicts divorce.* Hillsdale, NJ: Erlbaum.

Gottman, J. M., & Levenson, R. W. (1999). How stable is marital interaction over time? *Family Process, 38*, 159–165.

Greenberg, L. S., & Angus, L. E. (2004). The contributions of emotion processes to narrative change in psychotherapy: A dialectical constructivist approach. In L. E. Angus & J. McLeod (Eds.), *The handbook of narrative and psychotherapy: Practice, theory, and research* (pp. 331–349). Thousand Oaks, CA: Sage Publications.

Greenberg, L. S., Rice, L., & Elliott, R. (1993). *Facilitating emotional change.* New York: Guilford.

Greenman, P. S., & Johnson, S. M. (2013). *Process research on Emotionally Focused Therapy (EFT) for couples: Linking theory to practice. Family Process, 52*(1), 46–61.

Gross, J. J., & Levenson, R. W. (1997). Hiding feelings: The acute effects of inhibiting negative and positive emotion. *Journal of Abnormal Psychology, 106*(1), 95.

Guillory, P. T. (2021). *Emotionally focused therapy with African American couples.* Love heals. New York: Routledge.

Halchuk, R. E., Makinen, J. A., & Johnson, S. M. (2010). Resolving attachment injuries in couples using emotionally focused therapy: A three-year follow up. *Journal of Couple & Relationship Therapy, 9*(1), 31–47.

Hawkley, L., Masi, C. M., Berry, J., & Cacioppo, J. (2006). Loneliness is a unique predictor of age-related differences in systolic blood pressure. *Psychology and Aging*, 21(1), 152–164.

Herman, J. L. (1992). *Trauma and recovery.* New York: Basic Books.

Hesse, E. (1999). The adult attachment interview. In J. Cassidy & P. Shaver (Eds.), *Handbook of attachment* (pp. 395–433). New York: Guilford.

Izard, C. E. (1977). Differential emotions theory. In *Human emotions* (pp. 43–66). Boston, MA: Springer.

Johnson, S. M. (1996). *The practice of emotionally focused therapy: Creating connection.* New York: Brunner/Routledge.

Johnson, S. M. (2002). *Emotionally focused couple therapy with trauma survivors.* New York: Guilford.

Johnson, S. M. (2004). *Creating connection: The practice of emotionally focused couple therapy* (2nd ed.). New York: Brunner-Routledge.

Johnson, S. M. (2008). *Hold me tight: Seven conversations for a lifetime of love.* New York: Little, Brown Spark.

Johnson, S. M. (2013). *Love sense: The revolutionary new science of romantic relationships.* New York: Little, Brown Spark.

Johnson, S. M. (2017). An emotionally focused approach to sex therapy. In Z. Peterson (Ed.), *The Wiley handbook of sex therapy* (pp. 250–266). New York: Wiley.

Johnson, S. M. (2019). *Attachment theory in practice: Emotionally focused therapy (EFT) with individuals, couples, and families.* New York: Guilford Press.

Johnson, S. M. (2020). *The practice of emotionally focused therapy: Creating connection* (3rd ed.). New York: Routledge.

Johnson, S. M. & Campbell, T. L. (2021). *A primer for emotionally focused individual therapy (EFIT): Cultivating fitness and growth in every client.* New York: Routledge.

Johnson, S. M., & Greenberg, L. S. (1988). Relating process to outcome in marital therapy. *Journal of Marital & Family Therapy, 11*, 313–317.

Johnson, S. M., & Greenberg, L. S. (Eds.). (1994). *The heart of the matter: Perspectives on emotion in marital therapy.* New York: Brunner-Mazel.

Johnson, S. M., & Talitman, E. (1997). *Predictors of success in emotionally focused marital therapy. Journal of Marital and Family Therapy, 23*(2), 135–152.

Johnson, S. M., & Whiffen, V. E. (1999). *Made to measure: Adapting emotionally focused couple therapy to partners' attachment styles. Clinical Psychology: Science and Practice, 6*(4), 366–381.

Johnson, S. M., & Whiffen, V. E. (2003). *Attachment processes in couple and family therapy.* New York: Guilford.

Jordan, J. V., Kaplan, A. G., Miller, J. B., Stiver, I. P., & Surrey, J. L. (1991). *Women's growth in connection: Writings from the stone centre.* New York: Guilford.

Klein, M. H., Mathieu, P. L., Gendlin, E. T., & Kiesler, D. J. (1969). *The experiencing scale: A research and training manual* (Vol. 1). Madison, WI: Wisconsin Psychiatric Institute.

Klein, M. H., Mathieu-Coughlan, P., & Kiesler, D. (1986). The experiencing scale. In L. S. Greenberg & W. M. Pinsof (Eds.), *The psychotherapeutic process: A research handbook* (pp. 21–71). New York: NY. Guilford Press.

Lanktree, C., & Briere, J. N. (2017). *Treating complex trauma in children and their families: An integrative approach.* Los Angeles: SAGE.

Lebow, J. L., Chambers, A. L., & Breunlin, D. C. (2019). *Encyclopedia of couple and family therapy.* London: Springer.

Lee, N. A., Spengler, P. M., Mitchell, A. M., Spengler, E. S., & Spiker, D. A. (2017). Facilitating Withdrawer re-engagement in emotionally focused couple therapy: A modified task analysis. *Couple and Family Psychology: Research and Practice, 6*(3), 205–225.

Makinen, J. A., & Johnson, S. M. (2006). Resolving attachment injuries in couples using emotionally focused therapy: Steps toward forgiveness and reconciliation. *Journal of Consulting and Clinical Psychology, 74*(6), 1055–1064.

Mikulincer, M., Birnbaum, G., Woddis, D., & Nachmias, O. (2000). Stress and accessibility of proximity-related thoughts: Exploring the normative and intraindividual components of attachment theory. *Journal of Personality and Social Psychology, 78*(3), 509–523.

Mikulincer, M., & Florian, V. (2000). Exploring individual differences in reactions to mortality salience: Does attachment style regulate terror management mechanisms? *Journal of Personality and Social Psychology, 79*(2), 260–273.

Mikulincer, M., & Shaver, P. R. (2007). *Attachment in adulthood: Structure, dynamics, and change.* New York: Guilford Press.

Mikulincer, M., & Shaver, P. R. (2016). *Attachment in adulthood: Structure, dynamics, and change* (2nd ed.). New York: Guilford Press.

Mikulincer, M., Shaver, P. R., & Pereg, D. (2003). Attachment theory and affect regulation: The dynamics, development, and cognitive consequences of attachment-related strategies. *Motivation and emotion, 27*(2), 77–102.

Minuchin, S., & Fishman, H. C. (1981). *Family therapy techniques.* Cambridge, MA: Harvard University Press.

Nightingale, M., Ibilola Awosan, C., & Stavrianopoulos, K. (2019). Emotionally focused therapy: A culturally sensitive approach for African American heterosexual couples. *Journal of Family Psychotherapy, 30*(3), 221–244.

Palmer-Olsen, L., Gold, L. L., & Woolley, S. R. (2011). Supervising emotionally focused therapists: A systematic research-based model. *Journal of Marital and Family Therapy, 37*(4), 411–426.

Plutchik, R. (2001). The nature of emotions: Human emotions have deep evolutionary roots, a fact that may explain their complexity and provide tools for clinical practice. *American Scientist, 89*(4), 344–350.

Porges, S. W. (2011). *The polyvagal theory: Neurophysiological foundations of emotion, attachment, communication and self-regulation.* New York: Norton.

Porges, S. W. (2016, March). *The science of therapeutic attunement.* Keynote address presented at the Psychotherapy Networker Symposium, Washington, DC.

Ravitz, P., Maunder, R., Hunter, J., Sthankiya, B., & Lance, W. (2010). Adult attachment measures: A 25-year review. *Journal of Psychosomatic Research, 69*(4), 419–432.

Rheem, K. D. (2011). *Analyzing the withdrawer re-engagement change event in emotionally focused couple therapy: A preliminary task analysis* (Unpublished doctoral dissertation). Argosy University, Washington, DC.

Rice, L. N. (1974). The evocative function of the therapist. *Innovations in Client-Centered Therapy*, 289–311.

Rogers, C. (1961). *Client centered therapy.* Boston, MA: Houghton Mifflin.

Sandberg, J. G., Busby, D. M., Johnson, S. M., & Yoshida, K. (2012). The brief accessibility, responsiveness, and engagement (BARE) scale: A tool for measuring attachment behavior in couple relationships. *Family Process, 51*(4), 512–526.

Selchuk, E., Zayas, V., Gunaydin, G., Hazan, C., & Kross, E. (2012). Mental representations of attachment figures facilitate recovery following upsetting autobiographical memory recall. *Journal of Personality and Social Psychology, 103*, 362–378.

Shaver, P. R., & Brennen, K. (1992). Attachment styles and the five big personality traits. *Personality and Social Psychology Bulletin, 5*, 536–545.

Shaver, P. R., & Mikulincer, M. (2002). Attachment-related psychodynamics. *Attachment & Human Development, 4*(2), 133–161.

Simpson, J. A., & Overall, N. C. (2014). Partner buffering of attachment insecurity. *Current Directions in Psychological Science, 23*(1), 54–59.

Slootmaeckers, J., & Migerode, L. (2018). Fighting for connection: Patterns of intimate partner violence. *Journal of Couple & Relationship Therapy, 17*, 294–312.

Slootmaeckers, J., & Migerode, L. (2020). EFT and intimate partner violence: A roadmap to de-escalating violent patterns. *Family Process, 59*, 328–345.

Spanier, G. B. (1976). Measuring dyadic adjustment: New scales for assessing the quality of marriage and similar dyads. *Journal of Marriage and the Family, 38*, 15–28.

Stern, D. (1985). *The interpersonal world of the infant.* New York: Basic Books.

Tomkins, S. (1986). *Affect, imagery and consciousness.* New York: Springer.

Van der Kolk, B. (2015). *The body keeps the score: Brain, mind and body in the healing of trauma*. New York: Penguin Books.

Vangelisti, A. L. (2009). *Feeling hurt in close relationships*. New York: Cambridge University Press.

Wittenborn, A. K., Liu, T., Ridenour, T. A., Lachmar, E. M., Rouleau, E., & Seedall, R. B. (2019). Randomized controlled trial of emotionally focused couple therapy compared to treatment as usual for depression: Outcomes and mechanisms of change. *Journal of Marital and Family Therapy, 45*, 395–409.

Woolley, S. R., Faller, G., Palmer-Olsen, L., & Vitoria, A. D. (2016). Training the emotionally focused therapist. In K. Jordon (Ed.), *Couple, marriage, and family therapy supervision* (pp. 325–344). New York: Springer Publishing Company. ISBN 9780826126788

Yalom, I. (1989). *Love's executioner*. New York: Basic Books.

Zeytinoglu-Saydam, S., & Niño, A. (2019). A tool for connection: using the person-of-the-therapist training (POTT) model in emotionally focused couple therapy supervision. *Journal of Marital and Family Therapy, 45*(2), 233–243. https://doi.org/10.1111/jmft.12349

Zuccarini, D., Johnson, S. M., Dalgleish, J. A., & Makinen, J. (2013). Forgiveness and reconciliation in emotionally focused therapy for couples: The client change process and therapist interventions. *Journal of Marriage & Family Therapy, 39*(2), 148–162.

ABOUT THE AUTHORS

Brent Bradley, Ph.D., has a PhD in marriage and family therapy and a master's degree in theology. He is co-author of *Emotionally Focused Couples Therapy for Dummies* and many other chapters and professional journal articles on EFT. He is owner of The Couple Zone (www.couplezone.org), with couples counseling offices across the state of Texas. The Couple Zone serves couples online throughout the state as well.

Lorrie L. Brubacher is the founding director of the Carolina Center for EFT. A certified trainer with the ICEEFT, she has been an individual, couples, and family therapist since 1989. She is an adjunct faculty at University of North Carolina, Greensboro. She trains internationally and publishes on the topic of EFT and emotionally focused individual therapy (EFIT) specifically. She co-developed EFT's first interactive video training program on the EFT Attachment Injury Resolution Model (www.attachmentinjuryrepair.com) and has produced many EFT couples and individual training videos (https://steppingintoeft.com). Her book *Stepping Into Emotionally Focused Couple Therapy: Key Ingredients of Change* (Routledge, 2018) and her training videos have been translated into over 10 languages.

T. Leanne Campbell, Ph.D., is co-director of the Vancouver Island Centre for EFT and Campbell & Fairweather Psychology Group (a multi-site psychology practice) and is an Honorary Research Associate of Vancouver Island University. Initially trained by Dr. Sue Johnson, she has been working in the EFT model for the past three decades. Her clinical work focuses on loss and trauma across modalities, with individuals, couples and families. Dr. Campbell is an active ICCEFT-certified trainer, offering trainings in the areas of EFIT and emotionally focused couple therapy (EFCT) and trauma primarily, including relationship trauma and the AIRM. She also has been involved in the development of various educational materials and programs (see www.iceeft.com, www.eftvancouverisland.com). Most recently, she co-authored the first basic EFIT text with Dr. Sue Johnson, *A Primer for Emotionally Focused Individual Therapy: Cultivating Fitness and Growth in Every Client.*

James L. Furrow, Ph.D., is an author, researcher, and family therapist. He is an author of the original *Becoming an EFT Therapist: The Workbook* and co-author of *Emotionally Focused Family Therapy: Creating Connection and Restoring Resilience*; *The EFT Casebook: New Directions in Couple Treatment*; and *Emotionally Focused Couple Therapy for Dummies*, a practical resource for couples and therapists seeking an everyday understanding of emotionally focused therapy (EFT) principles and practices. Formerly

Freed Professor of Marital and Family Therapy and department chair at Fuller Graduate School of Psychology, he is a clinical fellow and an approved supervisor of the American Association for Marriage and Family Therapy, a Certified Family Life Educator with the National Council on Family Relations, and an International Centre for Excellence in EFT (ICEEFT)–certified EFT supervisor and trainer.

Susan M. Johnson, Ed.D., is a professor of psychology at the University of Ottawa and is involved in the ongoing supervision of clinical students in couple and in individual therapy. She teaches graduate courses in couples' therapy, trauma interventions, and experiential individual therapy. She is also director of the Ottawa Couple and Family Institute and conducts externships in EFT in Ottawa every year. Sue also serves as research professor at Alliant University in San Diego, where she conducts EFT training every January. She is the main proponent of emotionally focused couples' therapy and emotionally focused family therapy and received the American Association of Marriage and Family Therapy Outstanding Contribution to the Field award in 2000. Sue is also a fellow of the American Psychological Association and received the Excellence in Education award from the University of Ottawa in 2003. She received the award for research in family therapy from the American Family Therapy Academy in 2005. She is married with two children.

Veronica Kallos-Lilly, Ph.D., is a registered psychologist and a founding director of the Vancouver Couple & Family Institute (www.VCFI.ca) and Vancouver Centre for EFT Training (www.VCEFT.ca) in British Columbia, Canada. As a certified EFT trainer and supervisor, Veronica enjoys mentoring new and seasoned clinicians alike, both locally and internationally. She has been a member of ICEEFT since its inception and has been on the editorial board of the newsletter for the past ten years. Veronica was excited to co-author and publish the second edition of her book, entitled *An Emotionally Focused Workbook for Couples: The Two of Us.* To her delight, the first edition has now been translated into seven languages.

Gail Palmer, M.S.W., R.M.F.T., is one of the founding members of the Ottawa Couple and Family Institute and co-director of the International Center of Excellence in Emotionally Focused Therapy. She is one of the original co-authors in the first edition of *Becoming an Emotionally Focused Couple Therapist: The Workbook* and second author in definitive manual, *Emotionally Focused Family Therapy: Restoring Connection and Promoting Resilience.* Gail has a particular interest in applying EFT to the family context and offers trainings worldwide.

Kathryn Rheem, Ed.D., LMFT, directs the Washington Baltimore Center for EFT, the home of ICEEFT training in the Washington, D.C., area, and leads The EFT Café, an online interactive EFT course. She's written numerous chapters and articles and presents EFT internationally. As a trauma specialist, Kathryn has consulted for years with the US Army, US Marine Corps, US Department of Veterans Affairs and Veterans Affairs Canada. The restorative power of emotion, particularly from the experiences of those marginalized or traumatized, is the primary focus of her work.

Scott R. Woolley, Ph.D., holds the rank of distinguished professor at the California School of Professional Psychology at Alliant International University. He is a founder and director of the San Diego Center for Emotionally Focused Therapy and the Training and Research Institute for EFT at Alliant (TRI-EFT Alliant). Dr. Woolley has trained thousands of therapists in many areas of the world and is an ICEEFT-certified EFT trainer.

INDEX

Note: Numbers in **bold** indicate a table.

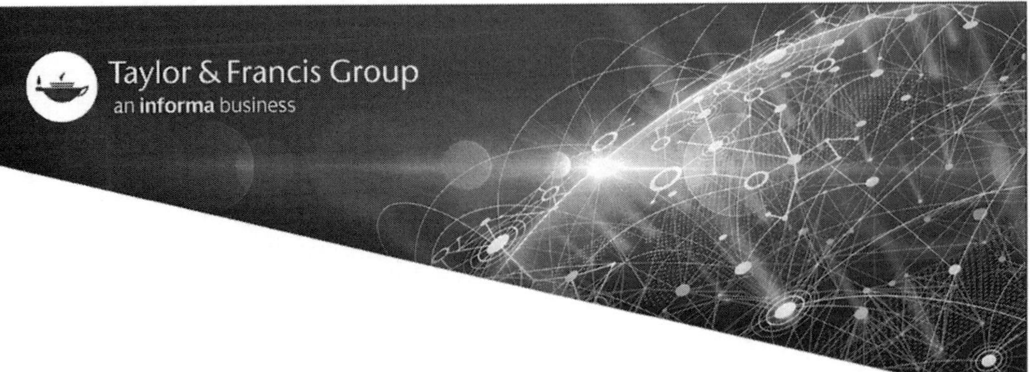
Taylor & Francis Group
an informa business

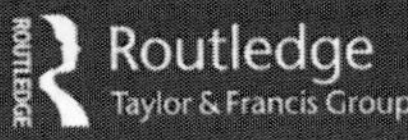
Routledge
Taylor & Francis Group

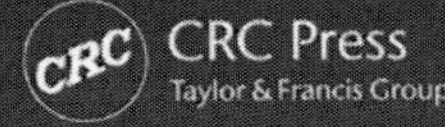
CRC Press
Taylor & Francis Group